THE
HOMEOPATHY BIBLE

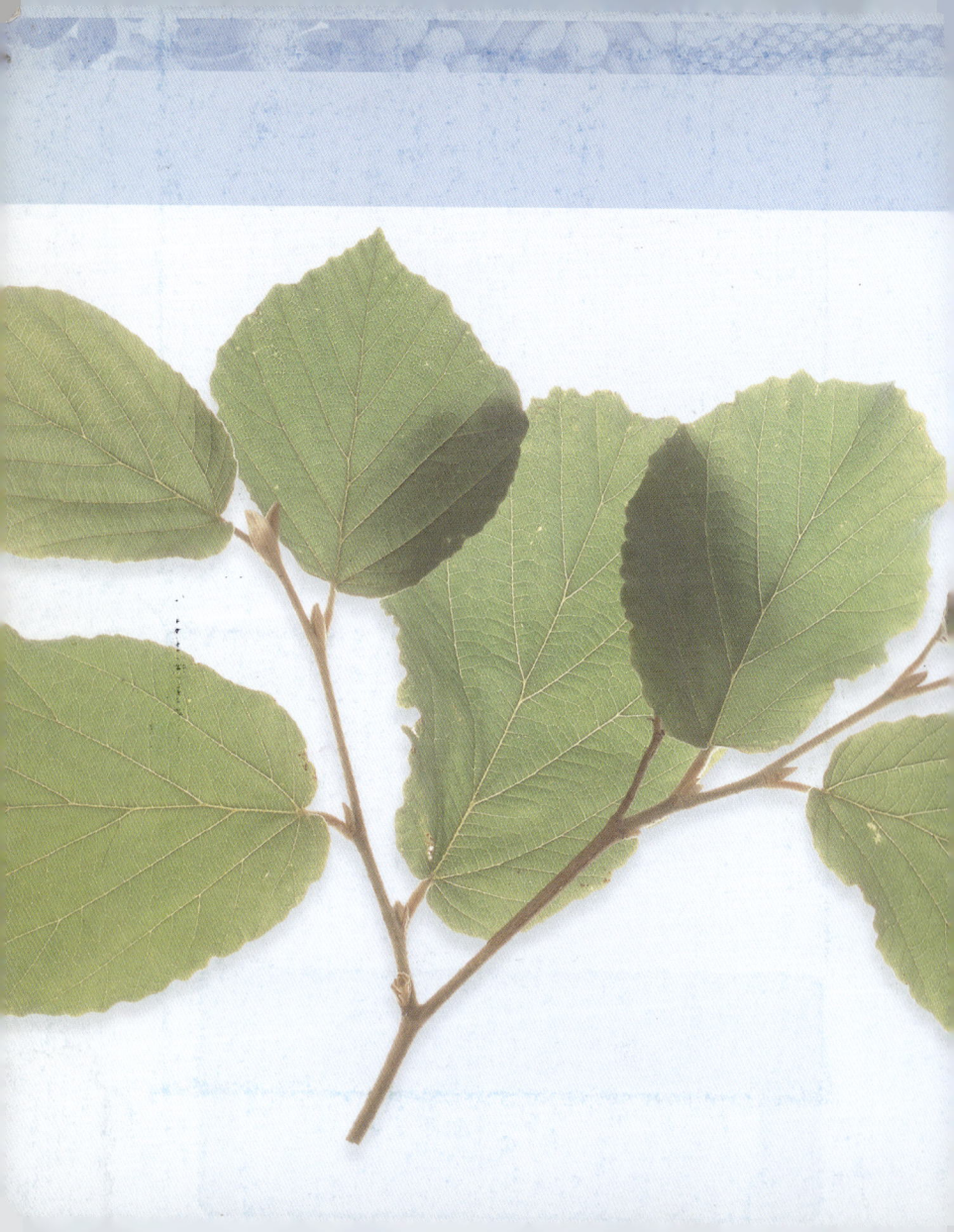

THE HOMEOPATHY BIBLE

THE DEFINITIVE GUIDE TO REMEDIES

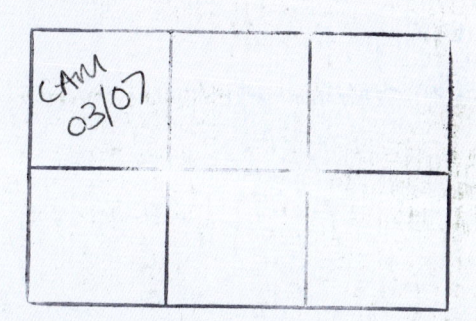

Ambika Wauters

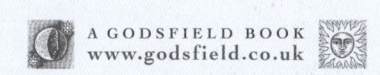

A GODSFIELD BOOK
www.godsfield.co.uk

CAMBRIDGESHIRE LIBRARIES	
9914	
Bertrams	15.02.07
615.532	£12.99

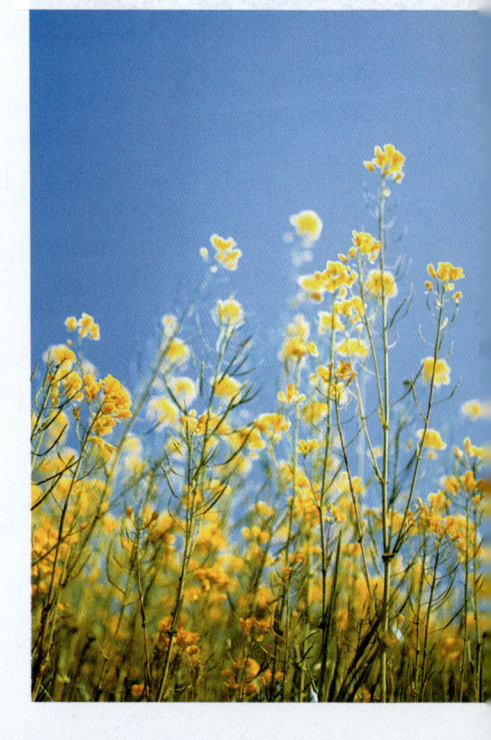

*First published in Great Britain in 2007
by Godsfield, a division of
Octopus Publishing Group Ltd
2-4 Heron Quays, London E14 4JP*

*Copyright © Octopus Publishing Group Ltd 2007
Text copyright © Ambika Wauters 2007*

*All rights reserved. No part of this work may be
reproduced or utilized in any form or by any means,
electronic or mechanical, including photocopying,
recording or by any information storage and
retrieval system, without the prior written
permission of the publisher.*

*ISBN-13: 978-1-84181-306-6
ISBN-10: 1-84181-306-0*

*A CIP catalogue record for this book
is available from the British Library*

Printed and bound in China

10 9 8 7 6 5 4 3 2 1

*DISCLAIMER
This book is not intended as an alternative to
personal medical advice. The reader should consult
a physician in all matters relating to health and
particularly in respect of any symptoms which may
require diagnosis or medical attention. While the
advice and information are believed to be accurate
and true at the time of going to press, neither the
author nor the publisher can accept any legal
responsibility or liability for any errors
or omissions that may have been made.*

CONTENTS

PART ONE
introduction • 6
what is homeopathy? • 8
the history of homeopathy • 10
the law of similars • 12
vital force • 14
differentiating systems • 18
case studies • 20
homeopathic dilutions • 24
homeopathic aggravation • 26
homeopathy and conventional medicine • 28
the practice of homeopathy • 30
genetic predisposition • 32
identifying the five miasms • 34
how to choose a remedy • 38
how to take a remedy • 40
contraindications • 42
keeping healthy • 46
avoiding common illnesses • 50

PART TWO
homeopathic *materia medica* • 54
understanding the *materia medica* • 56
first-aid remedies • 58
materia medica • 62

PART THREE
treating acute and chronic conditions • 292
how to self-prescribe • 294
circulatory and respiratory systems • 296
digestive system • 304
musculoskeletal system • 314
sensory and nervous systems • 320
skin • 330
moods and emotions • 342
reproductive system, pregnancy • 346
injury and surgery • 350
babies, children and immune system problems • 352

PART FOUR
support therapies and essences • 368
cell salts • 370
flower essences • 374
hormonal remedies • 378
homeopathic colour remedies • 382
gemmotherapy • 386
gemstone elixirs • 387

glossary • 388
index • 392
acknowledgements • 400

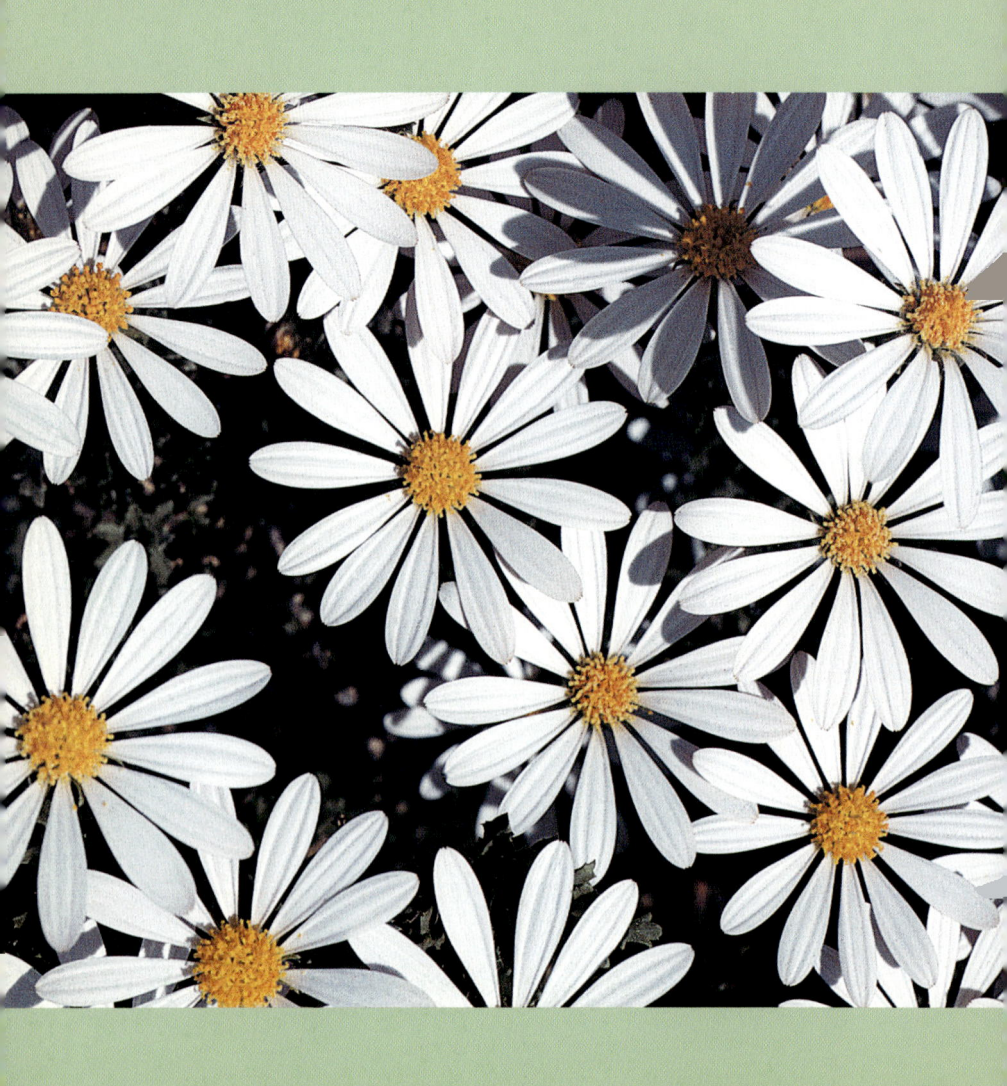

PART ONE

introduction

what is homeopathy?

Homeopathy is a gentle and effective medical practice that was first developed over 250 years ago and has been used in Europe ever since. Today, it is also gaining popularity throughout the United States, Australia and many other countries. As well as the many professionally trained homeopaths, there are growing numbers of people who are learning how to use homeopathy successfully by themselves to improve their health.

Homeopathy is based on the principle of 'like cures like' – that a substance that can make you ill in large doses can cure you if taken in small doses – which was first developed in 1796 by the German doctor, Samuel Hahnemann. Today thousands of people around the world have found that homeopathic remedies can help in the treatment of both acute and chronic conditions, from common colds and flu to eczema and asthma. People are successfully self-prescribing homeopathic remedies for a variety of common minor illnesses, such as colds, cuts, aches and minor accidents.

This book will help you to prescribe remedies for yourself and for your family, to alleviate the symptoms of many common minor illnesses. However, you should always consult a qualified homeopath before treating acute conditions, and always consult your doctor for anything other than minor conditions or for those conditions that do not respond to homeopathic treatment. Always consult your doctor immediately for serious medical conditions.

THE REMEDIES

Homeopathic remedies are created from animal, plant and mineral substances diluted many times so that less, or in the case of some dilutions, none of the original chemical substance is present. Although no one yet understands the precise science by which homeopathy works, it is believed that diluting the original substance creates an effective yet safe remedy that, when prescribed correctly, can cure a wide range of conditions. Furthermore, homeopathic medicines are less costly to produce and buy than conventional drugs, making them affordable, and an attractive form of alternative treatment for a variety of illnesses.

When a homeopath prescribes a remedy, he or she will look at every aspect of the patient, from their physical symptoms to their mental and emotional state. A basic tenet of homeopathy is that it treats the whole person, not just their symptoms; it is a holistic therapy.

Poisonous plants such as this fly agaric are often used for homeopathic remedies (left).

Little of the original substance remains after it has been diluted with water (right).

ABOUT THIS BOOK

This book will provide all you need to understand the basic features of homeopathy and its use for home prescribing. Part One explains the history and development of homeopathy from its beginnings in late 18th-century Germany to the latest research and practice. Part Two provides detailed information on the key remedies and the conditions and symptoms they address. Part Three features a reference guide to common ailments and conditions and Part Four describes the support remedies that can enhance your use of homeopathy.

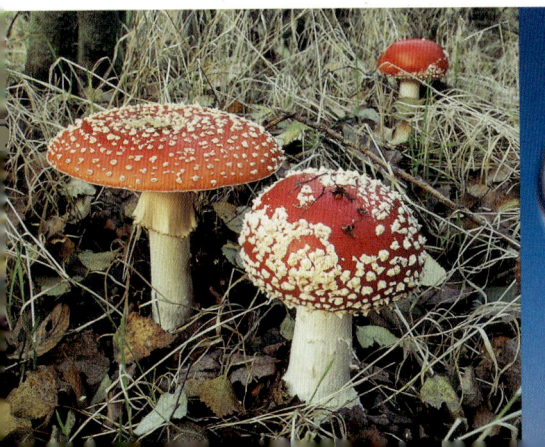

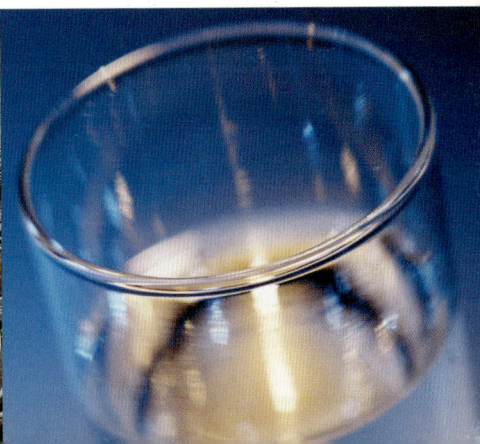

the history of homeopathy

In 1790 the German doctor Samuel Hahnemann (1755–1843) closed his medical surgery after 11 years of practice when he became disillusioned with the medical practices of his day. He began work researching and translating a wide range of books and treatises. Among them was the work of a Scottish doctor, William Cullen, on cinchona bark, a South American plant recently introduced as a medicine for the treatment of 'intermittent fevers' and malaria.

Hahnemann was sceptical about the claim and decided to test the efficacy of cinchona while he was healthy and without a fever. He found that cinchona produced symptoms identical to those of malaria and intermittent fever: trembling, a throbbing head and weakness in the limbs. In common with all physicians of his time, Hahnemann had studied the Law of Similars, written in the 5th century BC by the Greek physician Hippocrates (c.460–377/359 BC), and believed that in his test he had found proof of that ancient principle of 'like curing like'.

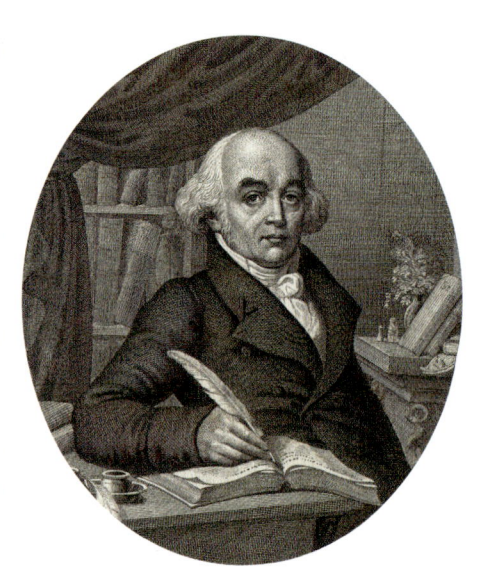

Dr Samuel Hahnemann (1755–1843), the founder of homeopathy, studied the principle of 'like curing like' over many years.

Hahnemann spent the next 30 years of his life cultivating, refining and studying this theory, convinced that by studying the physical and emotional effects of a substance on a healthy person he would discover its curative abilities.

DISCOVERING DILUTION

After 13 years of investigating toxic and non-toxic substances Hahnemann took the next step in developing homeopathy. He realized that substances could be diluted to remove their toxic effects and began experimenting with known poisons, diluting them to the point where they were no longer toxic and testing them extensively on people of all ages and from all backgrounds. He found that those substances that were highly diluted and shaken between each dilution had a more powerful healing effect than those that were less diluted and, therefore, shaken less. These tests formed the basis of his Homeopathic *Materia Medica*, a comprehensive list of symptoms and remedies. He named his new medicine 'homeopathy', from the Ancient Greek *homoios* (similar) and *pathos* (suffering). He also wrote the first edition of *The Organon of Medicine*, which described his theory and philosophy of homeopathy.

Hahnemann died in 1843, but his work was carried on by other practitioners, one of the most important of whom was the American physician Dr James Tyler Kent, who wrote the *Repertory to the Homeopathic Materia Medica*. This book is a guide to thousands of symptoms, their cures and aggravations and has been developed by homeopaths over many years.

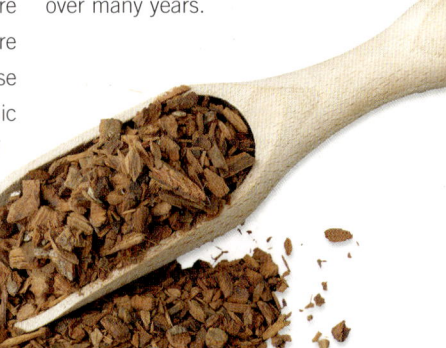

Cinchona bark, an anti-malarial treatment, was one of the first substances tested by Hahnemann on himself.

the law of similars

The Latin phrase *similia similibus curentur* (let likes be cured with likes), was coined by Hahnemann and describes his most profound discovery. This principle, embodied in the Law of Similars, states that any substance that can cause symptoms when given to a healthy person can help to heal someone who is experiencing similar symptoms.

THE ORIGIN OF THE LAW

Hahnemann first learned of the law from studying the work of the Greek physician Hippocrates. Born in *c.*460 BC on the island of Kos in Greece, Hippocrates became known as the father of medicine, basing his medical practice on observations and the study of the human body. He believed that the body must be treated as a whole and he recommended a healthy diet and lifestyle. Through his studies and practice Hippocrates noted that some individuals were better able to cope with

The fever inflicted by Belladonna (deadly nightshade) suggested to Hahnemann that it could be used to relieve similar symptoms.

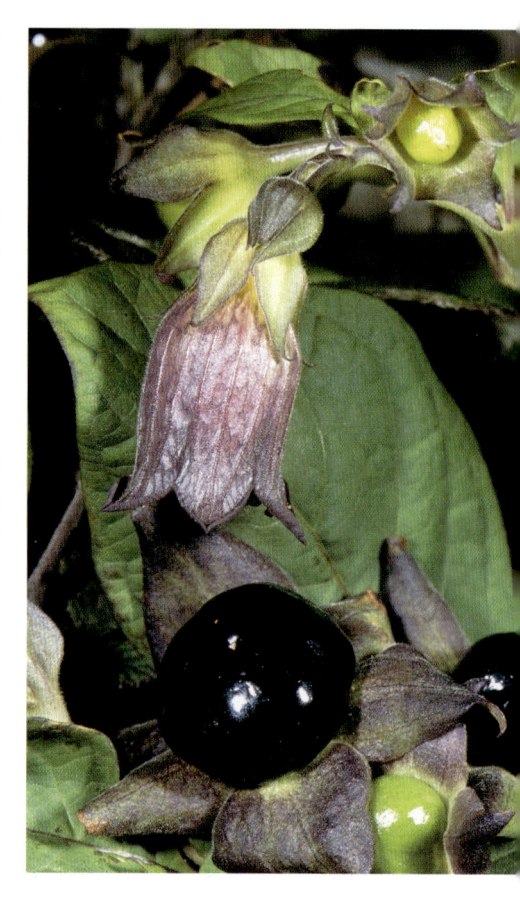

disease and illness than others. Famously he wrote, 'Through the like, disease is produced, and through the like, it is cured.'

FOLLOWERS OF HIPPOCRATES

The concept was developed by the physician Paracelsus (1493–1541), who stated: 'You there [sic] bring together the same anatomy of the herbs and the same anatomy of the illness into one order. This simile gives you an understanding of the way in which you shall heal.'

Two hundred years later a German doctor, Georg Ernst Stahl (1660–1734), also used the law when treating illness. He wrote: 'I am convinced that diseases succumb to substances that cause a similar ailment. This is how I succeeded in treating the predisposition to heartburn with very small doses of sulphuric acid, when a variety of absorbent powders had been used in vain.' Even today, we can find this principle in conventional medicine; for example, Ritalin is often prescribed for hyperactive children and yet is itself a stimulant. Radiation can cause cancer and yet is used in the treatment of the disease.

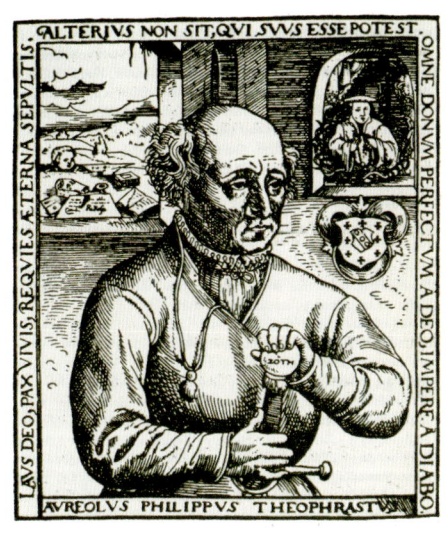

Engraving of Paracelsus (1493–1541), who also studied similars in illness and plants.

Despite this, we still do not understand the mechanism by which this law appears to work. Science may yet uncover the answer; meanwhile, millions worldwide attest to homeopathy's effectiveness.

vital force

When Dr Hahnemann worked with patients using homeopathy he became aware of the levels of inner strength and vitality that his patients were experiencing. People who had not been well for many years realized that they felt healthier than they could ever remember. It became apparent to Hahnemann that not only were their specific diseases cured but also an essential part of themselves had been healed, and this seemed to be part of the 'living presence' of that person.

In his book, *The Organon*, he suggested that this living presence controlled the physical, emotional and mental aspects of a person's well-being or illness and related to their spirit. He called this presence the 'vital force', and regarded this as the life force that distinguishes all living from non-living things.

A FINE BALANCE

He noted that the vital force, a kind of balancing mechanism, could become disturbed through large doses of medication and that it was also influenced by negative thoughts and emotions. Health, well-being and life itself would then be adversely affected. Hahnemann believed that by taking a particular diluted substance that was in harmony with the vital force it would restore balance where the vital force had become out of balance.

The vital force, then, is the living presence, or balancing mechanism, in a person, and can be recognized by the symptoms it manifests. These might be physical symptoms, which could become pathological if they remain untreated, or emotional symptoms, which would unbalance the health and well-being of the individual.

In order to study the effects of a particular substance he worked with healthy people who would then exhibit the physical, emotional and mental symptoms intrinsic to that substance. He recorded all his observations and shared them among his homeopathic colleagues, and

Hahnemann used healthy people whose 'vital force' was in balance, to test his diluted substances and recorded their reactions.

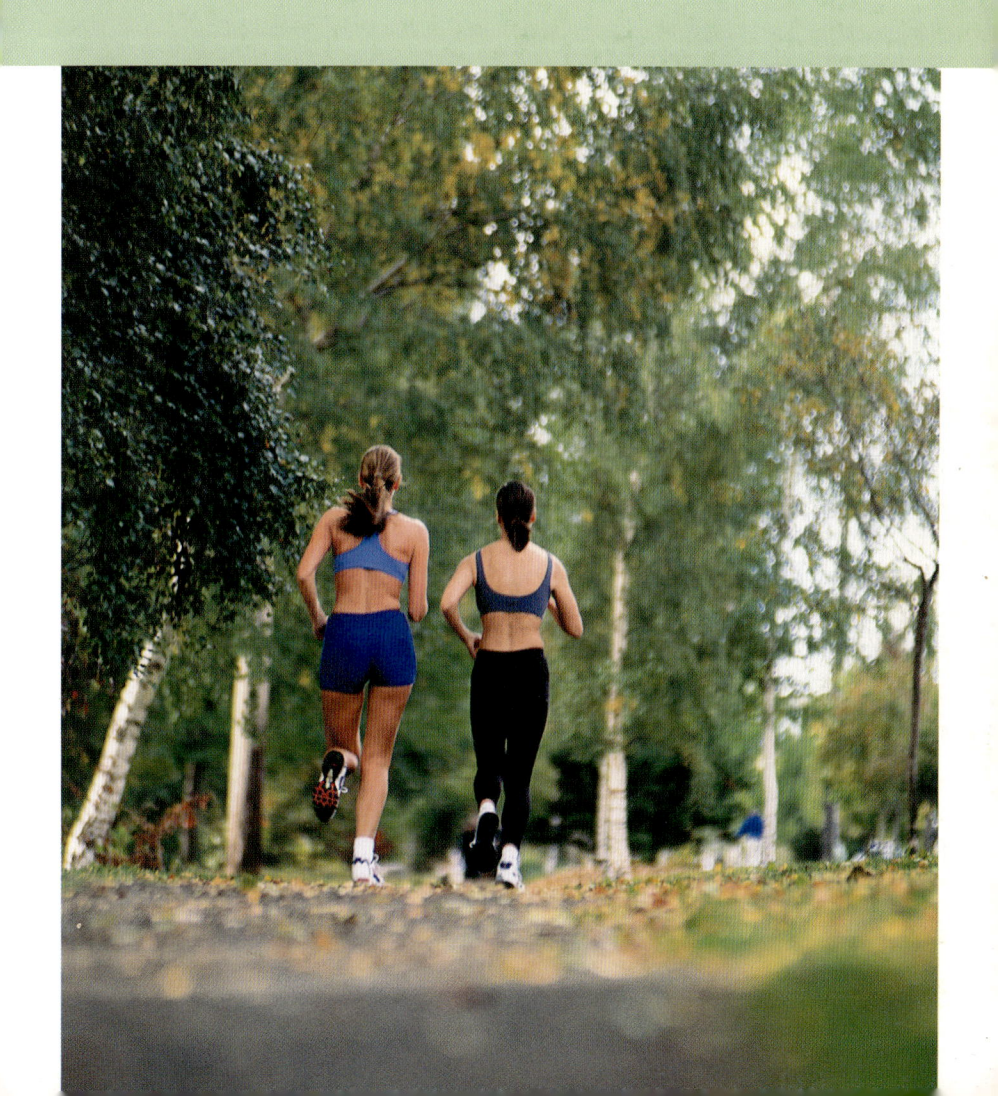

vital force 15

he also tested many of the substances on himself and his family, often achieving promising results.

MAINTAINING HARMONY

Hahnemann believed that the vital force should always be in harmony with its environment, and should remain stable and balanced through crises and challenges. If, at any point in a person's life, they suffered shock, trauma or injury then the vital force would do whatever was necessary to compensate for that experience, which would be depleting the person's energy; for example, when a person suffers a shock their core energy retreats to protect the heart and vital organs. Blood, energy and even consciousness will be slowed down so that life can be maintained and the metabolism stabilized. After the shock has subsided, the body regulates itself by increasing circulation and allowing blood to flow to the surface again and for consciousness to be awakened. Each time a person experiences shock the nerves are deadened and vitality diminished. In the case of a great shock this would be sufficient to overwhelm the nervous system; the energy would then be withheld from some vital organs and the senses would becomes less acute.

REPLICATING REACTIONS

Hahnemann discovered many substances that could produce shock-like states in the body. The plant aconite is one of these. It is toxic in its natural form but in a diluted form – known in homeopathy as 'potentized' – it has the ability to alleviate the symptoms of shock. Within a few moments of taking this remedy circulation will be restored and the signs of shock will lessen.

Understanding how the vital force protects and compensates itself for shock, trauma, injury, loss and separation, and matching those symptoms with the various substances – the remedies – is the basis of homeopathic medicine. It is able to relieve the stress of shock and its compensatory symptoms as well as dealing with long-term chronic conditions.

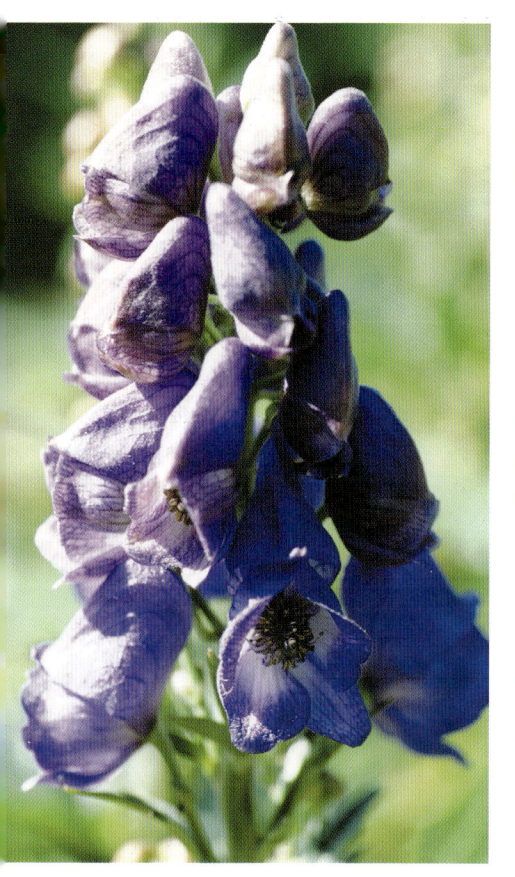

THE MINIMUM DOSE

While he studied the effects of his diluted substances it became clear to Hahnemann that the minimum dose was the best dose to stimulate the vital force in a patient. When he found the correct remedy that matched a patient's symptoms he would prescribe a very small amount. This stimulated the vital force to balance itself so that the symptoms would be alleviated. It took only a minimum amount of a remedy to move the vital force towards the direction of cure. However, if too much medicine was given, the vital force did not have to work to restore balance. Instead it became dependent on the constant input of medicines to 'fix' its problems. In doing this the organism became weaker rather than stronger. Providing the minimum dose to enable the vital force to respond without drowning in medication or being overwhelmed is an important principle in homeopathy.

Aconite (or monkshood) is a poisonous plant that produces shock symptoms if taken. The Aconite remedy alleviates similar symptoms.

differentiating symptoms

As homeopathy is a holistic medicine, physical, emotional and psychological symptoms must all be considered when deciding on the appropriate remedy. Hahnemann discovered that a condition might manifest itself in different ways with each patient and that no single remedy will cure the same disease in every patient. To decide which remedy is likely to be the most effective for an individual, the homeopath must carefully assess every aspect of their mental attitudes and emotional responses.

LOOKING AT A RANGE OF SYMPTOMS

Homeopaths define symptoms more broadly than is traditional in conventional medicine. In homeopathy a symptom will be any change that has been experienced or observed during the illness. This includes pain, physical changes, unusual reactions to heat or cold and the patient's mental and emotional state. The homeopath will take a detailed case history in order to get as full a picture as possible of the patient's symptoms, asking open rather than closed questions to focus on the individual's unique experience.

PARTICULAR AND GENERAL SYMPTOMS

Practitioners distinguish between 'particular' and 'general' symptoms. A particular symptom is something associated with a specific part of the body; for example, feet that are cold. General symptoms are those felt in the entire body, such as fatigue or restlessness. Emotional and mental states also fall into this category. A general symptom will reveal how the body is attempting to heal the disease. Homeopaths tend to find general symptoms to be most helpful in choosing the appropriate remedy.

MAKING A DIAGNOSIS

If you visit a homeopath, he or she will ask you to explain when the illness began and how quickly the symptoms developed, what the character of the symptom is (for example, does a pain feel sharp or dull?), where exactly the symptom is experienced, and any factors

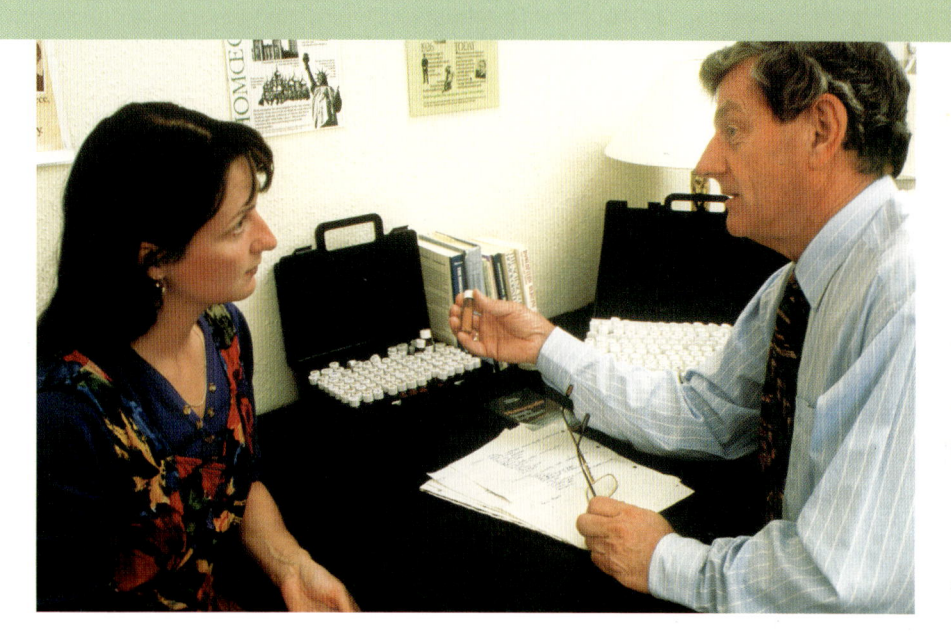

A homeopath will make a detailed case study of the patient, noting emotional as well as physical symptoms before prescribing.

that aggravate or improve each symptom. The more powerful the effect on the symptom, the more important this is in determining the correct remedy. The practitioner will also ask about general symptoms such as energy levels, sensitivity to temperature, changes in appetite and thirst, and changes in sleep patterns. When treating yourself with homeopathic remedies remember to observe these case-taking principles and note your own symptoms as thoroughly as possible.

It may be difficult to get a detailed history of symptoms from children or the very ill. In these cases your own powers of observation will be extremely important.

case studies

The following case studies illustrate how homeopathy can help both minor physical complaints and emotional problems. Sometimes self-medication is appropriate, but for more complicated conditions you may need to consult a trained practitioner. Remember that persistent or severe symptoms should always be referred to a doctor.

CASE STUDY: HARRY

Harry is a married 50-year-old father of three. He is the managing director of a successful export business and works long hours in the office. The business is growing and Harry has been travelling frequently to Europe to develop contacts there. His hectic lifestyle hasn't given him much time for exercise and he often overeats at business lunches. By the time he comes home from work the rest of the family has already eaten and Harry resorts to frozen meals for dinner. He is a little overweight as a result.

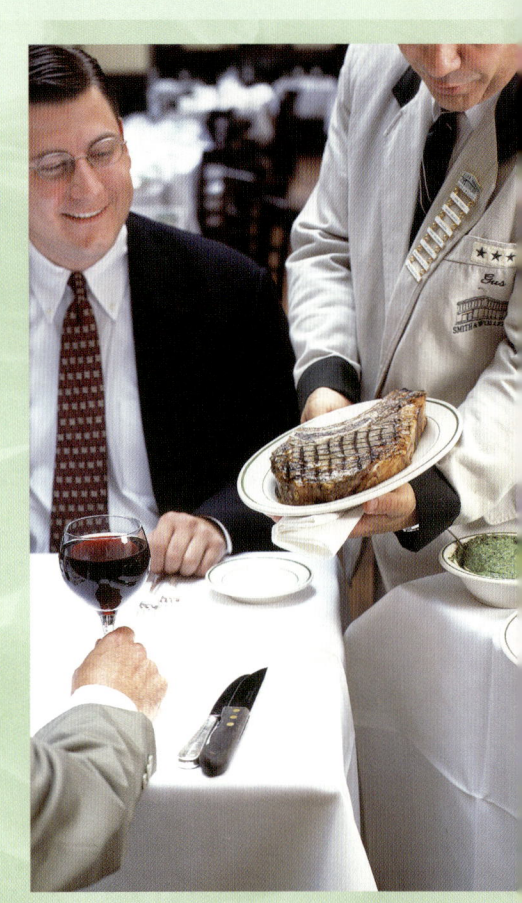

Harry's health problem Lately Harry has been suffering from constipation, accompanied by headaches and irritability. He has tried taking over-the-counter remedies but finds that his symptoms are not being relieved. His family are becoming increasingly exasperated with his bad moods, and stress levels in the household are high. Harry is also worried that his work performance is suffering and understands that he needs to address the problem urgently.

Home homeopathic care Harry's wife, Jean, has long been a fan of homeopathy and although Harry is sceptical he agrees to try a remedy. Jean gives him a dose of Nux vomica 30C. Her homeopathy guide recommends Nux vomica when digestive problems are associated with headache and irritability. She also noted that her guide recommends this remedy when symptoms are worse in the morning and are aggravated by eating – confirming the symptoms she has observed in Harry.

The result Harry found Nux vomica relieved his symptoms almost immediately, and he threw away the pills he had bought at the pharmacy. He also recognized that his diet and lifestyle weren't helping his condition and resolved to take a regular break each lunchtime to walk briskly for about 20 minutes. He paid more attention to his diet and aimed to eat easy-to-prepare yet nutritious salads if he was home late from work. Over the next few months his symptoms disappeared entirely and he has found he has more energy and has also lost weight.

Harry's health problems are typical of many who lead a hectic lifestyle, with frequent business lunches and little exercise.

CASE STUDY: MARY

Mary Smith is a 45-year-old mother of two girls aged 18 and 16. She has a responsible job as a legal secretary in a busy firm in the city and successfully juggles work and family commitments. Generally Mary has been fit and well, exercising regularly and eating a varied diet.

Mary and John separated three years ago after mutually agreeing that their marriage was at an end. The split was amicable and Mary felt sure that this was the right move for both of them. They had been married at a very young age and now that their children were nearing adulthood, they both felt the time was right to go their separate ways.

Mary's health problem Recently, Mary's divorce was finalized; at the same time she learnt that John had begun a new relationship. Despite her rational acceptance that this was inevitable she found herself deeply upset. She had been very distracted and forgetful at work leading to a rebuke from her boss. She had also been experiencing distressing bouts of uncontrollable crying and felt that her life had suddenly become directionless. She consulted her doctor who diagnosed mild depression. He felt that antidepressants would not be helpful and advised counselling. Mary was not keen to pursue this and turned to homeopathy.

The homeopath's analysis In her consultation with Mary, the homeopath observed that Mary was not keen to discuss her emotional state and she resisted the homeopath's attempts to console her. In fact, when the homeopath tried to help Mary acknowledge that the divorce had been for the best, Mary appeared to feel more distressed. Finally the homeopath noted that Mary sighed and yawned frequently – symptoms which are often a sign of suppressed feelings. All these symptoms together indicated that Ignatia would be the most beneficial medicine to treat Mary's grief.

case studies 23

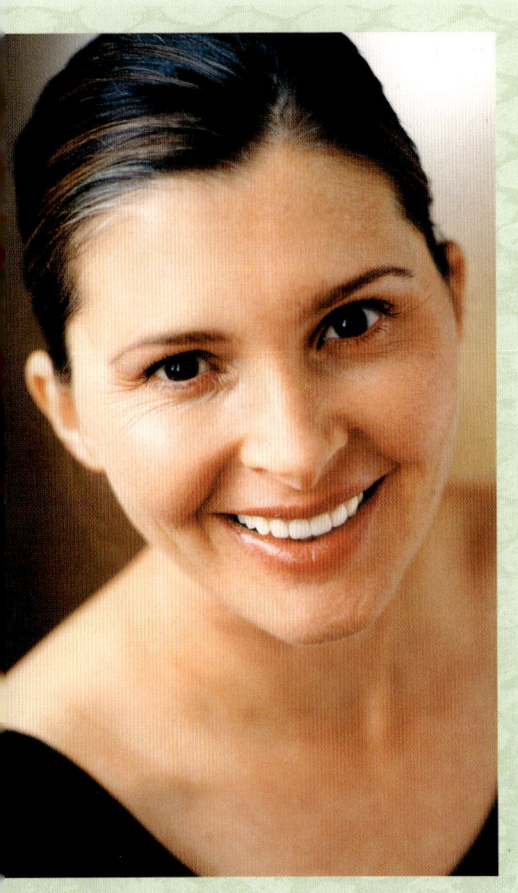

The result Mary took Ignatia 30C for a number of weeks. She found that she was better able to deal with her feelings, discussing her situation more openly with family and friends. Her two children in particular have been extremely supportive. Her bouts of crying diminished and she felt back in control at work. She decided to focus on building a new social network and joined a local tennis club where she has made new friends and enjoys the regular exercise. She now feels ready to pursue this new phase in her life energetically.

Mary found that after taking Ignatia her emotional problems improved so that she could enjoy life again.

homeopathic dilutions

One of Hahnemann's greatest discoveries was that of 'potentization' – a process where substances can be diluted to the point where any toxic properties are reduced and the healing qualities are increased.

For soluble substances the medicine is most often diluted in the ratio of 1 part to 99 parts of water or alcohol. The mixture is then vigorously shaken to mix. Some researchers have suggested that it is this mixing stage that releases the energy of the substance into the solution. For insoluble substances the medicine is finely ground and diluted with powdered lactose. The solution is then diluted again and again 3, 6, 30, 200, 1,000 or more times until the final potency is reached.

Centesimal potencies refer to remedies that have been diluted 1 part to 99 parts. They are usually labelled 6C, 30C, and so on, to indicate the number of dilutions. When the remedy has been diluted 1 part to 9 parts it is labelled 6X and 30X. A 1M remedy means a substance has been diluted, or potentized, one thousand times.

The higher the number of dilutions the stronger the medicine and range of action will be. The general rule of thumb in homeopathy is that a low potency works on the physical body. Dilutions of 6X or 6C are best used for minor problems that are related to physical symptoms. They need to be repeated in order for them to work effectively. A 6X remedy is generally repeated three to five times daily or until symptoms disappear. A 30C remedy is generally taken once or twice a day or until symptoms disappear.

A higher potency of a 200C, or above, works on the mental, emotional and physical aspects of an individual, and needs little or no repetition. These higher potencies should not be used by the home homeopath but may be prescribed by a professional practitioner.

When a substance is 'potentized' it is dissolved in water then diluted many times until the correct potency is reached.

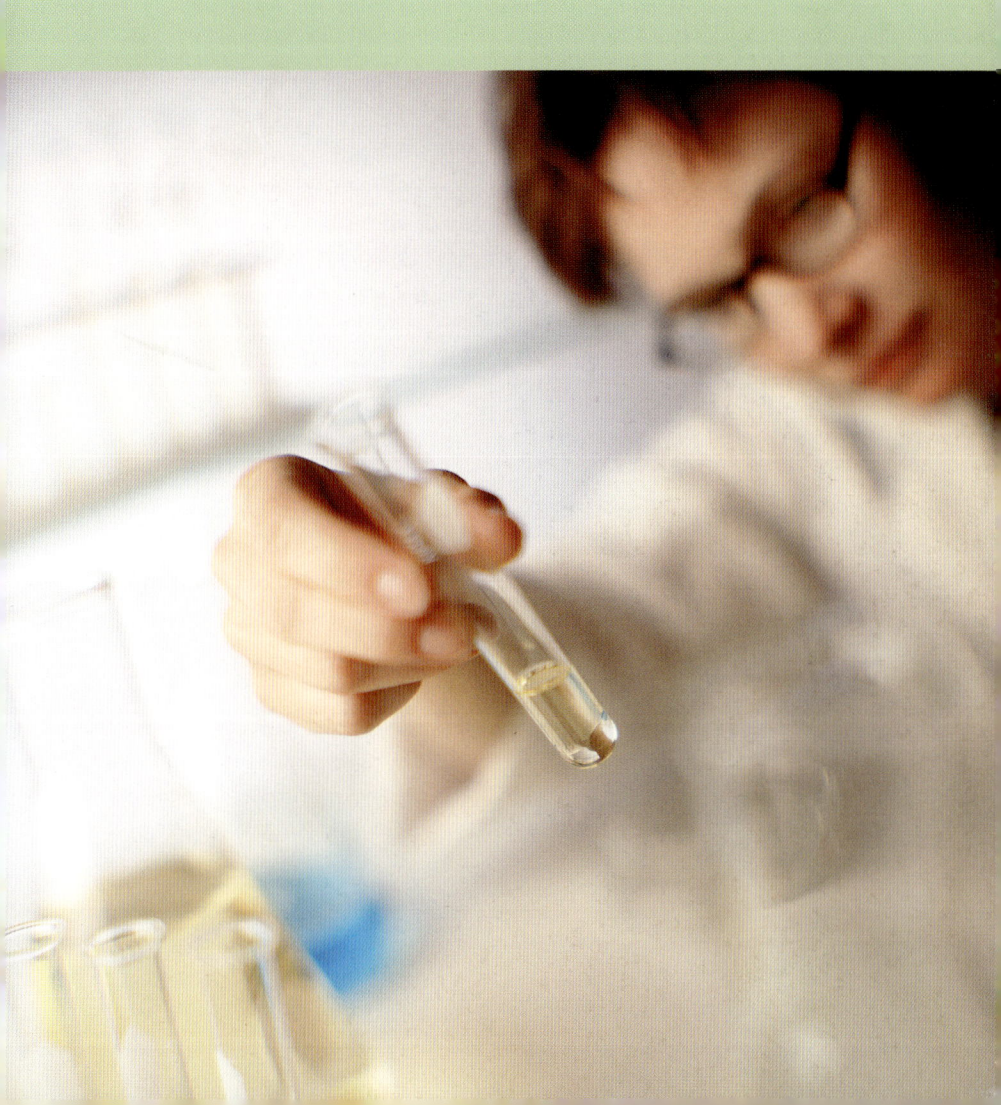

homeopathic dilutions

homeopathic aggravation

After taking a remedy some people experience what is termed a homeopathic aggravation. The aggravation might be on a physical level, causing the patient to experience symptoms that indicate their body is flushing out toxins, such as headache, flu, colds, discharges and diarrhoea, or it might be on an emotional level, causing the patient to become tearful. The aggravation occurs because the remedy has a temporary, but stronger, impact on the system than the natural disease, and it is just a sign that the remedy is closely matched to the patient's own symptoms and that the body is responding to the treatment. Aggravations are normally short-lived and may be more intense if the potency prescribed is high. Understanding how to manage these aggravations is the work of a skilled practitioner, as it is important not to create an overwhelming reaction in the patient, but to unfold the healing process gently with minor discomfort or reaction. These high potencies are not suitable for the home prescriber.

For the home user it is best not to use remedies above 30C. This is a safe, non-volatile potency that can be used for most common ailments. It is also the best potency to start with if you are new to using homeopathic remedies, as it works effectively and rapidly, and produces noticeable effects.

If you feel a higher potency might be appropriate, consult an experienced homeopath. He or she will be best placed to diagnose the most suitable remedy and will

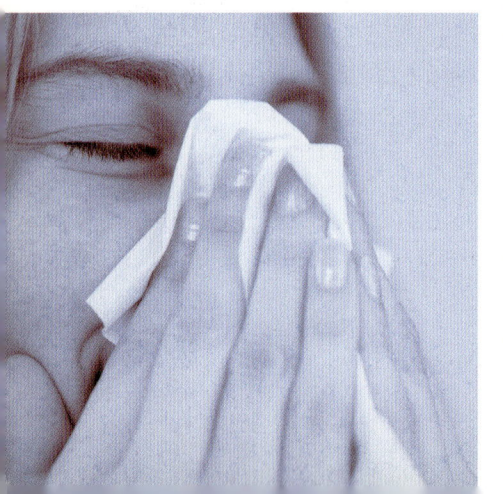

A cold can result after a homeopath has prescribed a high potency remedy, as the body begins a detoxification process.

Constantine Hering (1800–80) discovered three healing principles for all illnesses. These are known as Hering's Laws of Cure.

temporarily get worse. This healing process was first formally recognized by Constantine Hering (1800–80), a German homeopath who emigrated to the United States in the 1830s. He established certain healing principles that have become known as Hering's Laws of Cure. The three key principles are:

1 Healing begins from the inside of the body (including the vital organs as well as on a mental and emotional level) and then progresses towards the outside of the body via the surface of the skin. Eventually all symptoms will disappear.
2 As healing progresses symptoms appear and disappear in the opposite order to that in which they originally appeared.
3 Healing progresses from the upper to the lower parts of the body.

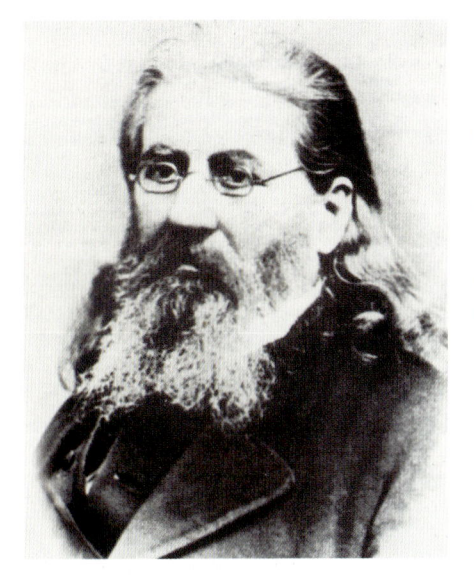

also be able to manage any detoxification process effectively.

HERING'S LAWS OF CURE

Homeopaths have found that in the treatment of chronic conditions the correct medicine tends to improve mental and emotional symptoms first while physical symptoms may

homeopathy and conventional medicine

Because homeopathic medicines contain no pharmacologically active agents they are generally recognized to be safe by many doctors. In France, approximately 32 per cent of doctors use homeopathic medicines and in the United Kingdom 42 per cent of doctors refer patients to homeopathic practitioners. Homeopathy, then, can work side by side with conventional medicine, but it is important to stress here that home prescribing is not appropriate for anything other than minor common ailments and first aid, and that a qualified homeopath should be consulted for more complicated conditions.

TREATING THE UNDERLYING CAUSE

It is in the treatment of chronic disease that homeopathy appears to be most successful. Conventional medicine acts on the symptoms of the disease itself, but often does not address the underlying cause of chronic conditions such as eczema and asthma. Because homeopathy is a holistic therapy it aims to restore the body to its natural state of health and uncover deeper issues that may be present, such as emotional and psychological problems, which can lead to imbalance.

WORKING TOGETHER

Many people are concerned that homeopathic remedies will not work in tandem with conventional medicines. In fact, there are only a few conditions where homeopathy is contraindicated if you take a specific medicine (see page 42). Never discontinue orthodox medication without discussing it with your doctor. In some cases, with careful monitoring, you may be able to reduce your medication while taking homeopathic remedies, but this should always be under medical supervision.

INFECTIOUS DISEASES AND ANTIBIOTICS

Although most people use homeopathy today to treat chronic problems, it gained its first success in the treatment of infectious diseases such as cholera and typhoid. Although the treatment of such serious

Overprescription of antibiotics can lead to a weakened immune system. Homeopathy aims to help the body to cure itself.

Homeopathy takes the view that infection arises due to both the germ and a person's compromised immune system. Homeopathic medicines aim to strengthen the body's own internal resources so that it is better able to resist infection in the first place, fight it more effectively if the body does succumb, and become more resistant to future infections.

Antibiotics are extremely effective at destroying an infective bacterial agent. However, we are now discovering that the overprescription of antibiotics can lead to bacteria becoming resistant so that any antibiotics subsequently prescribed will be less effective. Although antibiotics can be life-saving in the face of serious illness, you may choose to consider how necessary they might be when the condition is not serious. If you have been prescribed antibiotics, homeopathic remedies can help to strengthen your immune system during the recovery period.

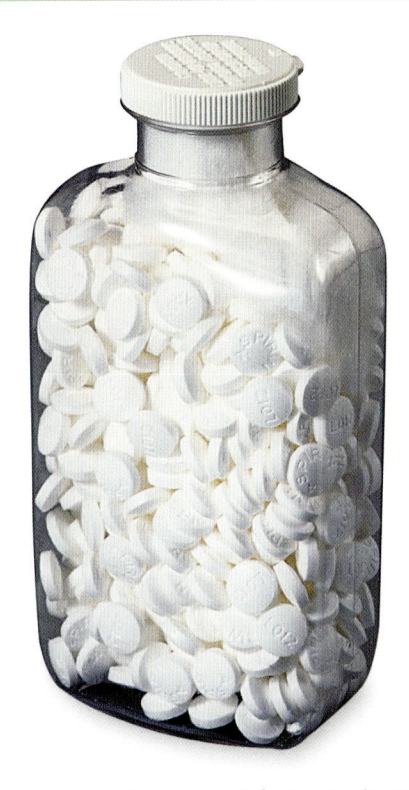

diseases is always best left to experienced medical staff, homeopathy can nevertheless be used to treat many types of infection with much success.

the practice of homeopathy

In classical homeopathy practitioners will generally use only one remedy at a time in the treatment of a condition or illness. They believe that using a number of different remedies within the body could produce unpredictable results and confuse the symptoms appearing in the patient. Classical homeopaths firmly believe in the unique pattern of illness found in every individual and, although they recognize that people want to be able to use over-the-counter remedies, they recognize that these may not be effective, as the cause of illness might be a much deeper problem that needs careful individual prescribing.

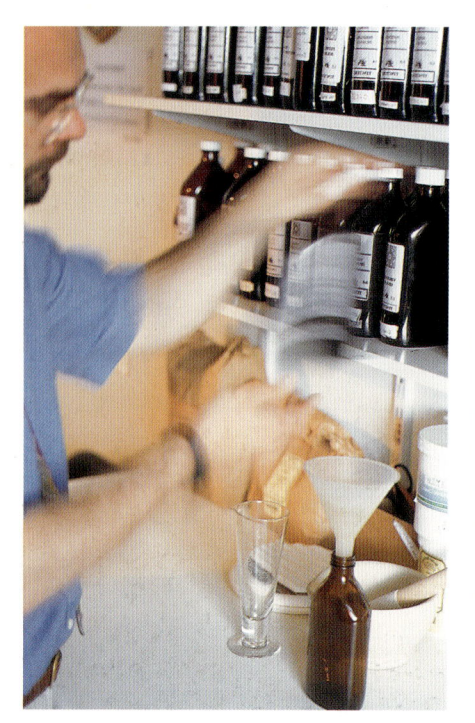

The practice of using complexes (which are multiple homeopathic medicines) is becoming increasingly popular in Europe and Latin America and many pharmacies and health food stores sell combination medicines for conditions such as headaches, colds and insomnia. For some people the process of carefully selecting the correct remedy is extremely difficult and they find this 'ready-made' approach very helpful.

Many people find complexes of different remedies work well in alleviating symptoms such as colds, flu and insomnia.

the practice of homeopathy

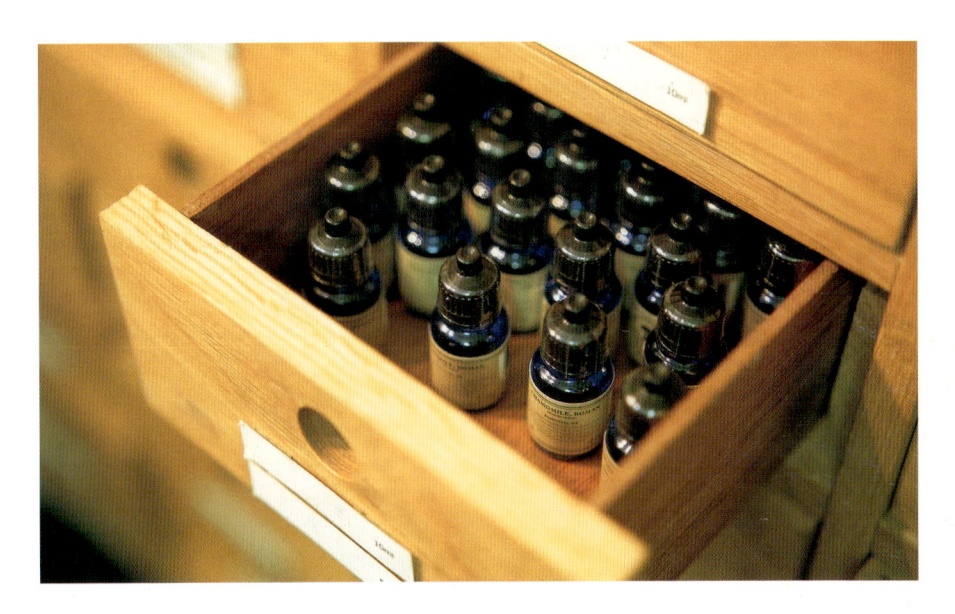

Homeopathic complexes may contain between five and ten remedies that are closely related in that they all work on a specific condition. They appear to be effective for acute illnesses but relatively ineffective for chronic conditions.

This book will help you to find a suitable remedy by using a methodical approach to

It is best to choose the single remedy most suited to your individual symptoms.

making your diagnosis, which will be more effective than using a homeopathic complex. If your condition does not respond to a remedy it may be time to seek the advice of a practitioner in selecting something more specific to your needs.

genetic predisposition

When Samuel Hahnemann treated chronic disease he found that there were people who were predisposed to specific weaknesses, never able to find good health no matter what their external life conditions were or what medications they took. Some people were prone to chest complaints; they suffered colds, lung conditions, bronchitis and pneumonia. Others were prone to constant catarrhal problems, and others developed skin irritations such as warts and moles.

Hahnemann believed that some illnesses were inherited. Today homeopathy aims to treat many of these kinds of symptoms.

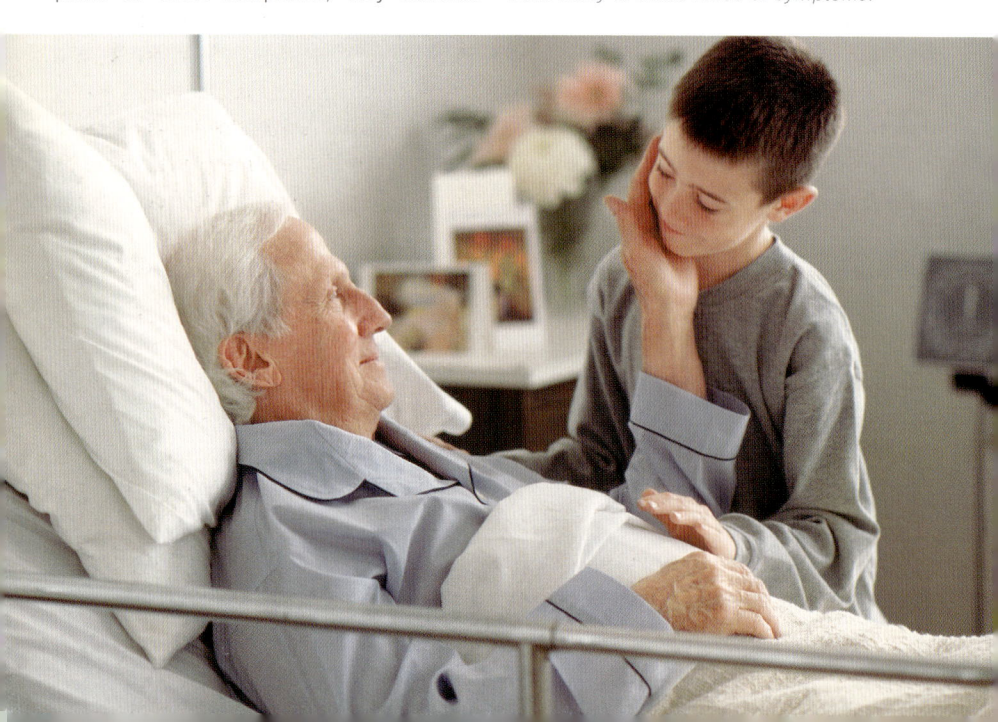

After 12 years of careful study Hahnemann came to the conclusion that previous infectious diseases were often the reason why people were not able to achieve good health, especially if the infectious disease had been treated with strong drugs that suppressed the disease in the body. He found that these people shared specific patterns of disease tendency, which he called 'miasms'.

The patterns Hahnemann identified related to the previous presence in a patient of scabies, syphilis or gonorrhoea and thus he identified three miasms. Moreover he was also able to identify the same patterns of disease or miasms in children who had not suffered with the infectious disease themselves but whose parents had been affected.

ILLNESSES THAT BECAME INHERITED

Hahnemann was able to trace the genetic patterns of disease through family lines to the time when a person was first afflicted with a disease and how it was suppressed. These three miasms – psoric, scycotic and syphilitic – formed patterns that Hahnemann was able to identify clearly and treat. In later years other homeopaths identified further miasms.

THE GENETIC LINK TO DISEASE

Subsequent homeopaths discovered that chronic broken-down states of health were genetically predisposed and could be treated following the principles of 'like cures like'. Hahnemann and his followers had outstanding success with their treatment and were able to eradicate many of the chronic symptoms of suffering they saw by following the basic principles of homeopathy.

This understanding of the principles of genetic predisposition has made the practice of homeopathy unique among other medicines. Being able to treat many of the problems that have been inherited from one generation to the next is one of the greatest gifts of the practice. It offers an individual the opportunity to release physical and emotional patterns of illness through treatment and the freedom to live healthily in a natural way.

identifying the five miasms

There are five widely accepted miasms that are treated in homeopathy today: the psoric miasm, tubercular miasm, sycotic miasm, cancer miasm and the syphilitic miasm.

THE PSORIC MIASM

Hahnemann believed that all humanity suffered from the psoric miasm, because it was a basic state of humanity. The psoric miasm manifests itself by a superficial itch on the surface of the body and this indicates that cellular activity is not functioning correctly. He believed that the psoric miasm was responsible for inactivity and stagnation in the system, resulting in chronic weakness and an inability to benefit from nourishment. This undernourished state affected the mind as well as the body.

The psoric miasm underlies all other miasms and can be seen in all people at some time during treatment. It manifests itself on a psychological level as a fear to go forward in life and an inability to take risks or to be assertive. On a physical level its symptoms appear close to the surface of the skin with rashes, psoriasis and skin infections such as boils. Although it is a chronic illness it is not destructive.

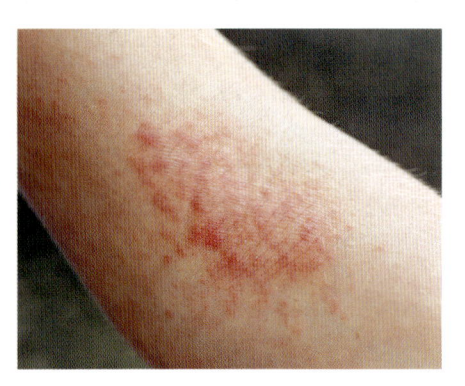

Physical symptoms of the psoric miasm are rashes, psoriasis and skin infections, from which Hahnemann believed everyone suffers.

THE TUBERCULAR MIASM

Dr Swan, who was a student of Hahnemann, identified the tubercular miasm, which has a destructive effect on the body causing weak lungs, bones and tissue. People who suffer with it are often restless and dissatisfied with

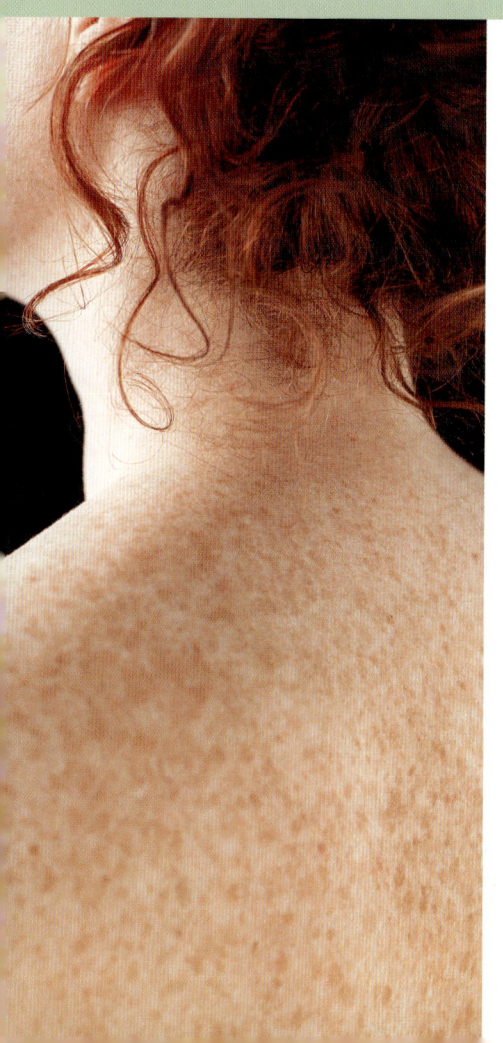

People with the sycotic miasm often have moles and freckles, as well as more troublesome conditions such as cysts.

where they live and what is happening in their lives, and they continually long for change. They frequently change jobs, relationships and circumstances, and are rarely peaceful or contented. This is reflected in their pathology. Because people with this miasm are intensely active they burn energy quickly. As with the wasting disease of TB itself, they always suffer with breathing, lung and bone problems.

THE SYCOTIC MIASM

The third miasm is called the sycotic miasm. It refers to the warty growths that appear on the surface of the skin, creating toxic deposits that form moles, freckles, cysts and tumours. The miasm is characterized by the overproduction of cells and tissue, and excess mucus.

People affected with this miasm are inclined to live excessively; for example, eating when they are full. They often have a tremendous amount of life force but this is often misdirected. Symptoms of this disease include excessive catarrh and tumours and fibrous tissue growth.

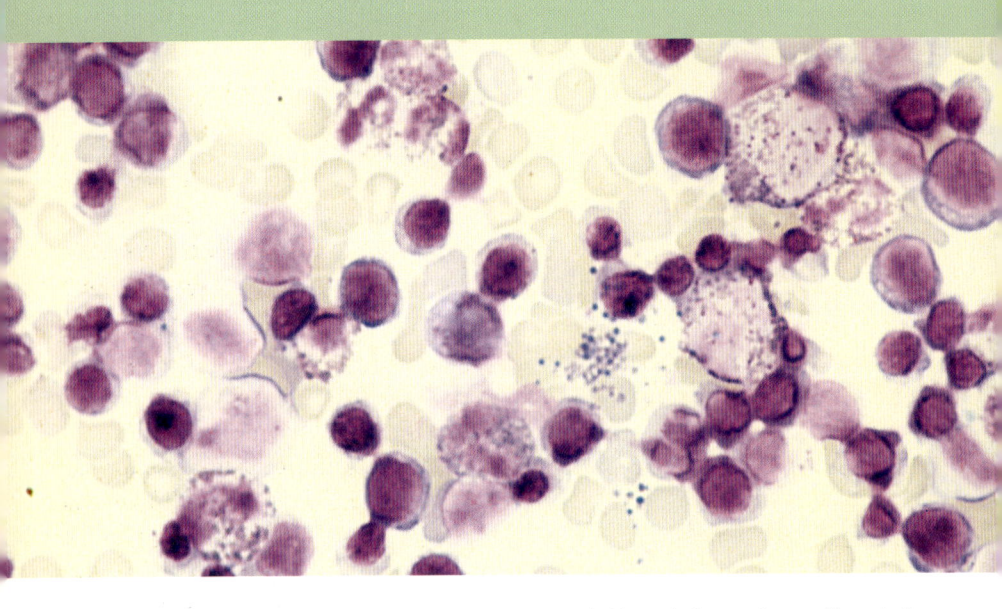

Sufferers with sycotic miasm can be aggressive and manipulative and this can emerge as a strong ego with leadership qualities, competitiveness and a passion for power. In contrast to the first two miasms people with the sycotic miasm are often physically strong. However, they often suffer with arthritis and rheumatism, although they usually respond well to homeopathic treatment and their aches and pains often disappear. After treatment they also become more balanced emotionally.

THE CANCER MIASM

Homeopaths believe a person's tendency towards cancer is generally inherited. Although there are many external and environmental

According to Hahnemann, when a person has the cancer miasm they have problems with erratic cell production.

factors that influence cancer, homeopathy believes that you do not contract it unless you are genetically predisposed to it. Whenever the immune response is weakened because of environmental factors or because of chronic, long-term unhappiness, this miasm takes hold and creates havoc with cell production.

Homeopathy treats both the miasm and the disease. It provides immune-building treatment as well as remedies that aim to treat the underlying cause of cancer.

THE SYPHILITIC MIASM

Hahnemann believed that through the common use of mercury to treat syphilis the illness became suppressed in a person's body. Although the disease would be cured externally, internally it would be pushed deeper into the cells of the body, which it would then destroy. This miasm would also be passed down through the generations.

The syphilitic miasm is destructive, affecting the centre of each cell. People with this miasm will suffer from insomnia and degenerative diseases such as cirrhosis of the liver, diabetes and colitis, as well as destructive behaviour and addictions. It can be deeply suppressed and then be brought to the surface in a person's life as the result of stress.

MIASMS IN GENERAL

All miasms lie just under the surface of our lives and emerge as the roots of disease. When we are confronted with shock, challenges or traumas these miasms appear and reveal themselves in states of health and in the way we respond to situations. Understanding miasms is one of the most complex aspects of homeopathy and their treatment is therefore highly unsuitable for home prescribing. If you feel that your homeopathic remedies might be blocked from working by a miasm, consult a qualified homeopath for treatment. The treatment might take a long time, often in excess of a year.

how to choose a remedy

To discover which remedy might best treat your ailment consult Part Three, Treating Acute and Chronic Conditions (pages 292–367). You will find a list of conditions that respond to homeopathy as well as a list of possible remedies that can be used for each condition.

FINDING THE APPROPRIATE REMEDY

Because of the individual nature of each person's case, a variety of remedies may be suitable to treat the condition. Choose only one remedy at a time for treatment, as homeopathy works best when just one remedy is used to address a condition. If you combine remedies you will not know which remedy is the one that worked for you. You may also create an aggravation, as explained earlier (page 26), with too much stimulation to your system. If the remedy you choose does not begin to work for you within a period of two to three hours you might consider discontinuing that remedy and instead take another remedy listed in the Treating Acute and Chronic Conditions section.

USING THE MATERIA MEDICA

Study the remedies as they are described in the Homeopathic Materia Medica section in Part Two (pages 54–291). See which symptoms best describe you and your condition. You may find that the mental symptoms apply but the physical conditions listed do not. Look at the other remedies in the Treating Acute and Chronic Conditions section listed under your condition and try to match the physical, mental and emotional conditions as best you can. The remedy that matches the closest to you, your condition and how you are feeling would be the best remedy for you to take.

THE CORRECT DOSE

Begin by taking a single dose of a 6C remedy. Wait a few hours to see if there is any improvement in your condition. If the remedy is working and you feel that there is a change do not repeat the remedy until its action has ceased working. If your condition is partially improved take another dose. When the symptoms you are trying to treat start to

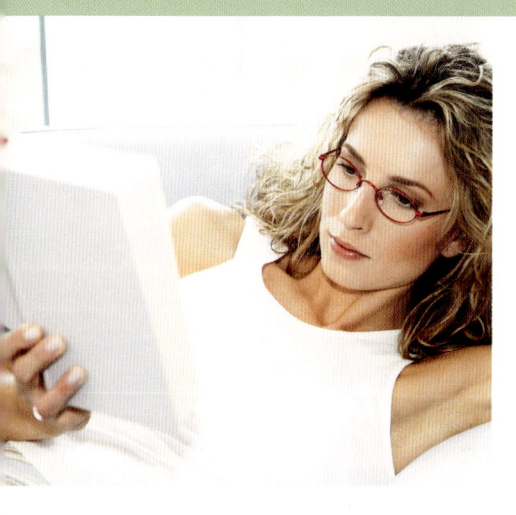

Match your symptoms as closely as possible to those listed in the Materia Medica to find an appropriate remedy.

improve, it's always best to stop the remedy. This way there will be no overstimulation to the system; it is always best to listen to your body than to be prescriptive.

For physical and emotional symptoms try using a 12C potency two times daily, or use a 30C remedy as a single treatment for symptoms that have a strong emotional element as well as physical illnesses.

HOW MANY TO TAKE

Homeopathy is not like allopathic medicine, which requires you to take a course of medication and to repeat it often. Homeopathy can work with one single dose of a remedy and does not have to be repeated until the symptoms return. This could be many weeks, months or even years.

USEFUL REMEDIES

When you know which remedies work for you and for your individual conditions then create a first-aid kit with the essential remedies that are best suited to you. You may find that remedies for such conditions as cramps, indigestion or headache work well for you most of the time. Keep these remedies in stock and take them when you need them.

On page 58 you will find a list of basic First-Aid Remedies that are useful for many of the conditions that people suffer from. Create a kit using these ten remedies and always have them to hand. They can be invaluable in treating the effects of accidents, injuries or shock.

how to take a remedy

Homeopathic remedies may come in drop form, as small tablets or as a powder. You should follow the instructions on the bottle as to how many drops or pellets are advisable to take. Most of the homeopathic remedies that you will need can be found at your local health-food store, but if you are unable to find them contact a homeopathic pharmacy, which will dispense low-potency remedies to you at minimal cost. You will find their name in your local telephone directory or on the Internet.

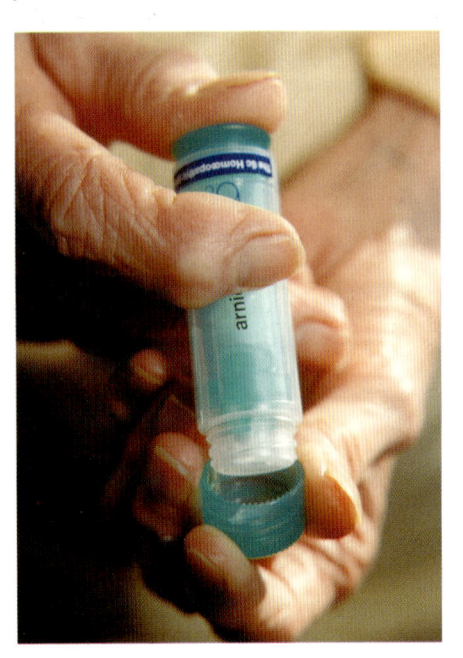

INSTRUCTIONS FOR TAKING THE REMEDIES

As your remedy will be affected by the flavours of food, drink or toothpaste, take it at least ten minutes after you have eaten, drunk or cleaned your teeth.

- **Drops** Drop the instructed amount directly onto your tongue unless other instructions are given.
- **Pills** Without touching the pill, shake it out of its container into the container cap. Tip the pill directly under your tongue and allow it to dissolve.

Take only one remedy at a time. Give it an opportunity to work in your system.

Tip the pill onto your tongue using the container cap and allow it to dissolve on or underneath your tongue.

BABIES AND CHILDREN

If you are administering a remedy to a baby or small child you can place the remedy inside their lip and hold it there for ten seconds. That is the length of time it takes for the remedy to enter the bloodstream. Alternatively crush big pills or dilute them in water. Always check with your doctor that it is safe to use a homeopathic remedy with babies and children.

If you are a nursing mother remember that any remedy you take will be passed on to your baby through your milk. If you are giving a remedy to a baby this is the best way to do it.

Strong aromas

Homeopathic remedies can frequently be affected by strong smells, so avoid drinking regular coffee and eating sweets or inhaling substances that contain mint, eucalyptus or camphor.

SAFE KEEPING OF REMEDIES

Homeopathic remedies will last a lifetime if you take care of them. Indeed, there are remedy kits that have been handed down from generation to generation that are over 150 years old and still work. Taking care of your remedies will provide you with inexpensive and quality care for you and your family for years to come, so always store them carefully. Keep them in a dark container or a dark space, as they will deteriorate in direct sunlight. They will also lose their effect if exposed to strongly scented odours such as camphor, eucalyptus or turpentine. Soaps, perfumes and tobacco will also affect their efficacy, so it is always advisable to store remedies away from any strong odours.

contraindications

It is wise to consult your doctor if you are in any doubt as to whether it is advisable to take a homeopathic remedy, but there are also particular instances when you should always consult your doctor before taking a remedy:

- If you are currently on medication that has been prescribed by your doctor, particularly medication for blood pressure, antidepressants or cortisone.
- If you are pregnant.
- If you have recently had surgery and are recovering.

If you have recently been taking antibiotics and then you begin a course of homeopathy it is likely that your old symptoms will return. Homeopathy works by discharging symptoms out to the surface of the body whereas antibiotics suppress symptoms by pushing them deeper into the body. It is therefore a good idea to wait several weeks after taking a course of antibiotics before starting a course of homeopathic remedies.

Some homeopaths give treatment to detoxify the system after antibiotics. They use Sulphur 6X and Nux vomica 6X, alternating each remedy every 2 hours for up to 3 doses of each remedy. This opens the bowels and purifies the blood.

SAFETY FIRST

Always be aware of situations where it is vital to seek immediate medical assistance. As a general guideline watch out for the following symptoms:

- Any unusual bleeding
- Rapid breathing, or difficult and shallow breathing
- Severe chest pain
- Convulsions
- Delirium
- A high temperature above 39.5°C/103°F
- A high temperature with a slow pulse (less than 60 beats a minute for an adult and 80 beats a minute in a child)

Homeopathic remedies can be used with many allopathic medicines. You should always check with your doctor first.

contraindications

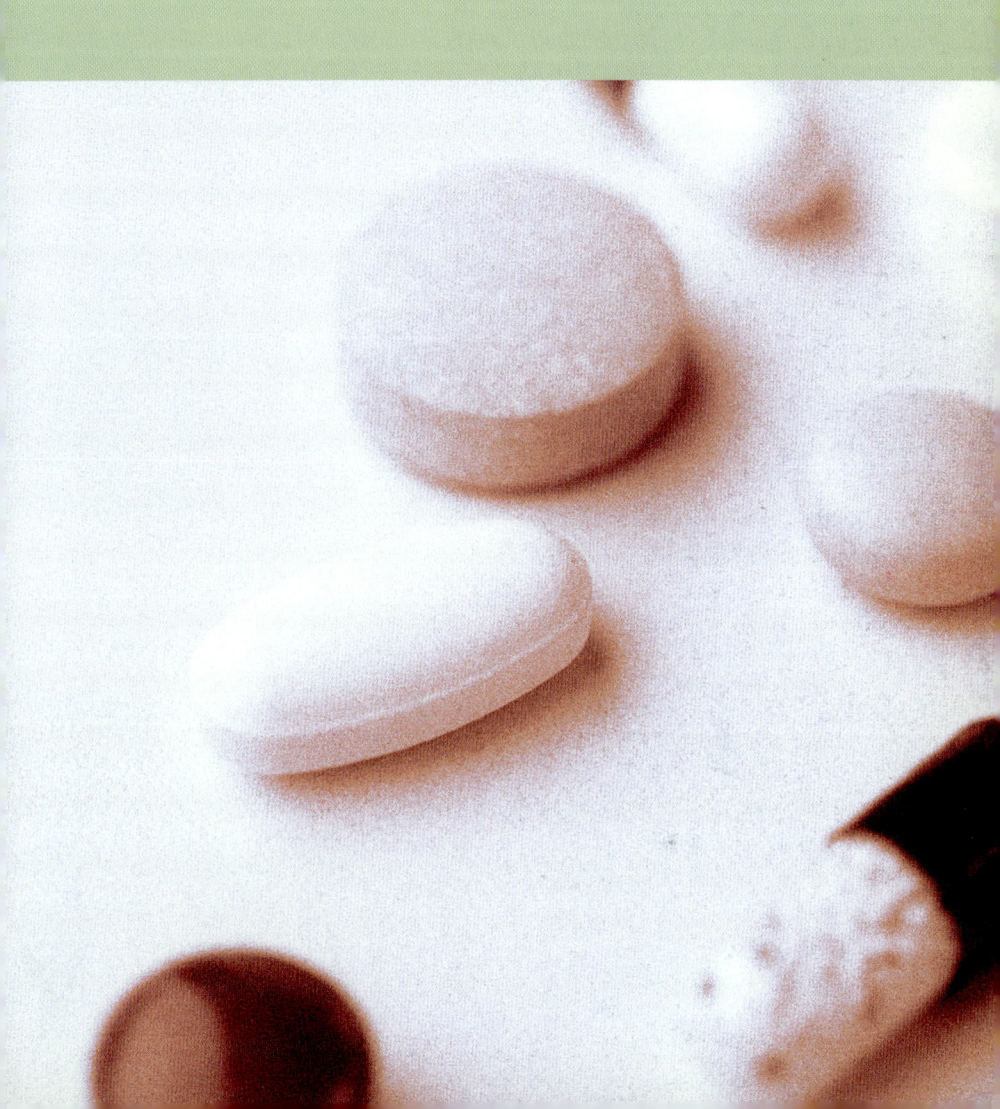

- Severe headache
- Uncharacteristic mental confusion
- Stiff neck
- Grey or almost white stools
- Profuse urination with a tremendous thirst
- Dark urine with blood, which has not been discoloured by eating foods such as beetroot
- Unexpected and repeated vomiting
- Extreme weakness
- Severe wheezing
- Yellowing of the skin or the whites of the eyes.

Meningitis

Early signs for meningitis are: leg pain, and cold hands and feet with pale or mottled skin. Later signs are: severe headache, stiff neck, a dislike of bright lights, fever and/or vomiting, drowsiness, a rash. This is a highly serious illness that needs immediate medical attention.

A high temperature above 39.5°C/103°F, especially in children, is a sign for concern and you should contact your doctor.

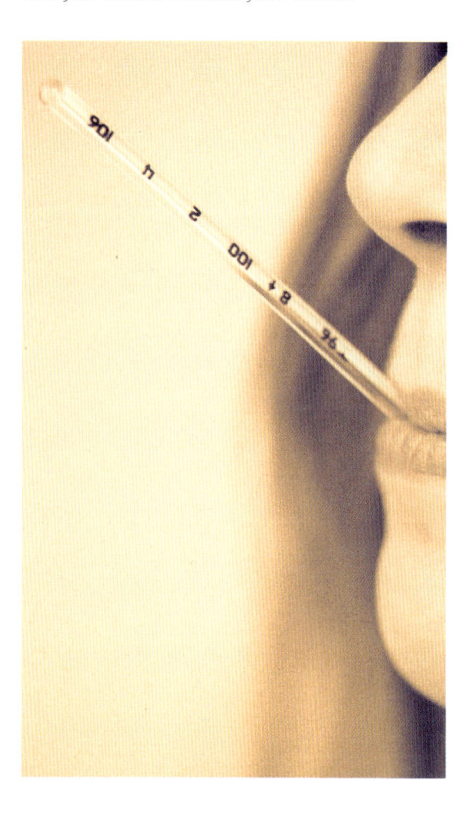

USING HOMEOPATHY WISELY

- Remember that although homeopathy can alleviate many conditions, if a person appears to be very ill it is essential to seek medical assistance.
- In a first-aid situation you might find a homeopathic remedy that can be used while you wait for medical assistance to arrive, but you should not rely on any homeopathic remedy in place of conventional medicine for anything other than common ailments and first aid.
- Homeopathic remedies can be used successfully to supplement medication prescribed by the doctor and can help the body to heal itself while using traditional medical treatment. However, always check with your doctor first. Many of the illnesses in this book are serious; do not home prescribe for any serious illnesses and always consider homeopathic remedies as support therapies to use alongside and not in place of medication and treatment prescribed by your allopathic doctor.
- If you or someone in your family shows signs of severe depression, is extremely unhappy or behaves in a way that makes them unable to take part in normal family life and society, you should speak to your doctor who can help by referring the patient to a suitably qualified professional. Similarly, someone showing signs of suffering from an eating disorder needs professional help, which is available through your doctor.
- A qualified homeopath can guide you in the correct use of remedies and can be contacted in an emergency to advise on suitable treatment. It is best to use a homeopath to help you achieve all-round good health in conjunction with following a healthy diet with plenty of exercise to help you to ward off illness. To find a qualified homeopath contact their governing body, such as the The Society of Homeopaths in the UK, The North American Society of Homeopaths (NASH) or the Australian Homeopathic Association.

keeping healthy

Homeopathic medicine aims to kick-start the body into healing itself. It will have more difficulty doing this if the body has been starved of good nutrition and is lethargic because of lack of exercise, so for the best results, practise homeopathy in conjunction with a healthy lifestyle.

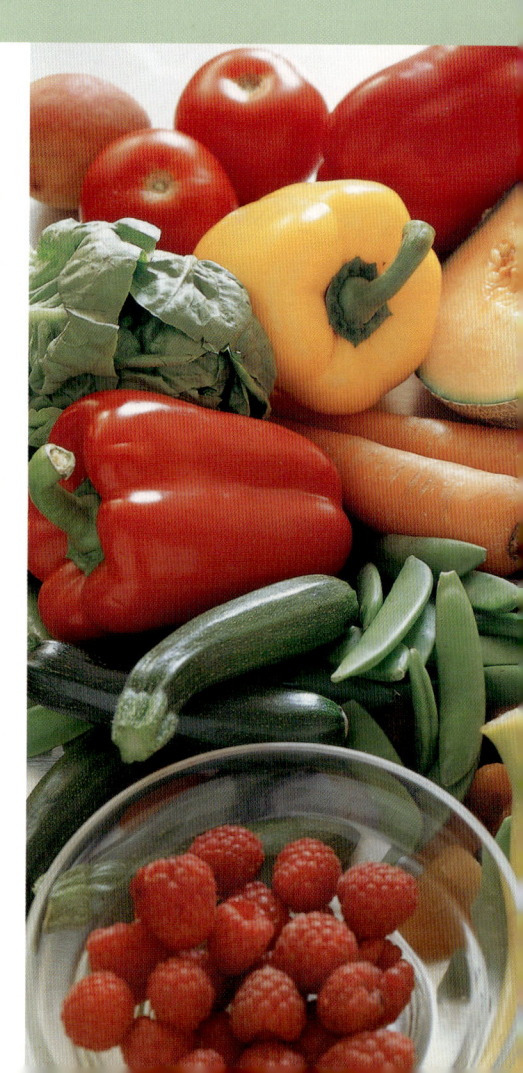

Eat plenty of fruit and vegetables and cut down on highly fatty foods and refined carbohydrates such as white bread and pasta. Eat red meat in moderation but eat plenty of lean meats such as chicken, oily fish, beans, peas and lentils, and whole grains, such as brown rice. Constipation need never be a problem if you are eating healthily and drinking plenty of water – try to drink at least eight glasses a day. This will also keep urinary infections at bay as well as keeping the skin plumped and fresh. If you do become slightly constipated you can usually resolve it by eating some dried fruit such as prunes, figs or dates. However, don't add bran to your meals, as it should always be eaten as part of the whole grain. If you have the symptoms of a urinary infection (a bearing-down feeling in the lower abdomen and discomfort when urinating) try drinking some cranberry juice or taking some cranberry capsules, which will alleviate discomfort and flush out the urinary tract.

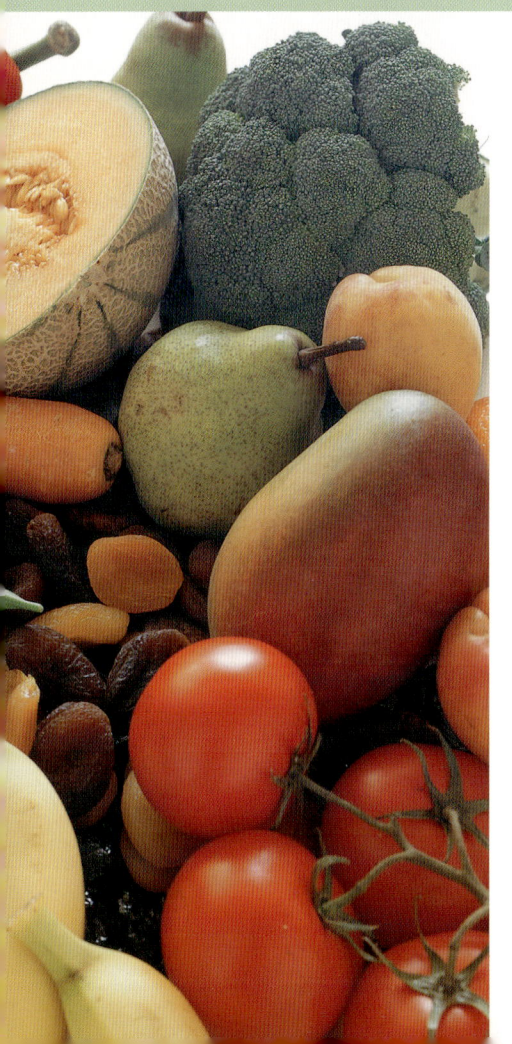

EAT YOUR GREENS

The recommended daily amount of five helpings of fruit and vegetables is really only a minimum and you should try to eat far more than this for optimum health. Organic produce is best, although it is more expensive. You will probably find this in your local supermarket or greengrocer or you might be able to join a scheme where you have a weekly box of vegetables delivered to your home. However, if organic food is too costly or unavailable it is better to eat non-organic produce than to limit fruit and vegetables in your diet; many common health problems, such as anaemia, can be helped simply by eating healthily.

Fresh fruit and vegetables are essential foods for good health and should be eaten plentifully every day.

KEEP ON YOUR TOES

Combine this healthy diet with plenty of exercise – walking is one of the best ways to keep fit – and always choose something that you will enjoy so that you will stick to it. If you dislike exercise, gradually build up walking from, say, 15 minutes a day to 30 minutes, and use as many opportunities to move around as you can, such as walking up the stairs instead of taking the lift. Don't sign up at the local gym unless you are sure you really want to exercise there regularly; it is better to fit in a few exercises at home than to give up altogether because you discover you don't have time for the gym. Yoga and Pilates are useful practices to help you to relax as well as strengthening your muscles and keeping your spine healthy and flexible. With a flexible spine you will avoid many health-related problems in later life and you will help keep yourself looking good. Both practices include exercises that you can use to loosen tension around your neck and head and therefore avoid stress-induced headaches.

ENJOY LIFE

Our lives are so busy these days that sometimes we forget how important it is to relax. Enjoy being with your family and friends – spending time playing with your children or just doing jobs around the house together. Go to the cinema, invite friends round for a drink or a meal, visit an art gallery or museum, or go for a walk in the park or the countryside. Never underestimate how important it is to spend time doing things that you take pleasure in with people you love and have fun with. It's the way to a healthy and happy mind.

Exercise every day for optimum health. A short, brisk walk is ideal, or find another form of exercise that you will enjoy.

keeping healthy 49

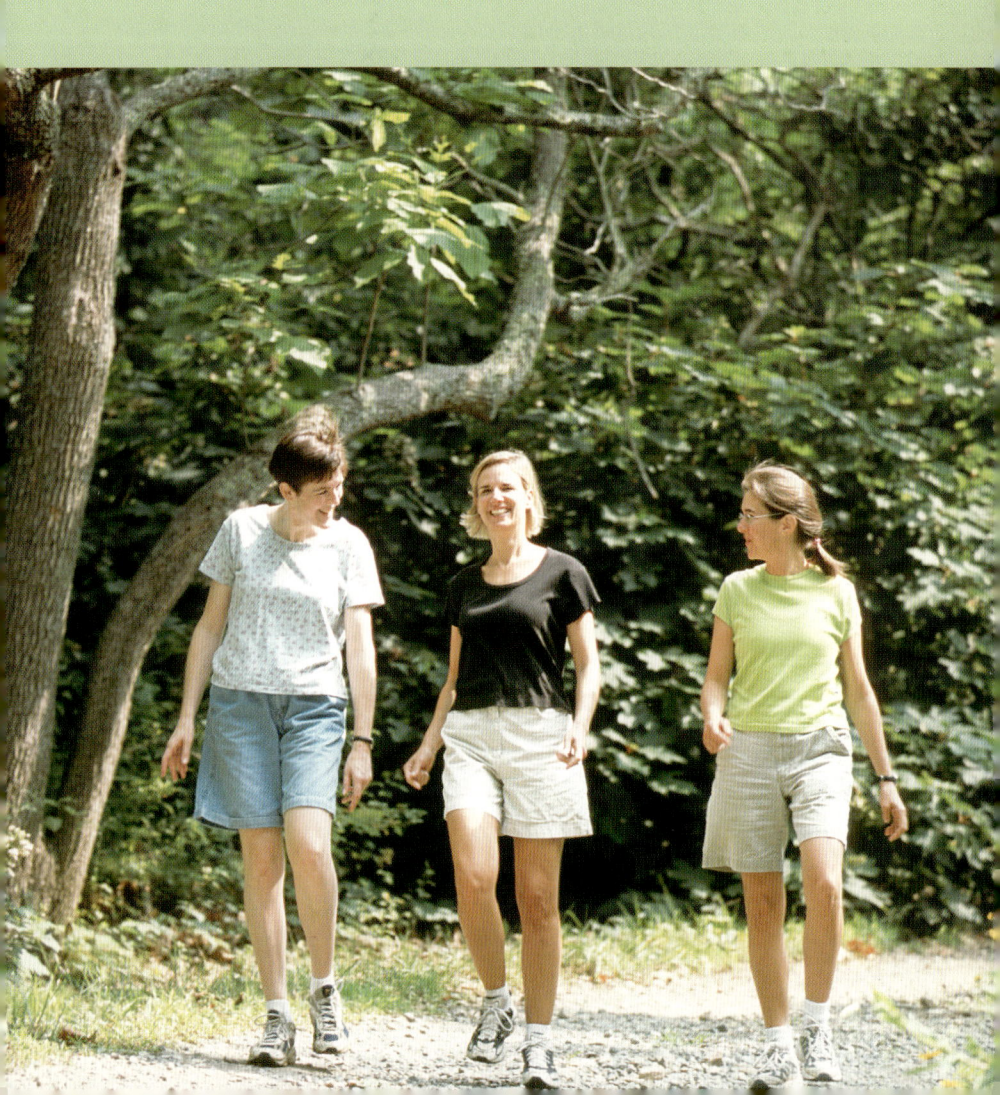

avoiding common illnesses

As well as taking the homeopathic remedies listed in the book, the following tips will help you avoid some ailments as well as making you or your patient more comfortable when you succumb to common illnesses.

BURNS AND SCALDS

For minor areas of skin that have been burnt, such as a finger or small part of the hand, immediately hold the burnt area under a tap of cold running water until it cools down. A few drops of essential oil of lavender can be applied to the area or gently apply some homeopathic burn ointment. If the burn becomes infected consult your doctor. Seek help for serious burns that cover an area of the body that is larger in size than half the palm of your hand.

COLDS, COUGHS AND FLU

If you catch a cold or flu or develop a cough it is especially important to keep your fluids up. Water is best and you might also like to add some squeezed orange or lemon juice. Always

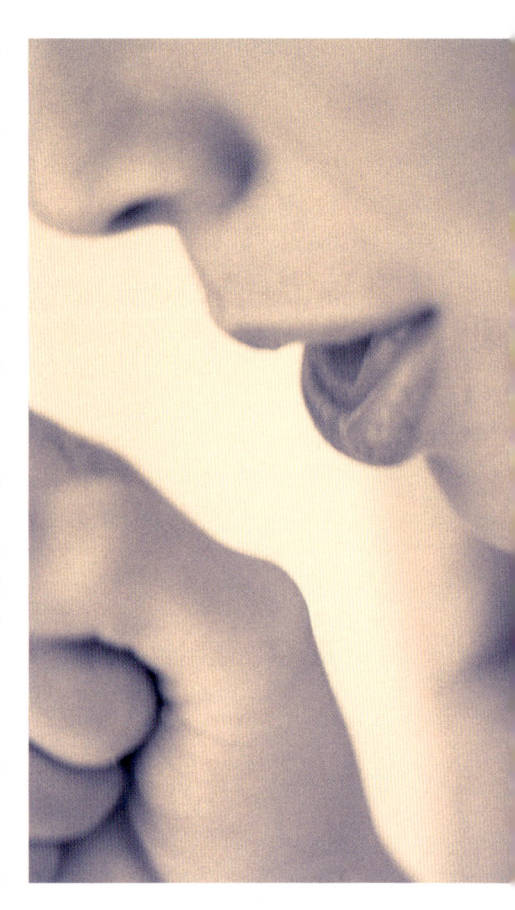

A tickly cough is one of the early signs of a cold developing. Simple home remedies can make you more comfortable.

drink plenty and rest as much as you can. Blow your nose gently to remove mucus and inhale steam from a bowl of boiling water to help dislodge thick mucus, if necessary. Try to avoid using the preparations that are advertised for relieving a cold as the only way to get over one is for your immune system to fight it. Also avoid cough mixtures as they can suppress the phlegm, which is better coughed up.

Always take to your bed with flu, as it is essential to have as much rest as possible. After a bad bout of flu take things easy for a while, as this is a time when the body is at its most vulnerable to catch other, possibly more serious, illnesses.

DIARRHOEA

Sip liquids to replace those lost through the diarrhoea, but limit food. Adults should avoid food for 24 hours. Avoid dairy products as these can aggravate the condition. When the patient feels better introduce light foods such as fruit juices and light vegetable soups, then try dry toast, bananas or white rice. Seek medical assistance for children who refuse to drink or if the patient is unable to keep liquids down, or if the diarrhoea lasts for more than a day or two or if the patient is in acute pain.

HEADACHES

Many headaches are caused by bad posture combined with stress. Try to sit and stand correctly and be especially aware of your posture if you work at a computer screen. Take plenty of short breaks away from the screen during the day, and try to stretch your whole body and loosen your shoulders if you can. Practising a few Yoga or Pilates exercises can end a stress headache in no time and are highly recommended. Also, help headaches by finding time to unwind and relax, perhaps in a hot bath or by going out for a walk in the fresh air. Practically any form of exercise will help a headache to subside that has been caused by stress.

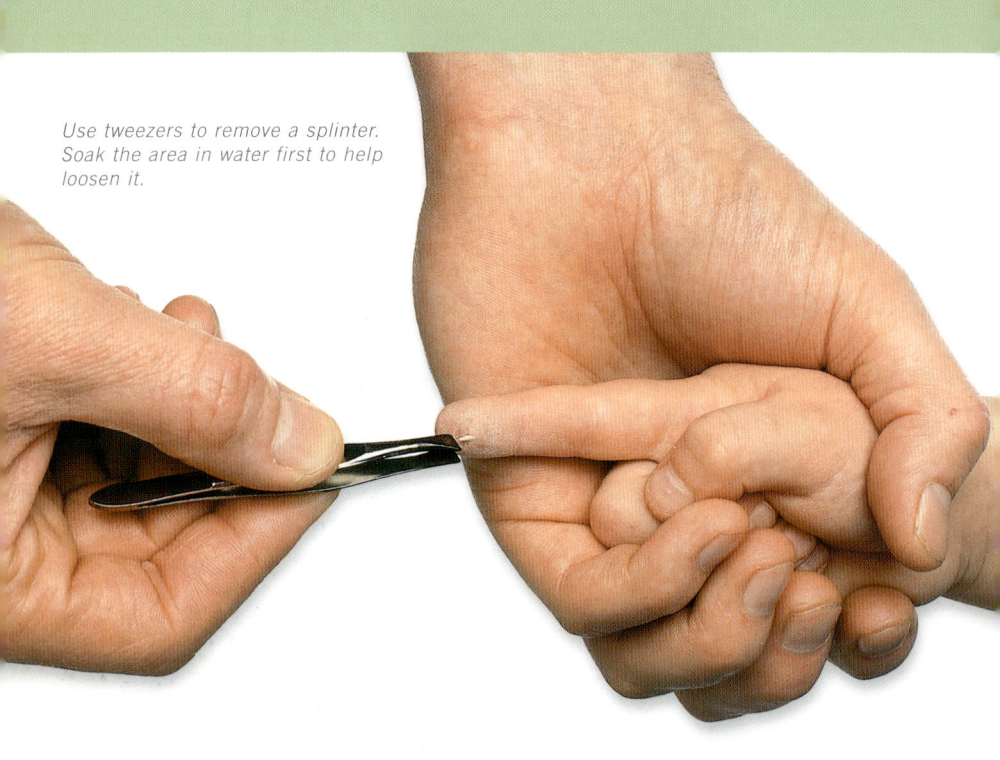

Use tweezers to remove a splinter. Soak the area in water first to help loosen it.

Eat regularly and sensibly, as some headaches are caused by a low blood-sugar level. If your headaches are severe or persistent, accompany a stiff neck, weakness or a rash, consult your doctor immediately (see also Meningitis on page 44).

SPLINTERS

Soak the area in warm water, which will help to loosen the splinter, then use tweezers to remove it. If necessary it can be loosened carefully using a sterilized needle. In time, the body will often reject and push out a splinter.

SUNBURN

Keep children, especially, covered up in the sun. You can buy sun lotions made with natural ingredients from your health-food shop. Always wear a hat in the sun. Avoid being in the sun during the hottest parts of the day, which are from 11.00 a.m. until 3.00 p.m., and keep spells in full sun to under 30 minutes. It is always best to sit in the shade if you are outside for long periods of time.

TEETHING

It's a good idea to keep teething rings in the refrigerator so that babies have something cool to chew on. Chamomilla granules are an easy way to administer the remedy, which soothes sore gums during teething.

TRAVEL SICKNESS

Have drinks handy, although avoid fizzy drinks. Chew some crystallized ginger or even a ginger biscuit, as ginger is especially good for helping nausea. Avoid reading or looking down while travelling.

NAUSEA AND VOMITING

Eat regularly if you are inclined to feel nauseous. Make a ginger tea by adding a little grated fresh root ginger to boiling water to help with nausea.

If vomiting occurs, take frequent sips of water and rest. Avoid food for several hours until the vomiting stops and avoid dairy produce until the vomiting has completely passed, as this can aggravate the condition.

Be careful to avoid dehydration; if the patient is unable to keep liquids down you will need to seek medical assistance. Also seek assistance if the vomit is dark or bloody or if the vomiting follows a head injury. Be especially cautious with babies and small children; seek help if a child is screaming, has projectile vomiting, or if the vomiting continues. If you think the vomiting is caused by food poisoning always contact your doctor immediately.

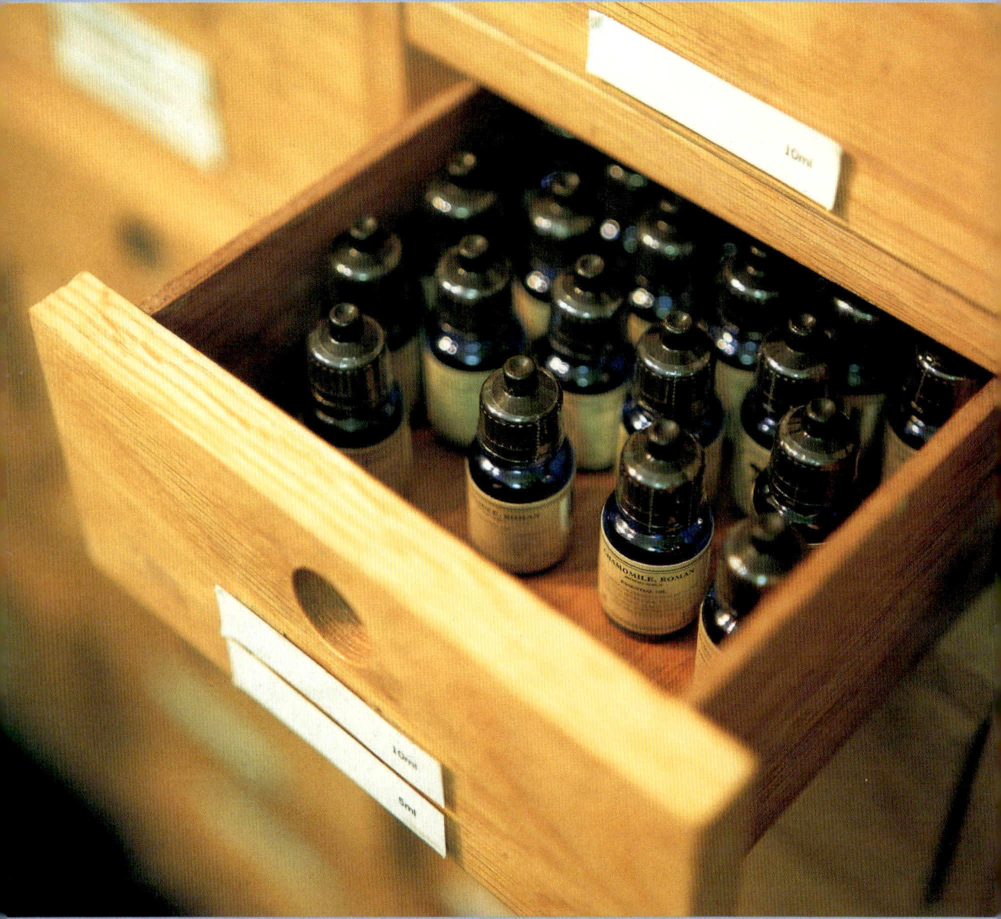
10ml
CHAMOMILE, ROMAN
ESSENTIAL OIL
10ml
5ml

PART TWO

homeopathic
materia medica

understanding the *materia medica*

When you are looking for a homeopathic remedy that will help treat your symptoms, check the basic First-Aid Remedies on page 58 before looking at other, less well-known remedies. However, if you have a medical emergency you should immediately contact your doctor or local hospital.

COMMON ILLNESSES

Conditions such as diarrhoea, constipation, headache, injury, some muscle pain, sprain, fever and flu in adults and small children can usually be treated with the ten basic First-Aid Remedies listed, so it is useful to keep them to hand. You can purchase these remedies at any health-food store. If you are unsure about the severity of your problems it is always best to consult your doctor.

The rule of thumb on selecting any emergency remedy is that if it does not act within two consecutive doses over a few hours you need to choose another remedy. If your symptoms persist after using two remedies you should consult your doctor.

HOW TO READ AN ENTRY

Each entry for a homeopathic medicine provides the following information:

1 The name of the medicine.
2 A list of codes for the remedy categories (see opposite), which tells you the specific use for each remedy.
3 The common name of the source of the remedy.
4 A general introduction to the main actions of the remedy.
5 An overview of the mental and emotional symptoms the remedy addresses.
6 A guide to the physical complaints.
7 The general complaints.
8 The key symptoms to look out for in the patient.

The remedies in the *Materia Medica* fall into the categories listed in the table opposite. You will find the following abbreviations with each remedy listed.

Homeopathic remedy categories

- **+FA** Homeopathic First-Aid Remedies. These can make all the difference at the very beginning of injury and illness. They can alleviate pain, distress and shock.
- **AA** Anti-ageing remedies and symptoms of age.
- **CB** Homeopathic remedies for childbirth. They can keep labour on course, prepare the cervix for dilation and ease pain and fatigue. They are good for mother and her new baby to help restore vitality and help the baby adapt to its new environment.
- **C-C-F** Remedies used for colds, coughs and flu.
- **CR** Children's remedies. These are specific to young children. They can help relieve fevers, colds, flu and injury. They can be used for babies and are effective for such things as constipation, diarrhoea, sore throat and earache. Remember that a high temperature is dangerous, especially in a child; if it reaches above 39.5°C/103°F you should seek medical assistance.
- **D** Remedies for the digestive tract that deal with nausea, constipation and diarrhoea.
- **F** Female remedies that relate to menstruation, childbirth, nursing and menopause as well as female sexuality.
- **GR** General remedy, used for constitutional treatment.
- **M** Mental states of anxiety, fear and anger. Symptoms that involve the mind. These remedies can alleviate tension and stress, but are not intended to be taken on a regular basis; continuing stress disorders need professional guidance.
- **Ma** Male remedies that relate to male sexual conditions. If the symptoms persist please consult your doctor.

first-aid remedies

A set of the following remedies will cover you and your family for most common illnesses and minor accidents.

ACONITUM NAPELLUS 30C
This remedy is to be used for the sudden onset of colds, flu or any illness. If taken within the first 12 hours it can stop symptoms from developing. It is also used for shock, trauma, injury and where the person feels fearful. This may be after an accident or having been exposed to extreme cold or heat.

ARNICA MONTANA 30C
This remedy is the premier homeopathic remedy for shock, injury or bruising when it has been necessary to react quickly. It is a useful remedy for when the patient feels pain. Arnica montana is suitable for use when the patient is not fearful and after an accident reports that they are feeling fine. Arnica montana is also useful for restlessness and sleeplessness, and after extreme exertion, such as physical workouts.

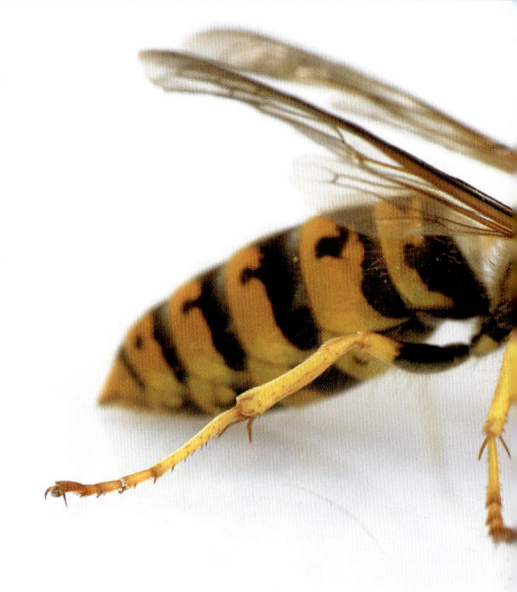

ARSENICUM ALBUM 30C
A remedy to treat food poisoning and to stop vomiting, diarrhoea, fever, flu and colds, asthma and sleeplessness. It is appropriate to use this remedy when symptoms are worse between midnight and 2.00 a.m. The remedy helps with restlessness and is a treatment for asthma attacks that occur between those hours.

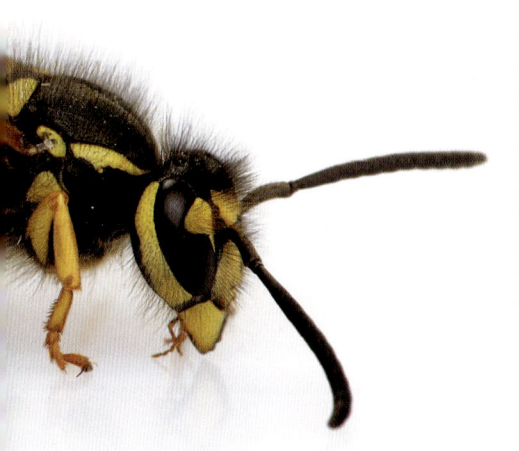

Protection from insects

Another useful remedy, especially if you live in the country or for times when you are holiday, is Apis mellifica, which is a first-aid remedy for stings, bites and rashes.

Painful wasp stings can be alleviated by taking Apis mellifica. It is a very useful remedy to keep in a first-aid kit.

BELLADONNA 30C

Use this remedy to relieve headache, fever with delirium, flu, inflammation and boils. Its use is indicated when the skin is red, dry and taut and the patient is not thirsty. Belladonna can bring down a high fever (sometimes after an initial increase) especially in children, and it also relieves many skin and internal symptoms where inflammation is involved.

BRYONIA ALBA 30C

Consider Bryonia alba first for headaches, coughs and colds, especially where the patient is thirsty. All symptoms are worse for movement and the patient prefers to be left to be still, quiet and alone. It is also a useful remedy for the relief of mastitis.

CARBO VEGETABILIS 30C
Use Carbo vegetabilis to relieve flatulence and stomach pain. It is also used for faintness and can revive someone who is unconscious by placing it just inside the lip (make sure that the patient does not choke).

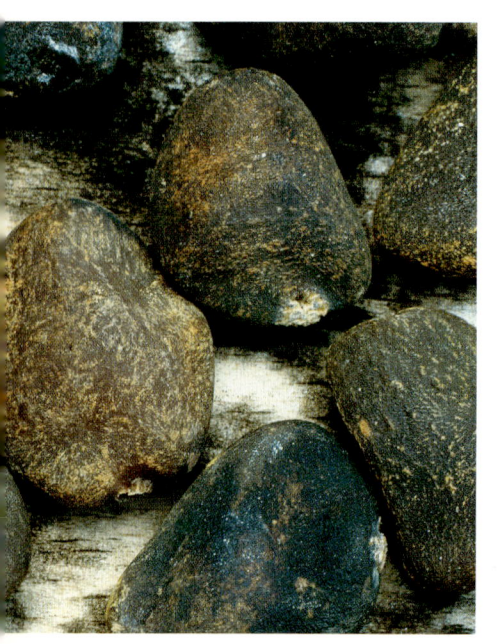

IGNATIA 30C
The remedy Ignatia is known as a grief remedy, as it can be used when the patient is emotionally upset – shocked through the news of death and for fear of loss or great disappointment. It also works for resulting sore throats and backaches.

NUX VOMICA 30C
Known as the hangover remedy, Nux vomica also fortifies the liver and helps relieve liver stagnation, which can lead to constipation. It is used when you eat excessively rich food, or after overuse of alcohol or tobacco. It is appropriate for those who have a sedentary lifestyle and rarely move enough to keep their liver active.

The bean from the Ignatia plant forms the basis of a remedy that is useful to give someone who is grieving.

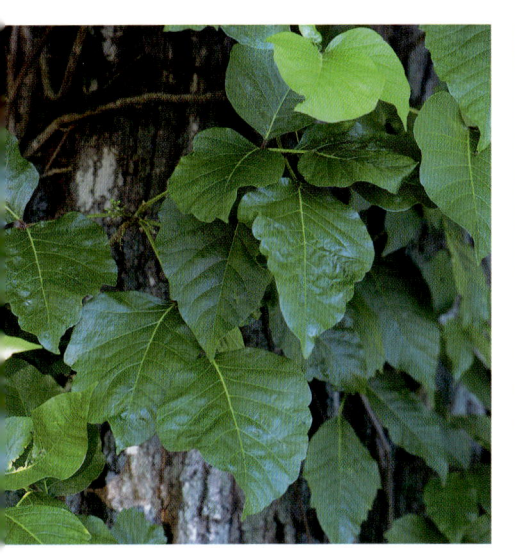

Poison ivy is the original substance used in dilution in the remedy Rhus Toxicodendron.

Useful ointments

Arnica, Rhus toxicodendron and Ruta graveolens are also available as ointments that can be used on the skin to work alongside the remedies.

RHUS TOXICODENDRON 30C

This useful remedy alleviates rheumatism, sore joints, pneumonia, colds and fever. It helps skin rashes and other skin irritations. It is often used when people complain of stiff joints and sore backs.

RUTA GRAVEOLENS 30C

Use Ruta graveolens for tendons and ligaments. It is excellent for sore hands, a sore and stiff back and for sprains. When combined together with Rhus toxicodendron 30C and Arnica montana 30C it can bring relief to painful parts of the body, especially the joints and a sore back.

Note: Throughout the Materia Medica an asterisk (*) denotes a first-aid remedy.

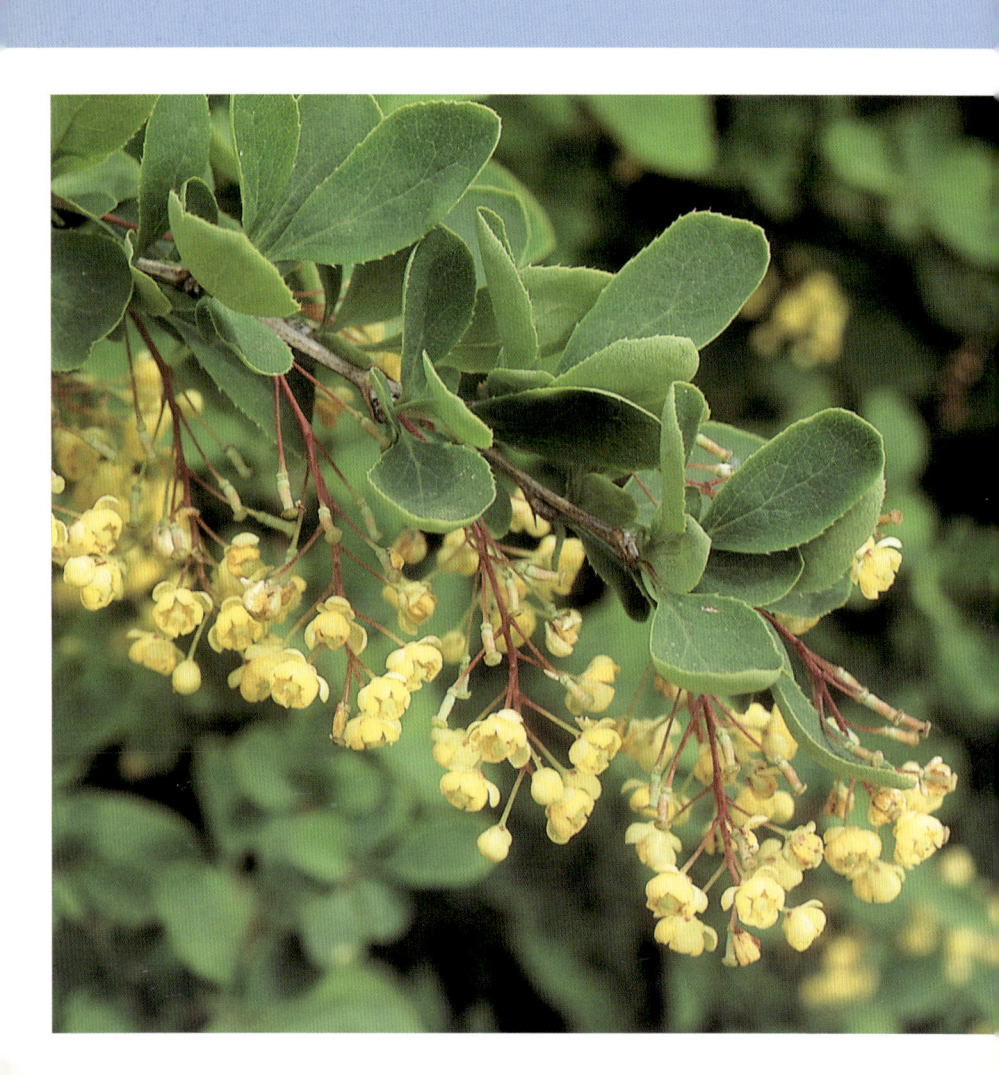

materia medica

ACONITUM NAPELLUS (ACONITE)

(+FA, C-C-F, CB, CR) monkshood *

Aconite addresses fear, anxiety and anguish. It is used to treat shock, injury and trauma which is accompanied by fear.

The symptoms that indicate the use of Aconite are acute and happen suddenly and violently, accompanied by fear, and with a fever, chill or a headache. The pains that accompany the illness can be intense.

The remedy is used for complaints that arise from exposure to cold, dry wind or to intense, dry heat. It works well for asthma, inflammations, bronchitis, pneumonia, fever and the onset of flu. Give Aconite within the first 12 hours of an acute illness, as it can stave off flu and cold, but it only works at the very beginning when symptoms first appear.

Mind and emotions

The patient feels great fear, anxiety and restlessness, fearing death, the future, a crowd or crossing the street.

> **Key symptoms**
>
> Extreme restlessness and fear • Panic attacks • Shock, injury and trauma accompanied by fear with a fever, chills or a headache.

Physical complaints

- A full, heavy, pulsating head that feels as if it is bursting and burning.
- Inflamed red eyes, which feel dry and hot, with an aversion to light. The eyelids are swollen, hard and red. The patient is also sensitive to noise.
- The face is red, hot and flushed. Where one cheek is red and the other pale, Aconite is an appropriate remedy.
- The face is extremely pale first thing in the morning. During the onset of a cold or flu

the throat is red, dry and constricted, with swollen tonsils.
- Stomach symptoms include vomiting accompanied by fear, profuse sweating and increased need to urinate.
- Respiration can be difficult with heaviness on the chest, a hoarse dry cough, accompanied by shortness of breath.

General symptoms

Excessive thirst. The patient feels better in the fresh air, and worse in a warm room; worse when hearing music, from tobacco smoke, and dry, cold winds.

Although the typical Aconite patient feels better in fresh air, their symptoms will be exacerbated in dry, cold winds.

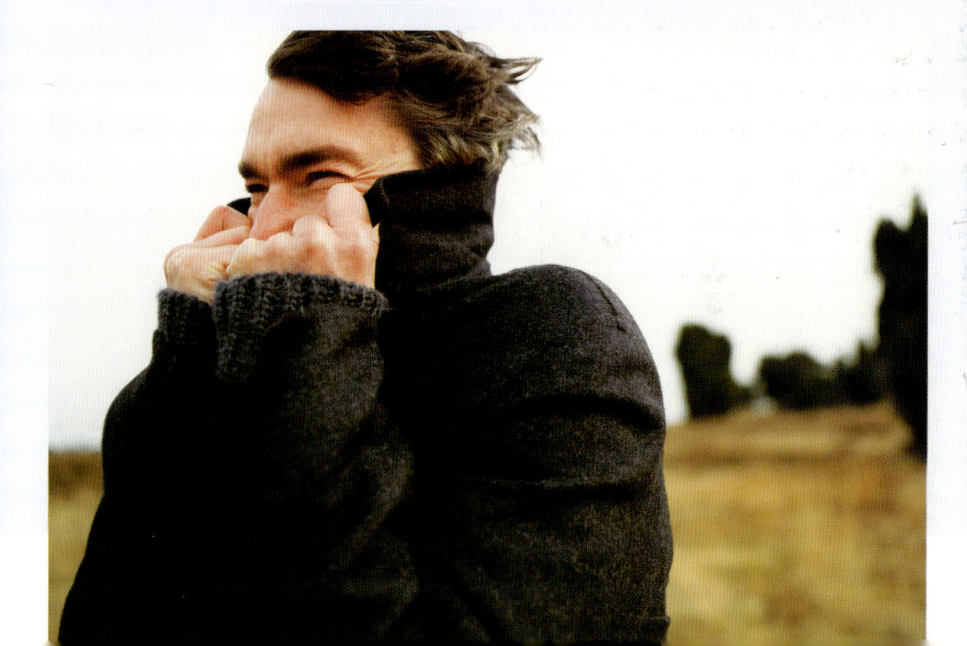

AGARICUS MUSCARIUS

(C-C-F, D, GR) fly agaric mushroom

A remedy for twitching, jerking and trembling; for neuralgia and spasmodic movements, and where patients are prone to headaches and sciatica. Agaricus is especially useful for treating chilblains. It works well for delirium, fevers, alcoholism and general paralysis.

Mind and emotions

The patient can appear delirious; talking but not answering questions. They may also express an aversion to work, act indifferent to situations and appear fearless. However, they may have worries about cancer and can be preoccupied with death.

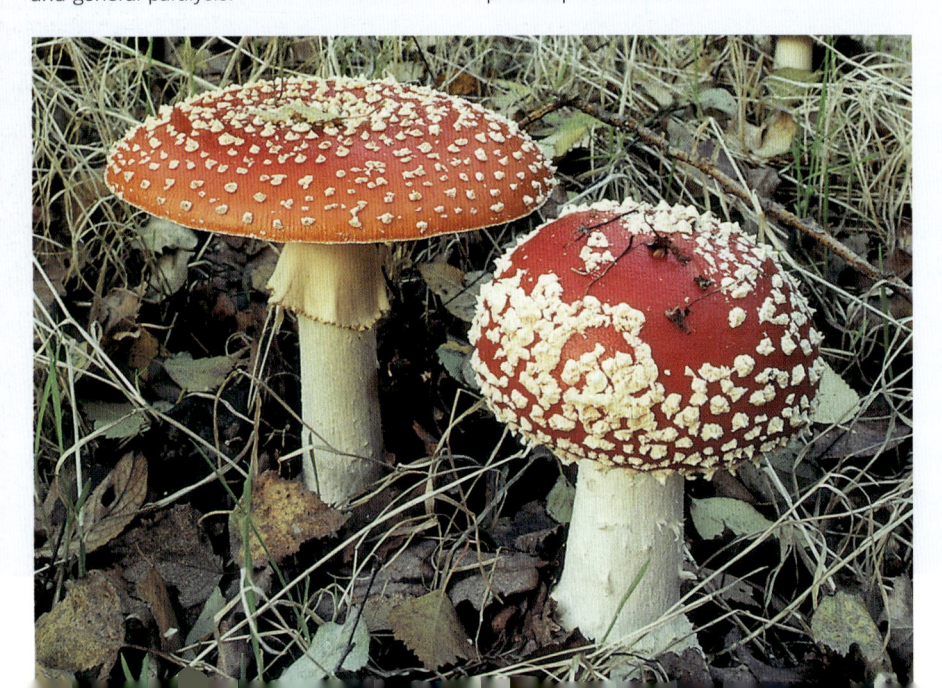

Physical complaints

- The patient may find reading can be difficult because the eyes are twitching; facial muscles will also twitch and burn.
- At times elderly people can experience nosebleeds or spasmodic sneezing after coughing, or spasmodic contractions in the stomach with a great, unnatural hunger that burns the stomach.
- A stitch pain might also be felt in the abdomen, with diarrhoea accompanied by wind, or gastric disturbances accompanied by a sharp pain in the liver.
- There might also be violent attacks of coughing that the patent attempts to suppress; spasmodic coughing at night after falling asleep.
- Chilblains that burn and are red.

The poisonous fungi fly agaric is used in dilution to relieve chilblains, as well as twitching and jerking movements.

Key symptoms

Twitching, jerking and trembling • Involuntary and exaggerated movements; awkwardness • Burning and itching • Chilblains.

General symptoms

During a fever the patient is very sensitive to cold air, and worse for pressure on their back. The remedy is suitable for people who are very chilly, even during warm weather, and who are worse for the cold. They can become disorientated and subsequently injure themselves. They are worse for exhaustion from mental activity, sex and alcohol. They appear better for gentle motion and in the evening.

ium medica

ALLIUM CEPA

(C-C-F, CR, M) common red onion

A remedy that is useful for colds with mucus streaming from the eyes and nose. It is useful in cold, damp climates with phlegmatic patients who have systems that have broken down due to life circumstances, illness or too much medication. The patient is worse from wet feet, dampness and for chilly, wet winds. This is also a good remedy for neuralgic pains following amputation of a limb or an injury to the nerves.

Mind and emotions
Patients are unable to think clearly or become open to new ideas or stimulation.

Physical complaints
- Ailments from eating cucumbers and salads, with an allergy to peaches, which make the nose run. There are watery discharges from the nose with a sensation of rawness and burning.

> **Key symptoms**
>
> Nasal discharge with burning •
> Sleepiness and difficulty concentrating.

- There can be coughing and tearing pains in the throat, and hay fever.
- For colic that begins after getting wet feet.
- Also good for the common cold when it moves down towards the chest, or for rawness in the throat when coughing.
- A remedy for men who experience pain in the prostate gland after sex.

General symptoms
For retention of urine that occurs after getting feet wet. The patient has a desire for onions, raw food and vegetables. Patient feels better for cold drinks; worse for wet feet.

allium cepa

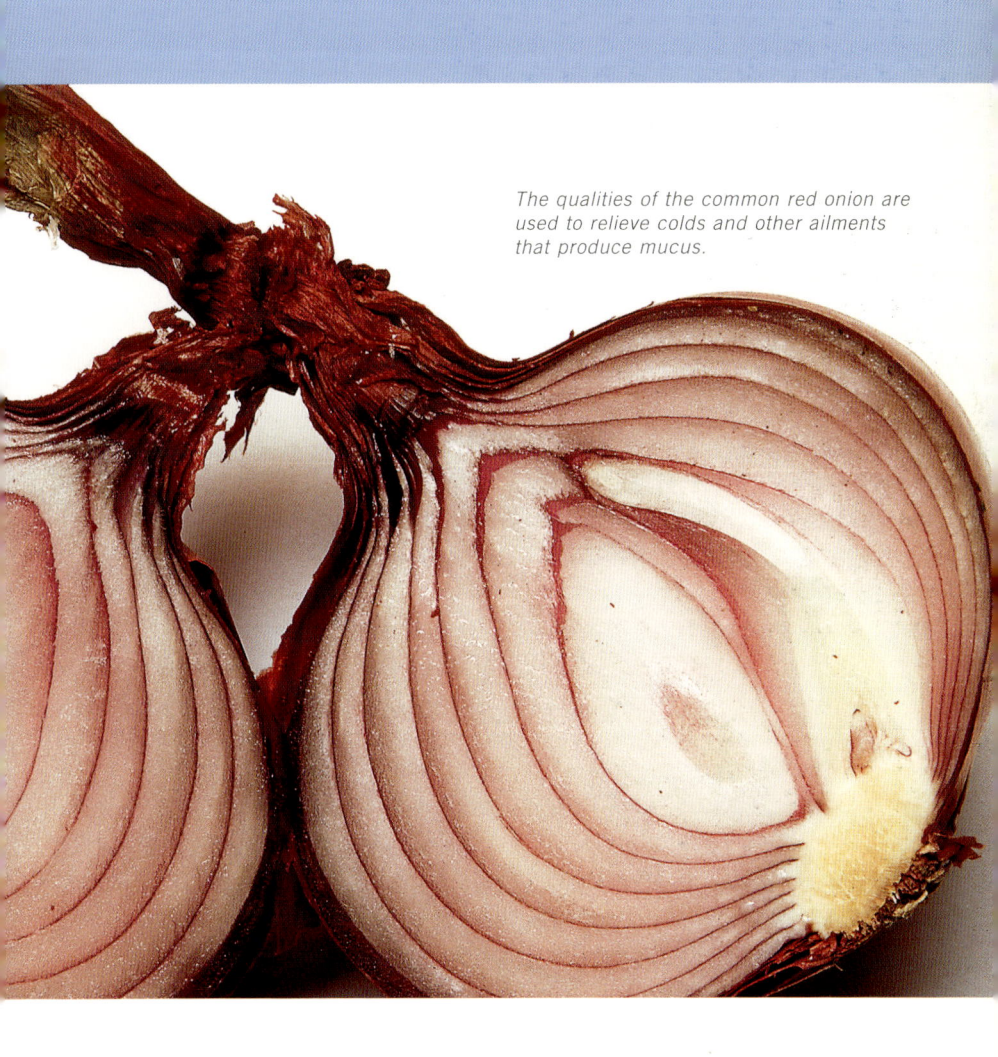

The qualities of the common red onion are used to relieve colds and other ailments that produce mucus.

ALOE SOCOTRINA

(AA, D, C-C-F, F, GR, M)
common aloe plant

An excellent remedy for digestive problems, Aloe socotrina is especially useful after too much medication. It is indicated for people suffering with a 'stagnant' liver (that is, those who have problems with anger, irritability and constipation) and also for people who have a sedentary lifestyle and so are not physically active.

Mind and emotions

The patient is angry and dissatisfied with him- or herself; weary and feeling aged. They will experience activity that alternates with laziness, and physical weakness will follow any mental activity.

Physical complaints

- The patient might experience headaches alternating with lumbago, where the body feels full, heavy, congested and dragging.

Key symptoms

Congestion and fullness, especially around the area of the liver • Involuntary stool • Headaches.

- There is heaviness in the eyes and a bitter taste in the mouth.
- The patient may cough up tough pieces of mucus and long for refreshing, juicy food.
- This is a remedy for nausea accompanied by fullness in the liver and with pains under the ribs. The stomach feels bloated, heavy and engorged.
- The patient feels weak, full of gas, and always ready to run to the toilet in fear of losing control of their bowels. There might be loose stools, with or without wind.

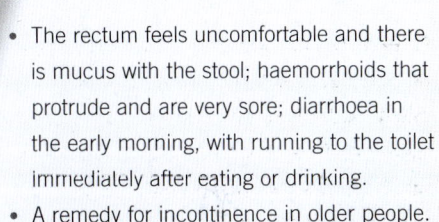

- The rectum feels uncomfortable and there is mucus with the stool; haemorrhoids that protrude and are very sore; diarrhoea in the early morning, with running to the toilet immediately after eating or drinking.
- A remedy for incontinence in older people.
- Use Aloe socotrina for women when they feel a bearing-down sensation in the rectum; worse when standing and during their periods; the uterus feels heavy.

General symptoms

The patient is worse in the early morning; during summer heat; in hot, dry weather; after eating and drinking in excess. Better for cold, fresh air that refreshes.

The curative properties of the aloe are well known and in homeopathy are especially useful for digestive and liver problems.

ALUMINA

(D, AA, C-C-F, F, GR)
oxide of aluminium

This remedy is used in digestive disturbances and is effective in treating persistent constipation where there is no thirst. It can also be used for treating premature ageing, especially when accompanied by dehydration and dryness.

> **Key symptoms**
>
> *Chilliness, confusion, retention and dryness • Slowness; patient easily feels panicked.*

Mind and emotions

The patient will be vague and hazy and have difficulty expressing him- or herself. Or they will have an active mind but be slow to act. The patient will also make mistakes in speech and writing; they will feel that time passes too slowly or, alternatively, can feel hurried; they are better when allowed to move at their own pace and worse when dealing with time constraints; they easily feel panicked and take a long time to do what is needed.

This is also a remedy for disappointment, violent anger and prolonged mental exertion.

The patient might be easily confused. They also fear pointed, sharp objects, such as knives, as well as the sight of blood.

Physical complaints

- Dryness is a keynote symptom of Alumina and this is reflected in an inability to think through one's conditions so that the patient is unable to move forward in life. This is a remedy for the aged.
- It is also good for girls who have a dry appearance, making them look older.

- Use for delicate children who are weak, particularly if they frequently eat convenience food and don't eat enough fruit and vegetables. Suitable for anybody who has had a poor diet or for those who have too much aluminium in the body due to eating too many canned foods, using deodorants with aluminium, and using aluminium utensils exclusively for cooking.
- It is also good for people who have taken too much medicine.
- Suitable for patients who find digesting grains and potatoes difficult.
- Alumina is a remedy for constipation that is accompanied by straining, even when the stools are soft; water retention, when water is held in the system and not released through sweat, urine or periods.
- It also can be used for a chronic, dry sore throat with frequent coughing.

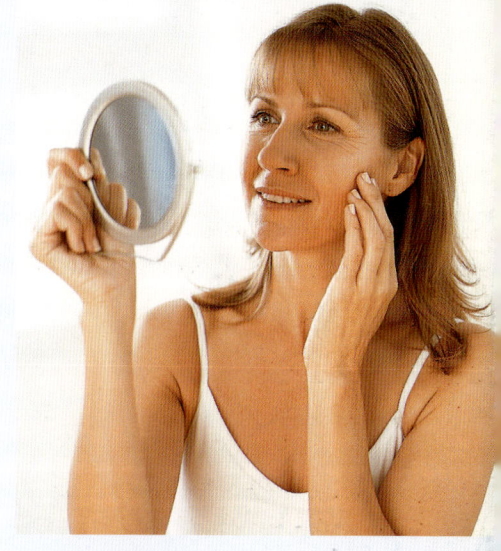

Skin that is dry and dehydrated might show symptoms of premature ageing. These symptoms can be treated with Alumina.

General symptoms

The patient's mucous membranes tend to be dry, resulting in stagnancy where nothing is able to move smoothly from the body. This also affects the mind working smoothly.

ANACARDIUM ORIENTALE

(AA, GR) cashew nut

This remedy is used primarily for mental symptoms that affect the nerves. It is useful for adolescent boys and girls who have become hardened and unkind due to difficult childhoods and who often act extremely, sometimes even violently. This is a good remedy for people who tend to be insulting and unkind to others.

Mind and emotions

The patient lacks confidence, and feels helpless and that they are not worthy or good enough; they wish to prove their worth, but have a fear of exams or being tested in any capacity. They can be angry and unkind and dislike to be contradicted. They take everything badly, and anger can cause them to become violent. Patients who would benefit from Anarcardium orientale are sometimes abusive and can feel extreme hatred, acting hard-heartedly and

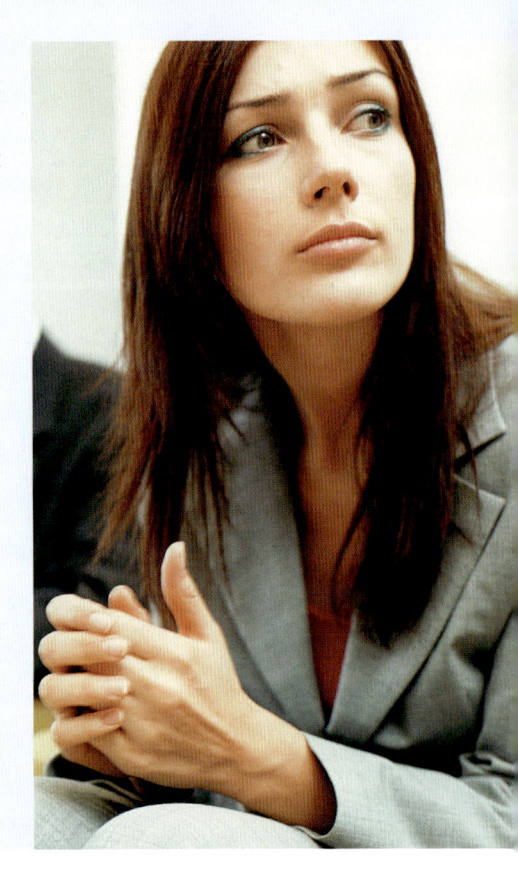

Anacardium orientale can be used to treat a patient who is lacking in confidence, particularly when faced with a test or exam.

maliciously, with cursing and swearing. They can also be fastidious, unable to rest if things are not in their proper place.

Physical complaints
- Headaches and eczema.
- The patient might experience constipation and is better for eating. Although their symptoms might disappear during meals they may reappear afterwards. They may also experience a sensation of constrictions inside as if there is an internal band around the affected part.
- The patient can be worse for lying on their side and find that symptoms are felt on one side only.
- External numbness is sometimes experienced.

Key symptoms

Lack of confidence, patient needs to prove him- or herself to others • Prolonged mental exertion • Sensation of a plug or band around the parts of the body that hurt • Symptoms are better for eating.

General symptoms
Numbness in parts of the body and often a plug-like sensation in the eyes, ears and abdomen. Their headaches are better for eating. They can suffer eczema with excessive itching that is better for immersion in very hot water.

ANTIMONIUM CRUDUM

(CR, D, GR) sulphide of antimony

This is a remedy to be used for problems of the stomach, digestive tract, the mind and skin. The symptoms appear predominantly on the left side of the body.

Mind and emotions

The patient detests being looked at, touched or washed. The remedy is suitable for sulky children who do not wish to speak or be spoken to, and who are angry at the slightest attention. It is also suited to adolescent girls who are sentimental and suffer from affection that is not returned, girls who are dreamers, and those who can become depressed after disappointment in love.

Physical complaints

- The patient suffers from digestive disturbances and gout. Gastric disturbances will be caused by eating too much farinaceous food, such as bread and pasta, from bathing in cold water, or from overheating and hot weather.
- They can be sensitive on the soles of their feet, finding walking difficult and painful.
- Cracks at the corners of the mouth, the nose and the eyes, and even horny or split nails would indicate the need for Antimonium crudum.
- The patient might have headaches from taking cold, alcoholic drinks and rich food.
- They feel better for vomiting, diarrhoea and sneezing.

> **Key symptoms**
>
> *Sulky, easily angered at being looked at or touched • Romantic, sentimental adolescents • Ailments from digestive disturbance • Nail and skin problems.*

- The tongue will be coated milky-white due to indigestion.

General symptoms

The patient feels worse for heat during the summer, and becoming overheated at any time. They love acidic foods, and often desire large quantities of food, but this frequently leads to emotional, gastric and skin problems. The symptoms often change: gastric symptoms change to gout; symptoms go from one side to another or change locality. Perspiration will be experienced at the slightest exertion. The patient suffers ailments due to sunburn, overheating or warm weather.

Antimonium crudum is a useful remedy for digestive and skin problems, and is suited particularly to children who are sulky.

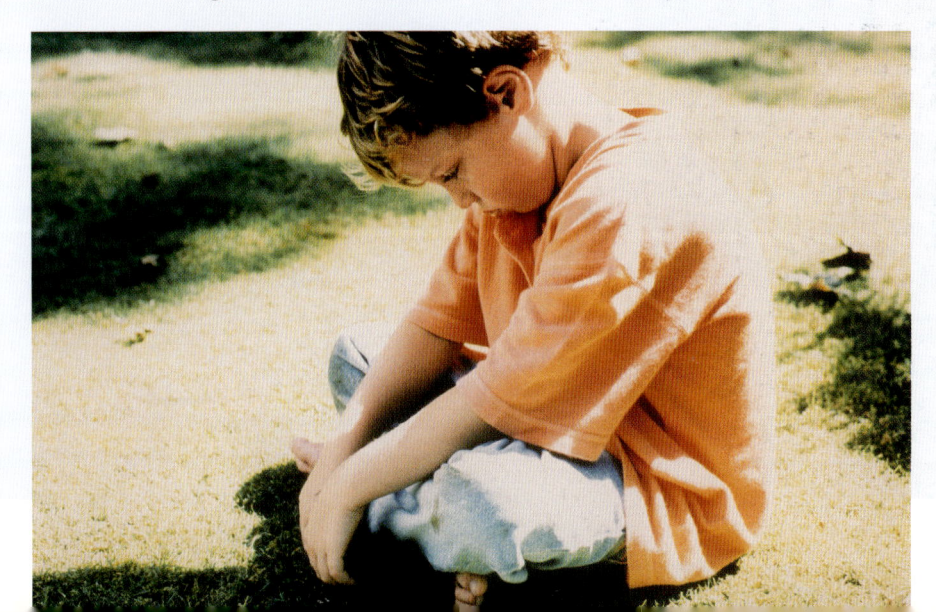

ANTIMONIUM TARTARICUM

(C-C-F, CR, GR) tartar emetic

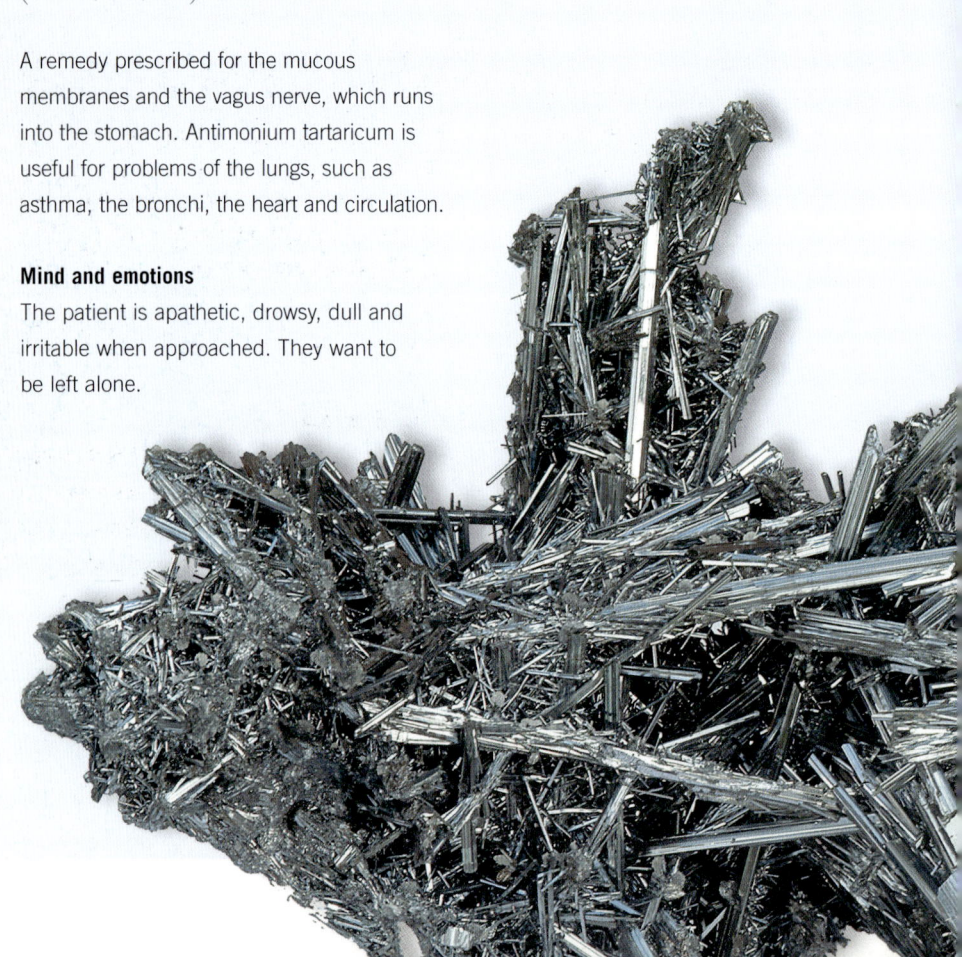

A remedy prescribed for the mucous membranes and the vagus nerve, which runs into the stomach. Antimonium tartaricum is useful for problems of the lungs, such as asthma, the bronchi, the heart and circulation.

Mind and emotions

The patient is apathetic, drowsy, dull and irritable when approached. They want to be left alone.

Physical complaints
- The patient becomes increasingly weak, drowsy, sweaty and lacking in energy. They are sleepy.
- This remedy is particularly useful for children with a milk allergy, and it is also suitable for a bad reaction to vaccination.
- Suitable for conditions where the patient experiences large amounts of mucus with rattling in the chest.
- It is also a remedy for nausea.

Tartar emetic, the source mineral for this remedy that is useful for chesty illnesses in drowsy and irritable patients.

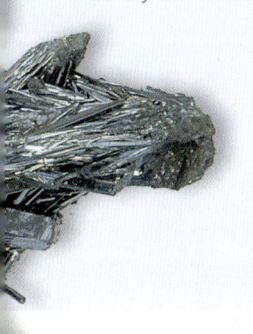

Key symptoms

Patient dislikes being looked at and wishes to be left alone • White tongue • Rattling in the chest, but patient is unable to cough up the phlegm • Drowsiness and weakness.

General symptoms
A useful remedy for shortness of breath that alternates with coughing that is loose and produces a rattling sound but with no phlegm. Also for nausea that comes in waves, accompanied by weakness, a cold sweat and anxiety.

APIS MELLIFICA

(F, AA, GR) honey bee*

This remedy has many uses, including first-aid for stings, bites, rashes and irritable skin.

Mind and emotions

The patient suffers from ailments related to receiving bad news, grief, anger and fright. It is appropriate when there is jealousy, fury, sexual excess and mental shock. It is suitable for nervous, irritable people who are difficult and hard to please. It is also useful for when people are clumsy, either physically or mentally; particularly children or women who, although generally careful, become awkward and let things fall out of their hands.

Physical complaints

- A remedy for people who are always warm and have swellings.
- The symptoms are burning and stinging pains that are better for cold applications. The skin is very sensitive to the touch.
- It is a good remedy for the bad effects of measles, mumps or scarlet fever.
- Useful for varicose veins that swell, and for puffy swelling under the eyes as well as for styes.

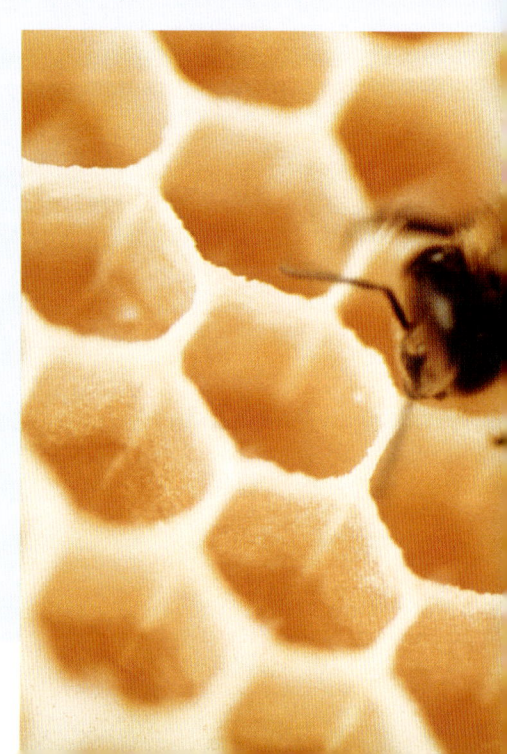

- Also for rashes or asthma due to a change in the weather or during a fever, or from heavy perspiration.
- It can be used successfully for water retention and diarrhoea.

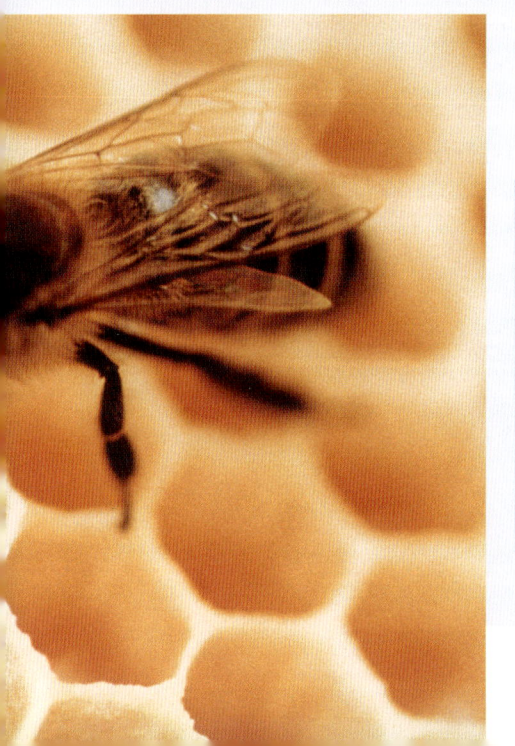

General symptoms

An effective sore-throat remedy when the throat feels constricted and burning. Good for rashes of all kinds. Apis mellifica is indicated for warm-bodied people.

The remedy Apis mellifica is derived from the honeybee and is used for illnesses accompanied by stinging pains.

Key symptoms

Jealous, busy, fidgety and clumsy • Burning and stinging pains that are worse for the heat and better for the cold • Swellings that are extremely sensitive to touch and pressure • Little or no thirst.

ARGENTUM NITRICUM

(M, C-C-F, Me, F, GR) silver nitrate

The remedy Argentum nitricum is excellent for anxiety and nervous tension.

Mind and emotions

The patient is nervous about their health but reserved when expressing their feelings. They try to compensate for their lack of self-confidence with good behaviour. They seem soft and yielding, but there is a hidden side where they can be bossy and difficult, usually when at home. They might fear high or narrow places and crowds. They are worse when anticipating events; even catching a train or bus can provoke anxiety. They can be close to nervous breakdown, so affected are they by the stress in their life, and their suffering has weakened the ability of their

A remedy for nervous tension, Argentum nitricum, is derived from the pure crystals of silver nitrate.

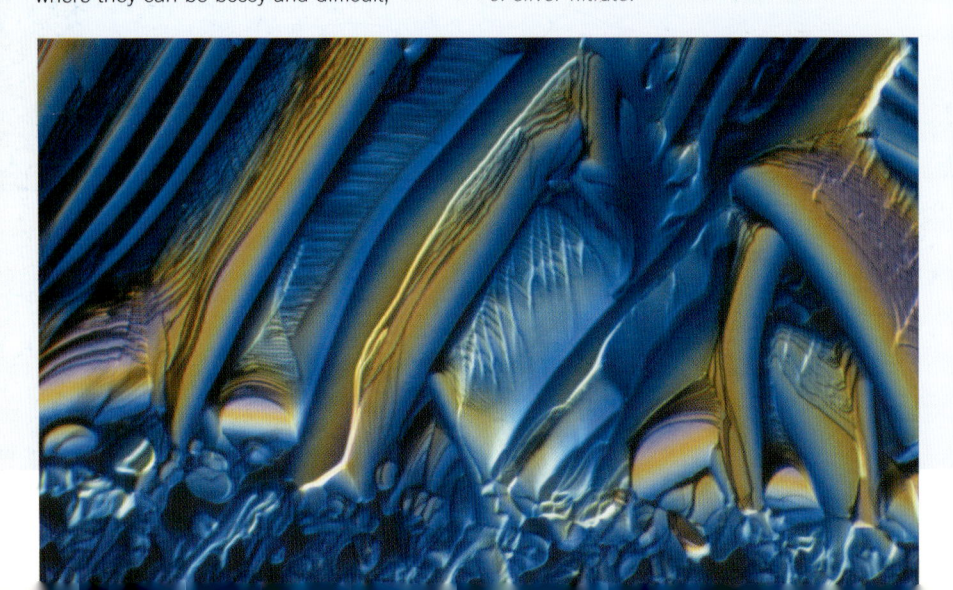

muscles to function properly. They may also tremble with anxiety.

Physical complaints

- The patient will be chilly and weak from pain.
- Thick secretions, such as mucus, cause them to become tense, tight and stiff.
- Argentum nitricum is a good remedy for inflammation of the cartilage, swelling, sensitiveness and soreness.
- It is also good for injuries to the eye.
- This is a specific remedy for hoarseness and is especially appropriate for professionals, singers and public speakers, who are worse from talking, singing or reading aloud; they can sometimes experience a total loss of voice.
- Also a remedy for testicles that are sore from having been hurt or crushed; worse on the right side.

Key symptoms

Symptoms usually found in warm-bodied people who crave fresh air • Anxiety when anticipating events • Injuries to the eye • Fear of high or narrow places • Hoarseness • Desire for sweet things, but these upset the stomach.

General symptoms

Pressing pains in the body, ulceration of the mucous membranes and blotchy skin. Diarrhoea as a result of eating sweets. Convulsions that occur after periods of extreme restlessness or after fright, during a menstrual period or from experiencing nervous tension.

ARISTOLOCHIA CLEMANTIS

(F, GR) flowering aristolochia plant

Specifically a female remedy. Its name means *aristo* (better), *locheria* (delivery). Used in childbirth and afterwards, Aristolochia clemantis can also help with the emotional conditions that are related to childbirth.

> **Key symptoms**
>
> *Urinary tract problems in women*
> * *Female problems, especially in pregnancy* • *Menopausal problems*
> * *Mild eczema and dermatitis.*

Mind and emotions

Mentally depressed, with loneliness and a fear of the future, often refusing to participate in society.

Physical complaints

- The patient has never been well since she began taking the birth control pill. She can experience lack of periods, altogether absent or short lasting, or they might be late with heavy clotting. Symptoms include psychosomatic conditions related to her menstrual cycle.
- The remedy works well for minor uterine problems following a sore throat, and for pains and hardness in the breasts and heaviness in the legs during periods. The fingers and legs will be swollen before the onset of periods, and varicose veins are worse before periods.
- Aristolochia clemantis is effective in the treatment of eczema of the vulva, which is accompanied with intense itching. It can also be used for premenstrual aggravation where the patient improves during her menstrual bleed.

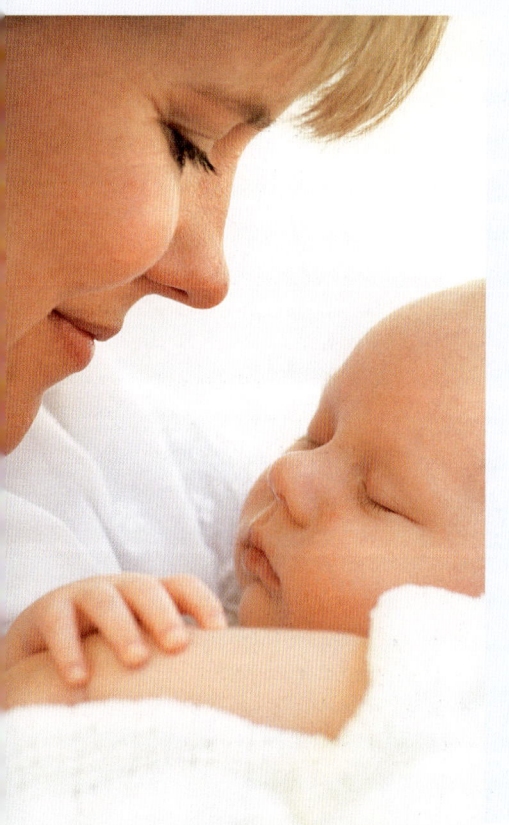

General symptoms

It can be used when there are the following symptoms: irritation and inflammation of the urinary tract and mild cystitis. Mild eczema and dermatitis. Where there are female problems such as lack of periods, menopausal arthritis, sterility, ovarian difficulties and problems in pregnancy, the remedy can support conventional medicine. Similarly, for prostate problems in men.

Aristolochia clementis can be used to alleviate problems occuring with pregnancy and childbirth as well as other specifically female conditions.

ARNICA MONTANA

(+FA, C-C-F, CR, GR, M)
leopard's bane, sneezewort plant*

The premier remedy in homeopathy, Arnica montana is best known for the treatment of shock, injury and trauma. It is different from Aconite, although it is used for the same conditions. A person requiring Arnica montana never outwardly shows fear but is always fearful. It alleviates bruising, bleeding and pain; it is also a good remedy for aiding recovery from jet lag.

Arnica flowers, shown here dried, make a useful remedy for bruises.

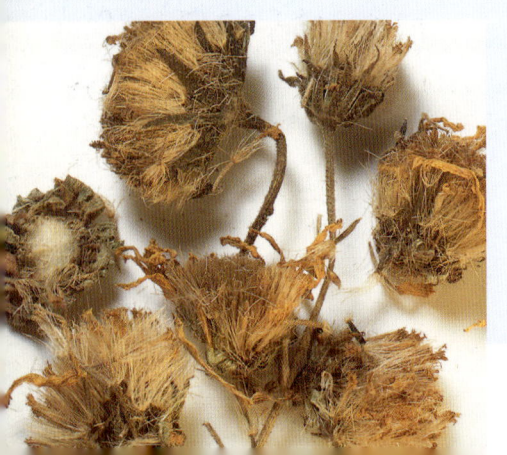

Mind and emotions

Patient starts from sleep, caused by disturbing dreams after an accident or injury. Their fear manifests itself while asleep and they awake in terror with a horror of death. Arnica montana is good for patients who worry over and exaggerate trivial symptoms. Also useful for people who have ailments from injuries, either physical or mental, such as grief, remorse, sudden financial loss, fright and anger. The whole body might feel oversensitive; the patient wants to be left alone and tells you they are just fine.

Physical complaints

- Useful after suffering from injury, or before and after surgery or dentistry, or for the trauma of past experiences.
- The patient feels a sore bruised feeling all over, as if they have been beaten. They will

arnica montana

> ### Key symptoms
>
> Sore and feeling bruised. Patient does not want to be touched • Injuries, accidents, or after surgery or dentistry • High fever with a cold body and a hot head.

have a sensation that the bed is too hard, and will be so sensitive that they do not want to be touched.

- The patient will suffer from offensive belching, vomiting, gas, stools and sweat, and may have bad breath and an unpleasant taste in the mouth.
- This is a useful remedy to stop bleeding from a cut or injury.
- It is also useful for violent coughs, and for muscular pain due to sports activity or overdoing a physical activity such as dancing or gardening.
- Use for a high fever with a red, hot head and a cold body.
- It is also good for gout or rheumatism where there is a fear of being touched.

General symptoms

Patients are worse at night, and for being heated; better for cold bathing. They may become overly tired but unable to sleep. The remedy is for the bad effects of mechanical injury, even for things that happened in the distant past. The patient is extremely sensitive all over the body and dislikes being touched. They have offensive discharges. There is pain in the body, as if being beaten. For backaches and people who bruise easily; there can also be a tendency to haemorrhage.

ARSENICUM ALBUM

(+FA, M, D, CR, GR) arsenic trioxide*

This is a remedy used for a variety of symptoms that work at many different levels.

Mind and emotions

The patient feels insecure and afraid of being alone, having a constant desire for company. They can be very restless and have many fears: for example, of disease, cancer, robbery, poverty, death and being alone – they are preoccupied with death. They are fastidious and critical and might dress and groom themselves immaculately and be obsessive in their behaviour. They can also be miserly and are careful about taking risks. They might be a collector, who likes valuables and antiques. They find comfort and security important. They can be possessive about their belongings as well as selfish.

Arsenicum album patients can experience sleeplessness, with all symptoms worse between midnight and 2.00 a.m. They can become anxious when things are expected of them and might suffer with anxiety about their health, often exaggerating their symptoms. They are dependent on others, particularly their doctor or health-carer.

Physical complaints

- The patient will feel strong pains, like fire, sparks or hot needles, which are better for warm applications. They may also suffer from cramps.

> **Key symptoms**
>
> *Restless and fearful • Burning pains that are better for heat • Patient hates to be alone and has a strong desire for company • All symptoms are worse between midnight and 2.00 a.m.*

arsenicum album

Burning pains that are worse during the early hours of the morning can be relieved by taking Arsenicum album.

- Use Arsenicum album when the patient is exhausted after a sickness.
- For a nasty cough that will not go away, where the patient is worse after midnight.
- They might also constantly crave food but be unable to eat it.

General symptoms

The patient suffers from ailments where they suddenly feel weak, accompanied by fear and restlessness. They are chilly and can suffer from heartburn, gastroenteritis, food poisoning, vomiting and diarrhoea, a burning thirst, burning pains and physical weakness.

This remedy also treats asthma, which is worse after midnight. It is good for treating hay fever, skin eruptions and also for eczema that is worse in winter and better in summer.

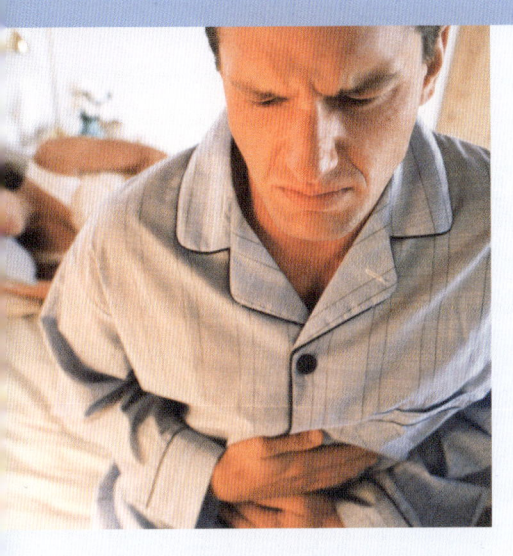

- There is a sudden loss of vitality where the patient feels helpless very quickly. They are worse after physical exertion and from fast, energetic walking.
- They can experience thin, unpleasant-smelling or burning discharges.
- During a fever or flu there is a burning, unquenchable thirst, with a strong desire for sipping cold drinks.

AURUM METALLICUM

(GR, Ma, M) gold

This remedy is good for depression, despondency and despair.

Mind and emotions

This remedy is used for extreme cases of depression, when life seems unbearable and there is great despair. It is for those who are upset and feel that all their hard-earned efforts amount to nothing.

The Aurum metallicum personality can be oversensitive to contradiction, resulting in fits of violence and rage, perhaps thinking of throwing themselves from heights. They tend to drive too fast. Although they love music they fear the least noise. Aurum metallicum is a remedy for ailments that occur due to fright, anger, contradiction, wounded pride and loss of property; also for people with too many responsibilities. It helps hard-working people who are weighed down by guilt and who feel remorseful.

Often the patient will pray obsessively for relief during their bouts of depression. They can suffer from low self-esteem, and are overly sensitive to the opinions of others. This is a remedy for serious people who are reserved and alone.

Physical complaints

- Symptoms include suffering violent pains and the despair caused by pain.
- The symptoms are worse at night with a desire for the fresh air.
- The pains are often worse for warmth.
- The patient can experience trembling after anger, fright or upset. The patient might also experience bad pains in their bones, especially at night, as if the bones were actually broken.
- Aurum metallicum is also useful for eye problems such as double vision or problems with the cornea.

aurum metallicum

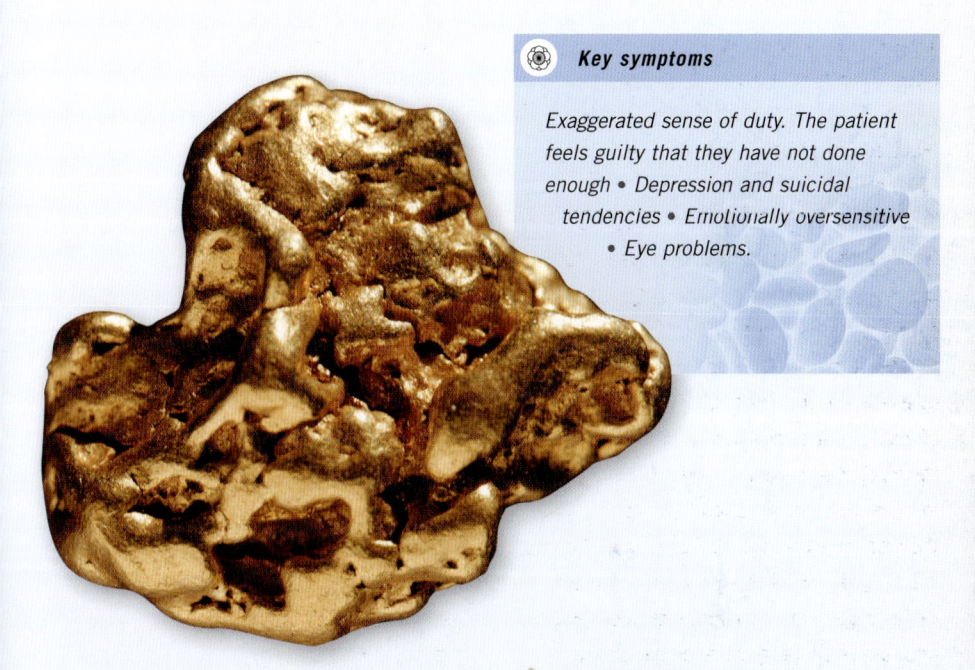

Key symptoms

Exaggerated sense of duty. The patient feels guilty that they have not done enough • Depression and suicidal tendencies • Emotionally oversensitive • Eye problems.

Gold is the mineral from which this remedy is derived. It is suitable for people who are oversensitive and depressed.

General symptoms

The patient is worse for becoming emotional when depressed, and for mental exertion.

BARYTA CARBONICA

(C-C-F, CR, GR) barium carbonate

This remedy works on nutritional deficiency and swollen glands, and it helps the heart and nerves.

Mind and emotions
This remedy is characterized by problems relating to weakness. It is useful for young children whose development is slow and for old people who are mentally regressing into their second childhood so that they are becoming physically dependent on others to look after them. It is also for people who are weakening with age and therefore need their vitality reviving.

Baryta carbonica people will suffer from weak bones and tendons. The patient can appear slow to comprehend and also slow in their movements, inept as well as bashful and timid. They can feel inefficient and unworthy of what they want, insecure at school or with friends.

This is a good remedy for bedwetting and other problems with toilet training where there is a lack of confidence and a feeling of uncertainty. This remedy is also used for mental slowness after a serious illness, such as measles, typhoid, mumps or scarlet fever.

Physical complaints
- The patient is very sensitive to cold, and susceptible to becoming cold.
- They also suffer from enlarged glands, especially in the throat, and physical weakness in general.

General symptoms
The patient is worse when they think about their symptoms, and for cold, damp and pressure. They are better for warm wraps, walking in the fresh air and being alone.

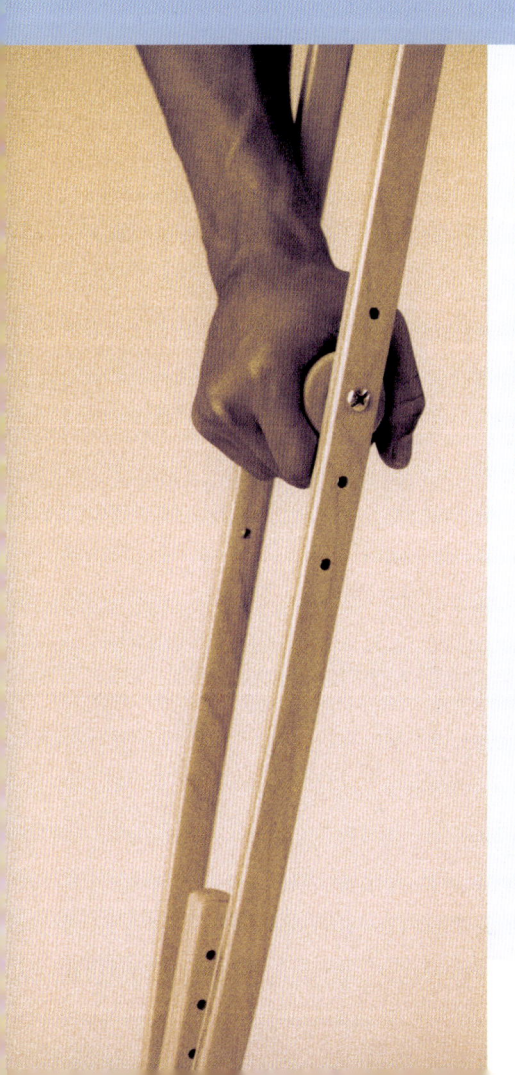

Key symptoms

Slow development in children and older people who are mentally regressing • Bashful and timid • Weak bones and tendons • Lack of confidence • Sensitivity to cold.

For people with weak tendons and bones, which are easily damaged, Baryta carbonica might be a helpful remedy to take.

BELLADONNA

(+FA, CR, C-C-F, GR)
deadly nightshade*

The remedy Belladonna has many uses. It is useful where the symptoms are heat and dryness with a lack of thirst.

Mind and emotions
The patient can experience violent mental symptoms, with a terrible rage and delirium when ill. Adults who are suited to Belladonna can be lively and entertaining but become violent when sick and delirious; Belladonna children will throw tantrums. They can strike, bite and pull hair, and they suffer from hallucinations during a fever. They develop illness due to excitement, fear, grief, disappointed love and anger. The patient

Atropa bella-donna *(deadly nightshade) is used in a remedy for a high temperature.*

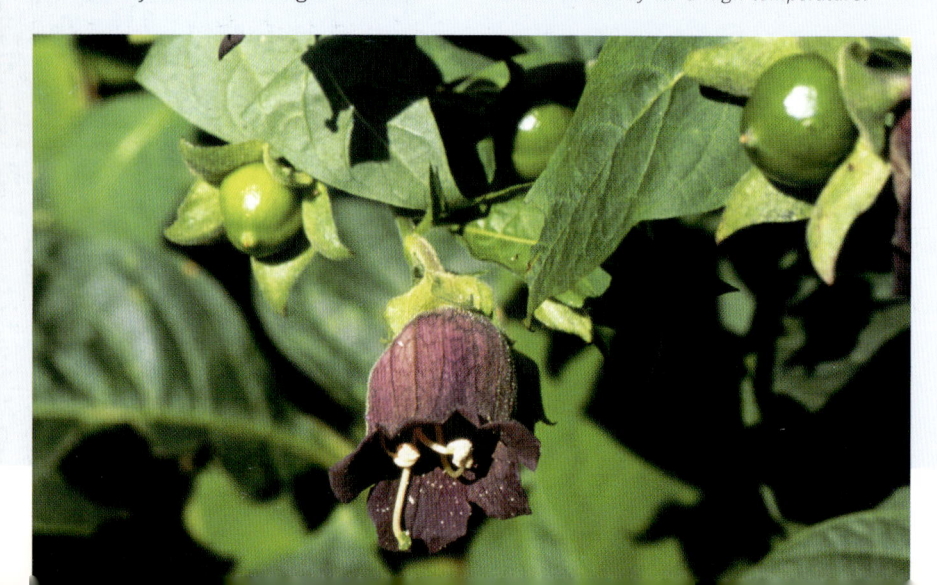

Key symptoms

Sudden and violent onset of all symptoms • Redness, burning and heat. Patient is hot to the touch • Extreme sensitivity to touch, light and noise • Illness makes them bad tempered.

lives in a world of his or her own, sometimes seeing ghosts and having visions, such as seeing monsters, which they are frightened by. They experience acute senses where everything is heightened.

Physical complaints

- Symptoms are acute and violent, and appear suddenly.
- The patient is oversensitive to sounds, sights, taste and touch.
- Symptoms are found in parts of body that are red, dry and very hot. There is a high fever with no thirst.
- Belladonna is a remedy for swollen eruptions and skin complaints such as boils, styes and carbuncles.
- It also works well as a remdey for sunstroke and scarlet fever.
- Patients can have dilated, shining pupils, indicating delirium in fever. Babies can suffer convulsions due to teething.

General symptoms

Air sickness, headaches, and swollen and painful joints. Patients are worse for the heat of the sun, draughts to the head, noise and jarring. They are better for rest in bed, in a dark, warm room.

BELLIS PERENNIS

(CB, F, GR) daisy flower

The remedy Bellis perennis is good for all injuries to soft tissues. It is similar to Arnica montana but specific to soft-tissue injury or pain to soft-tissue areas. It is excellent after surgery and dentistry.

Mind and emotions

This is a remedy for resilient people who always recover well after disasters.

Physical complaints

- The patient is bruised and sore, but is better for rubbing the injured parts.
- This remedy is indicated where there is deep trauma to the body, especially useful after dentistry or invasive surgery to soft tissue. It helps to heal wounds.
- It is good for people who have done hard physical labour or who are weary from travel.
- Use for sudden earaches, where the face is red and swollen, and the ear throbs.
- It also helps in pregnancy when it is uncomfortable to walk because the abdominal muscles are under strain, or when the baby kicks too hard and injures internal tissue.
- It is also useful for injury to the soft tissues of the breasts.
- Use Bellis perennis as a support therapy for cancer of the breast, where there are hard areas or nodules on the breast.
- Note that all symptoms are worse from weight and pressure.

Key symptoms

Sore, bruised feeling; better for rubbing
- *Swelling remains after injury*
- *Problems with soft tissue, such as the breasts* • *A fall, accident or strain or after surgery.*

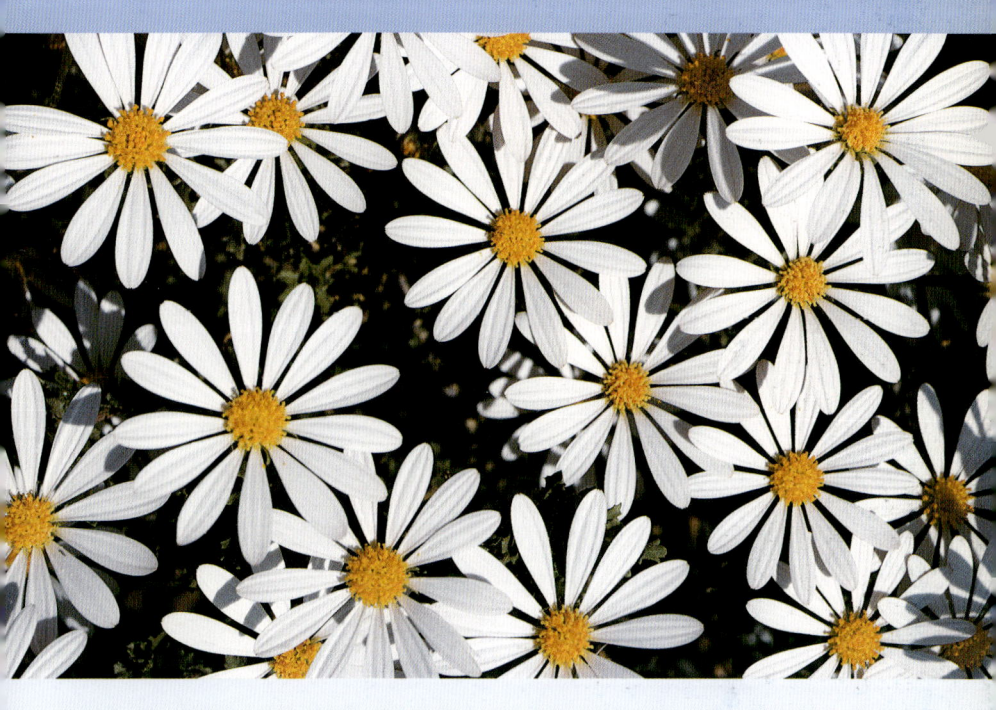

General symptoms

Where there has been an injury resulting in swelling, this is an indication for using Bellis. Think of this remedy for the treatment of the effects of blows, falls, accidents or strain.

The dainty daisy Bellis perennis *is used in homeopathy to make a remedy for bruises and where there is swelling.*

BERBERIS VULGARIS

(CR, CB, F, GR) bark and dried root of the barberry plant

This remedy is a specific kidney tonic after assault, injury or great fear.

Mind and emotions
No symptoms.

Physical complaints
- All the symptoms rapidly change and alternate and feel as if they are shooting outwards from one point.
- This remedy is useful for pains in the kidneys and loins, which will feel like boiling water, with gurgling, jarring, numbness and stiffness.
- Berberis is a remedy for weakness in the kidneys. Used for any time the kidneys have been forced to release adrenalin into the system because stress has caused the 'fight-or-flight' reaction in the body and they have therefore become drained of energy. Also where weakness in the kidneys has been caused by chronic fatigue, auto-immune deficiency or exhaustion.
- It can be useful for women who experience a lack of sexual pleasure, or for a dry vagina.

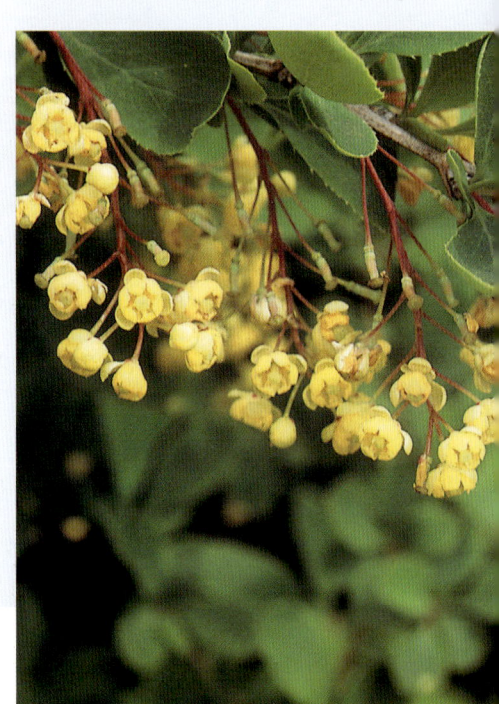

berberis vulgaris

- It is also useful for back pains where there is numbness and the patient has difficulty standing up from sitting, with pain extending down the legs to the pelvis. It is good for stiffness in the lower back.

General symptoms

Used for radiating pains, external numbness, twinges of pain. The patient is always worse for motion, jarring, stepping hard, rising from sitting, and from fatigue.

> **Key symptoms**
>
> *Radiating pains • Pain and stiffness in the small of the back • Sensitivity in the area of the kidneys.*

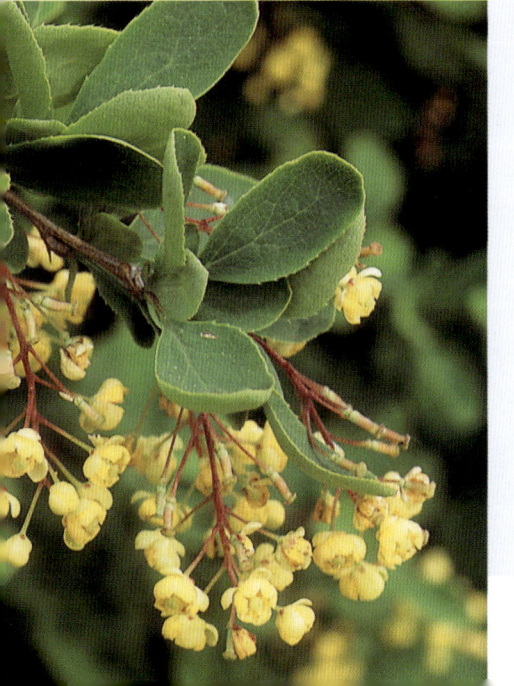

The barberry plant is used to prepare a remedy for disorders with radiating pains and stiffness in the back.

BORAX

(CR, GR) sodium borate

The remedy Borax works on nutrition, skin, kidneys and bladder.

Mind and emotions

The patient experiences fears and aggravations of their symptoms, which are worse with any downward motion such as elevators, or walking down stairs or hills. Borax is a remedy for children who are anxious about sleeping, who are crying, clinging without cause or when terrified. It is useful for nervous, anxious people who have a fear of falling, and is especially useful for easily frightened children.

Physical complaints

- Infants with pale faces, who refuse to eat or who have little appetite.
- Symptoms relating to the head are congestion, vertigo, impaired vision and flickering lights before the eyes.
- The patient suffers from dry skin, which festers easily and will not heal. There are mouth ulcers that will not heal.
- The patient has a congested nose, and their eyes become sticky with hot mucus.
- Female symptoms are profuse whitish or yellowish discharge from the vagina; sore mucous tissues in the mouth, eyes, nose, anus and vagina. For childbirth this remedy is used for ailments experienced by breastfeeding mothers and their babies.

General symptoms

The patient is worse from downward motion, sudden noises, breastfeeding. The slightest injury suppurates. This is a good remedy for babies and young children.

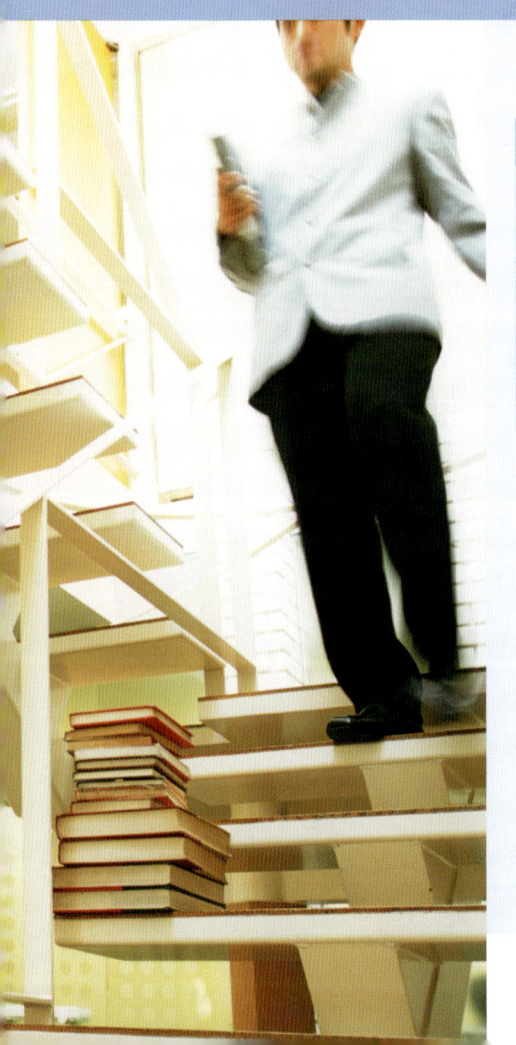

Key symptoms

Worse for downward motion • Nervous adults and easily frightened children. • Waking from sleep horrified and crying • Ailments in mothers and babies that relate to breastfeeding.

Where the symptoms include vertigo or are worse when walking down stairs Borax might be an appropriate remedy.

BRYONIA ALBA

(+FA, CR, CB, C-C-F) wild hops*

This remedy is used for problems with circulation and the liver. It is also excellent for headaches, joint aches, mastitis and the abdomen.

Mind and emotions
The patient has money worries and fears poverty. They wish for security, and they try to find this through property and money. This is good for people who are slow to change, methodical, censorious, reliable and economical. The constant money worries, constant distress and problems use up their energy. They are very irritable when ill and want to be left alone.

Fruit can cause digestive problems in the Bryonia alba type of person who also suffers from headaches and joint aches.

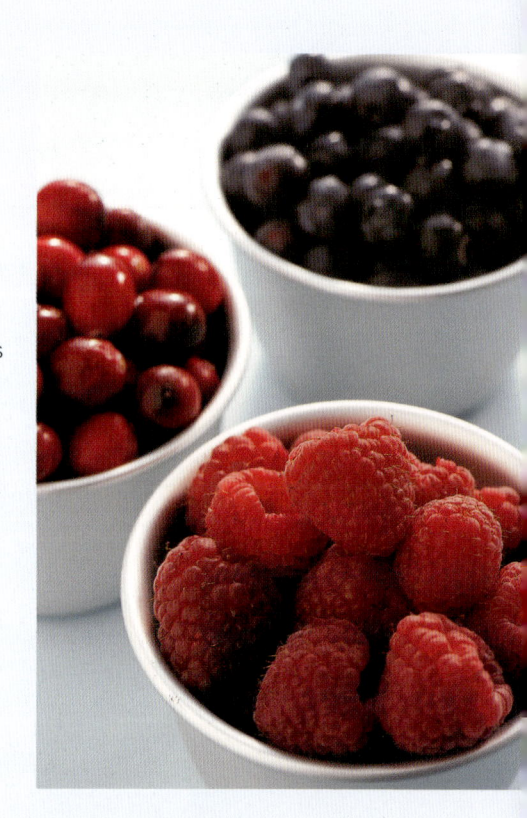

Key symptoms

Dryness of mucous membranes and a great thirst • Terrible headaches with indigestion • Digestive problems • Fear of poverty; talking constantly about business.

Physical complaints

- All the conditions are worse for movement.
- The patient suffers ailments from being overheated, such as a skin rash that burns, and will become slow and languid.
- They have digestive problems from fruit and food that makes them flatulent. Food can feel heavy in the stomach. There may also be vomiting.
- Mucous membranes are excessively dry.
- The patient is thirsty, especially for cold water, and can have constipation.
- They suffer from terrible headaches that come from indigestion and a weak liver.
- Patients can also have dry, painful coughs or chest colds with a cough. They can also suffer from pneumonia.
- They suffer from lumbago in bed when they cannot turn because they are so stiff.

General symptoms

All movement makes symptoms worse.

CACTUS GRANDIFLORUS

(+FA, GR, M,)
night-blooming cereus plant

This remedy works on the heart, circulation and chest, and can work alongside conventional medicine to help a heart attack.

Mind and emotions
The patient wakes frightened, and suffers from sadness and ill humour. They can be very anxious about death.

Physical complaints
- The patient can have severe headaches, with a sensation of weight on the crown of the head. Also congestive headaches where the head feels as if it is in a vice.
- Profuse nosebleeds may occur as well as constriction in the throat, or a feeling of a band around the chest. The breathing is affected.
- Immediate medical attention is required for these following symptoms: there is heart constriction, with a sensation of an iron band gripping the chest. There are palpitations, with pains shooting down the left arm, swelling of the arms and legs, and numbness of the left arm.
- The patient can be sleepless from a throbbing sensation in their body or without apparent cause.

> **Key symptoms**
>
> *A constricted feeling in the chest. A sensation as if the heart were clutched and released by an iron band. Swelling of the left hand. (Seek emergency help if you have these symptoms.)*
> - *Bad headache on the crown of the head* • *Frightened and anxious.*

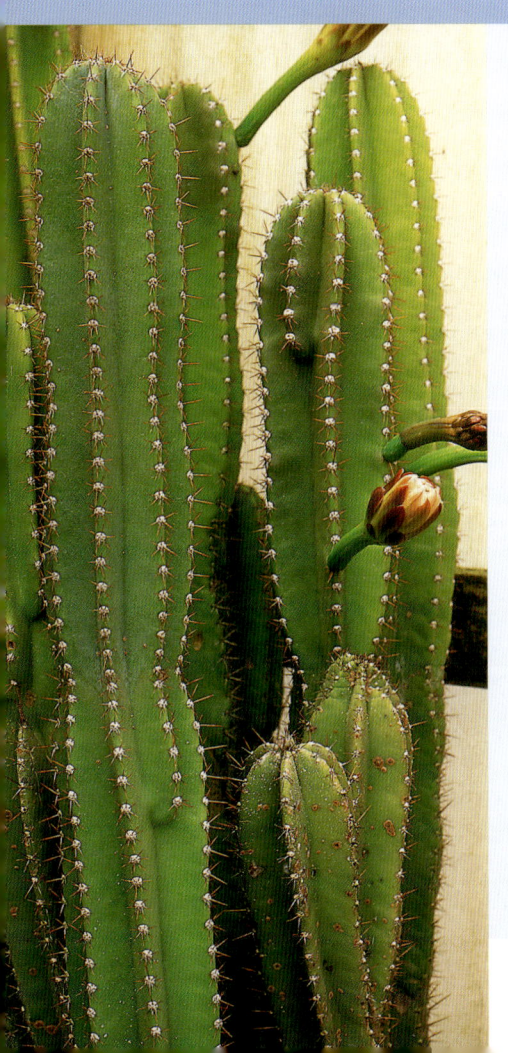

- This remedy can be used to strengthen a heart weakened by tobacco or arteriosclerosis. It is a good support therapy for angina where there are feelings of suffocation, a cold sweat and tightness in the arms or chest. Can be used alongside conventional medicine for constrictions of the heart, with a weak pulse, and painful stitching pains.

General symptoms

The patient's symptoms are worse when lying on their left side. They may have suffered from exposure to the sun, disappointed love, or may feel worse after eating or fasting. They feel better for fresh air, sitting and rest.

Cactus grandiflorus (night-blooming cereus plant) is the source of this remedy for the heart, circulation and chest.

CALCAREA CARBONICA

(CR, GR, M)
calcium carbonate, carbonate of lime

This is a remedy needed by 90 per cent of the population at some time in their healing process. It works on warts and where the body is insufficiently nourished, and is specifically for glands, skin, bones and exhaustion due to overwork. Useful also for strengthening teeth and preventing tooth decay. It is also known to increase pituitary and thyroid function.

Mind and emotions
The patient can be apprehensive and dislike the attention of others focused on them. They are shy, timid and slow, and often seek protection. They seek stability and like order. The patient has many fears and anxieties.

This remedy can give people who are unable to find their inner strength the courage to live their lives, giving them both stamina and grit emotionally, mentally and physically.

Calcarea carbonica is also for people who dislike being observed and have a fear of being judged. Patients are also terrified of cruelty and deeply affected by external traumas. Patients, especially children, have a noticeable fear of animals. The patient loves to be touched. This remedy is especially useful for children.

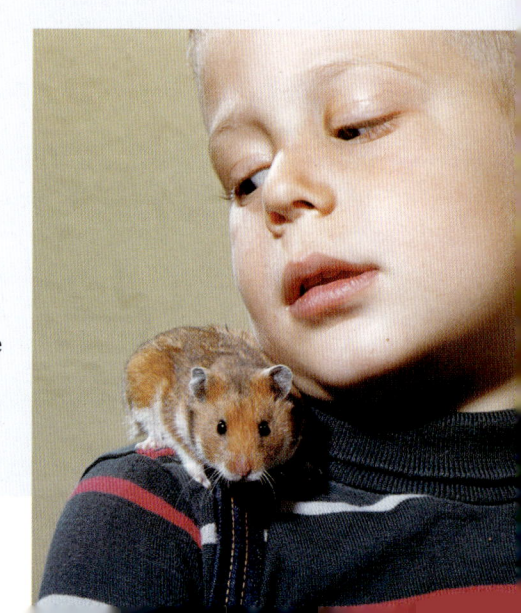

Physical complaints

- The patient is inclined to get fat and flabby, especially children. Also prone to diarrhoea, weakness and dizziness.
- It is indicated for children whose fontanelles are late to close, who can also be late walkers and talkers as well as slow in developing their teeth.
- It is a remedy for children who have large heads, a hard stomach and enlarged glands.
- They are often very chilly, and worse in cold, damp weather.
- They can be averse to physical activity and love sweets and eggs.
- Often they perspire on the back of the head, particularly when emotional, and have a tendency to be constipated.

Calcarea cabonica is a remedy especially useful for children, particularly those with a noticeable fear of animals.

> **Key symptoms**
>
> *Slow or delayed development in children, who have a tendency towards overweight • Many fears and anxieties • Chilly and worse in cold, damp weather • Tendency to perspire and be constipated.*

- Also suitable for women who have breast tenderness prior to a menstrual period.

General symptoms

Use for ear infections. The patient has cold hands and is worse for cold, raw air, bathing and a change of weather. They do not cope well with mental or physical exertion, puberty, overstimulation or mental pressure. They are better in warm, dry weather.

CALCAREA FLUORICA

(GR, Ma, M)
calcium fluoride, fluoride of lime

When used in low potency, Calcarea fluorica works well for bone spurs and hard tumorous growths. In high potency it works on delusions about glamour and what glitters.

Mind and emotions

The patient fears poverty, has a love of luxury and of material possessions, and values the importance of looking good to others. They can become extremely depressed and have groundless fears about money. They long for guidance and seek support.

Physical complaints

- The patient's limbs are overflexible, lacking coordination with over-relaxed ligaments and muscles. This is a remedy for gymnasts, dancers, ballet dancers and sportsmen who have strained and overstretched ligaments.

Key symptoms

Tooth enamel that is weak or premature dental cavities • Overstraining and overstretching of muscles and joints, especially in active loose-limbed people • Extreme fear of poverty.

- The patient is chilly. There can be hard, stony growths in the muscles and tendons.
- It is used for lumbago and pain in the small of the back, and is helpful for cramps in the calves at night.
- It can also be used for premature decay in teeth where the enamel is discoloured or deficient.
- Use for a head cold with thick, yellow discharge, and for a croup-like cough.

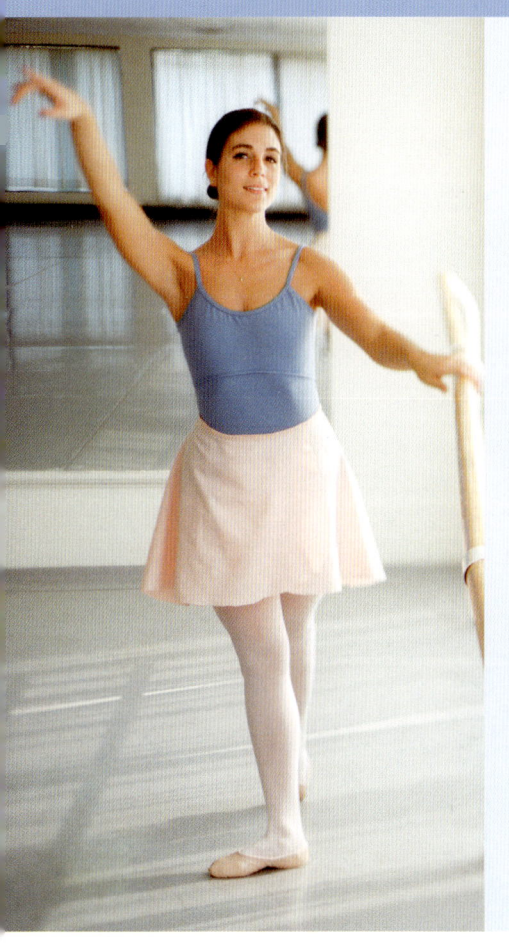

Ballet dancers, gymnasts and sportsmen who have strained ligaments might benefit from the remedy Calcarea fluorica.

General symptoms

Strain and overstretching of ligaments, muscles and joints that occur in gymnasts, dancers and sportsmen. The patient feels chilly, and needs to be warm. Hard stony glands, tonsils, neck and haemorrhoids; nodes on breasts. Hardening of muscles; swelling and hard nodes in the ligaments, muscles and tendons. Birthmarks, varicose veins, varicose ulcers. Slow development of bones; slow in learning to walk.

CALCAREA PHOSPHORICA

(CR, GR, M)
calcium phosphate, phosphate of lime

Use Calcarea phosphorica for problems with bones, growth, tardy development of the teeth and anaemia.

Mind and emotions

The patient is forgetful, never satisfied with anything, peevish and has a weak memory following grief. They are extremely restless, always wanting to go somewhere. However, they have little motivation due to lack of energy.

This remedy is good for treatment after acute diseases, injury, disappointment, unhappy love, grief or too rapid growth. The patient suffers from fear after hearing bad news. A change in the patient's situation temporarily brings back motivation but then the old symptoms return.

Babies who crave feeding but are intolerant of their mother's milk might benefit from Calcarea phosphorica taken by the mother.

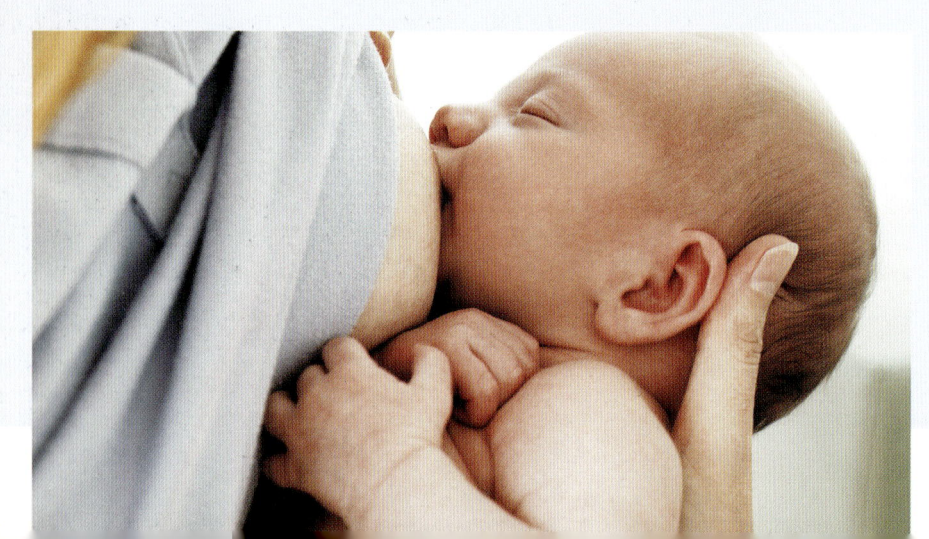

Physical complaints

- The patient suffers from swollen tonsils and adenoids, and has problems with teeth developing slowly and decaying easily.
- An infant craves nursing continuously, and yet it is intolerant of its mother's milk, which causes vomiting with colic and diarrhoea. Calcarea phosphorica is an appropriate remedy for children who vomit easily.
- It is also good for rapid growth in children, when long bones grow too fast, causing growing pains.
- Also suitable for females when their period comes too early, is accompanied by headaches or is excessive in young girls.
- Good for rheumatic pains caused by draughts, which produce a stiff neck.
- The patient suffers soreness in the sacroiliac joints, feeling as if they were broken in two.
- Calcarea phosphorica assists with curvature of the spine.
- The remedy also helps relieve headaches in students that have become worse from too much mental activity.

General symptoms

Sore chest; suffocating cough. Patient is better lying down. Stiffness and pain with a cold, numb feeling that is worse for any change of weather. Pains in joints and bones.

Key symptoms

Dissatisfaction • Over-rapid growth in children, who suffer growing pains and weakness • Headache caused by mental exertion • Stiff neck caused by a draught.

CALCAREA SULPHURICA

(GR, CR)
calcium sulphate, plaster of Paris

The remedy Calcarea sulphurica works on connective tissues, glands, bones and skin.

Mind and emotions
Fear of birds.

Physical complaints
- The patient suffers from eczema and glandular swellings.
- A remedy for cystic tumours and fibroids.
- It works for wounds where there is pus and for abscesses. There is a constant discharge of thick yellow pus.
- Works well for boils, wounds, sinuses, tonsillitis, and inflammation of the middle ear, diarrhoea, carbuncles, pneumonia, glandular swellings and ulcers.
- Useful in all cases where there is pus, when the discharge continues for too long and when the skin is slow to heal.

> **Key symptoms**
>
> *Tendency to have wounds or ailments that become infected • Thick yellow pus • Good for warm-bodied people.*

- It also works for cold, foul-smelling foot sweat that burns the soles of the feet.

General symptoms
The patient is worse for getting wet and physical exertion. They suffer from heat flushes while eating. They crave sour fruit and are worse for milk.

Prescribe Calcarea sulphurica for warm-bodied people who crave sour fruit if they suffer from wounds that become infected.

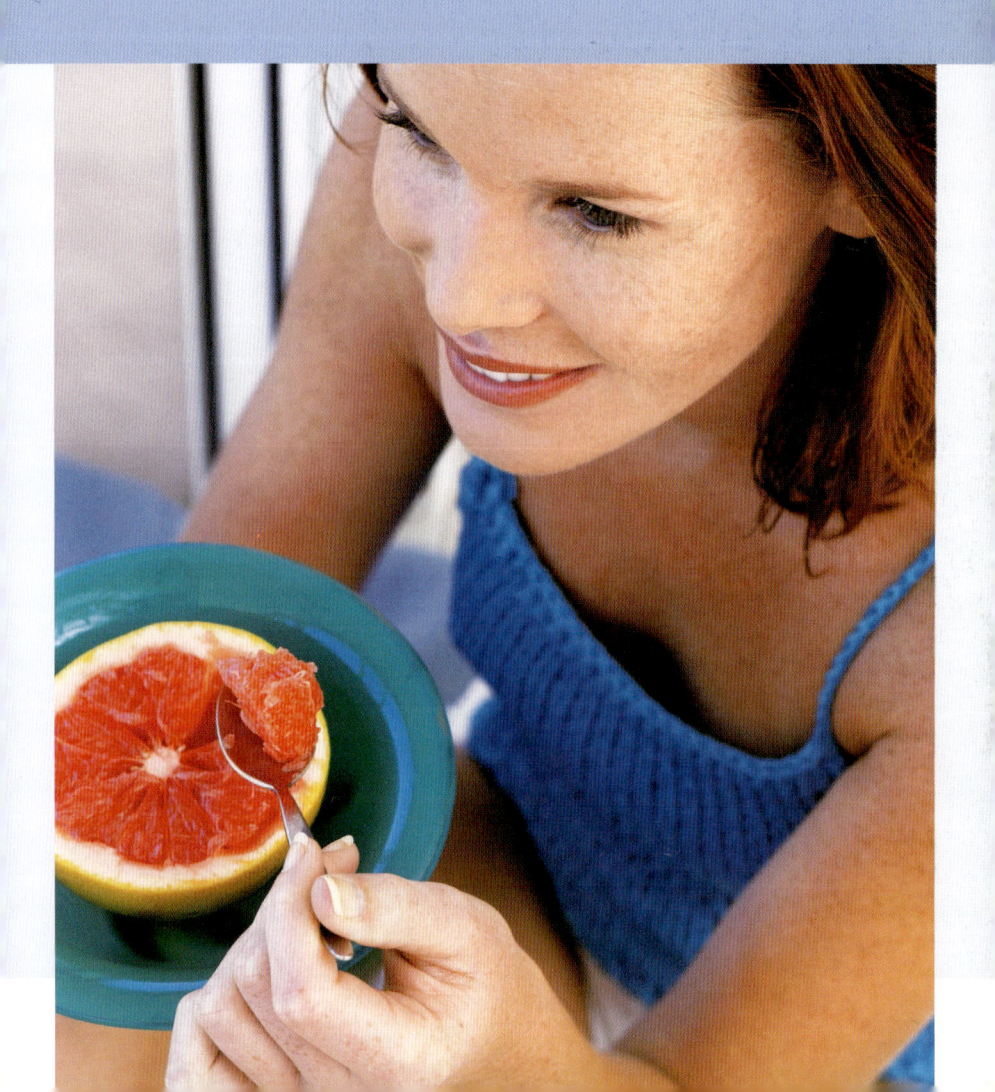

calcarea sulphurica 113

CANTHARIS VESICATORIA

(+FA, CB, F, GR, Ma)
Spanish fly (beetle)

Use Cantharis vesicatoria for urinary tract infections with pain, bleeding and irritation as well as for sunburn. It can also be used for blisters caused by hiking or poorly fitting shoes.

Mind and emotions

The patient can experience anger and delirium, and also feel anxious and restless. They can be very distressed, especially about sex, and can act as if in an amorous frenzy. There can be raging and crying, or even loss of consciousness.

Physical complaints

- The patient can experience burning sensations, as if the brain is full of boiling water or the eyes or skin feel as if they are burning. There will be difficulty swallowing, with a scalding feeling in the mouth, or from actually burning the mouth on too hot food.

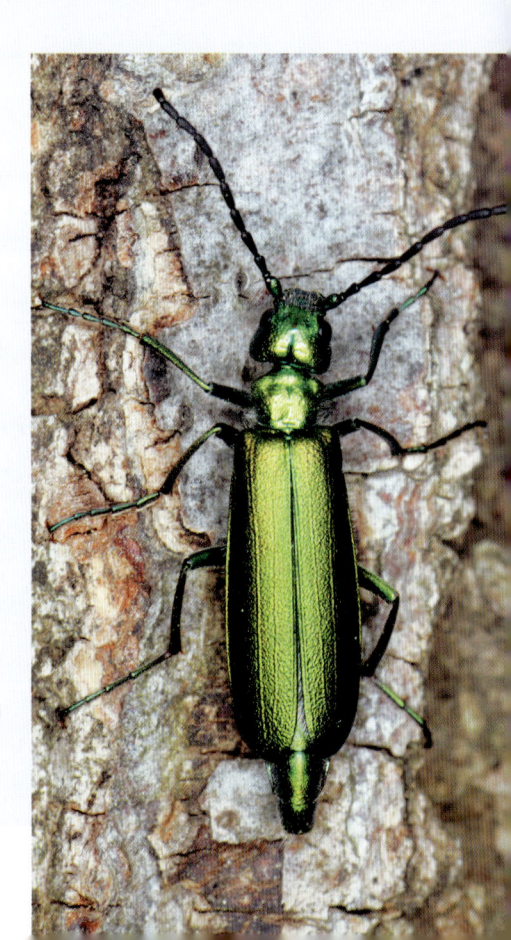

The Spanish fly beetle (Cantharis vesicatoria) is the source for a remedy to soothe burning and cutting pains.

- Other symptoms are mouth ulcers, pleurisy, with frequent dry coughing. There are burning pains in the throat, stomach and oesophagus.
- The patient also experiences a burning thirst, with aversion to all fluids.
- They can feel a cutting and burning feeling in the whole kidney and bladder area.
- There is a constant desire to urinate, and a scalding sensation when passing urine.
- Men's symptoms include painful erections.
- Women experience a strong sexual desire, with burning in the ovaries, back pain and a strong need to urinate.
- Stomach and liver complaints are aggravated by drinking coffee.
- Feeling of vertigo that is worse in open air.

Key symptoms

Burning and cutting pains during and after urination • Bladder symptoms and and excessive sexual desire • Patient is worse for drinking coffee or cold water • Anxiety and restlessness.

General symptoms

The patient is worse from touch, urinating, drinking cold water or coffee. They are better for being firmly rubbed but are oversensitive in all parts of the body. Raw, burning pains characterize all aspects of this remedy.

CAPSICUM

(M, CR, F, GR, Ma) cayenne pepper

This remedy is made from pepper and it heats people up. It also dilates the blood vessels in the mucous membranes and helps release hardened mucus in the digestive tract. It is also known as an effective remedy for homesickness.

Mind and emotions

The patient is peevish and irritable, and suffers from homesickness accompanied by depressed thoughts. They want to be left alone. People who are suited to Capsicum are irritable and get angry easily.

Physical complaints

- The patient suffers from headaches, and has a hot face and red cheeks, although they are cold to the touch.
- There are swelling pains behind the ears, and inflammation of the mastoid bones, which are found behind the ear.
- This is a good remedy to work alongside conventional medicine for otorrhoea in children (when the ears become inflamed with mucous and the mastoid bones swell before pus forms), which can cause deafness, tinnitus and vertigo.
- It is useful for subacute inflammation of the Eustachian tubes, when the patient is in great pain.
- It is also a remedy for a sore throat in smokers and drinkers.
- The patient has a fetid mouth odour and women might suffer from genital herpes. They have an intense craving for stimulants. They suffer from bloody mucus with a burning feeling in the rectum and bleeding haemorrhoids (piles).
- Females may have menopausal symptoms.
- Male symptoms are coldness of the scrotum accompanied with impotency and atrophied testicles.

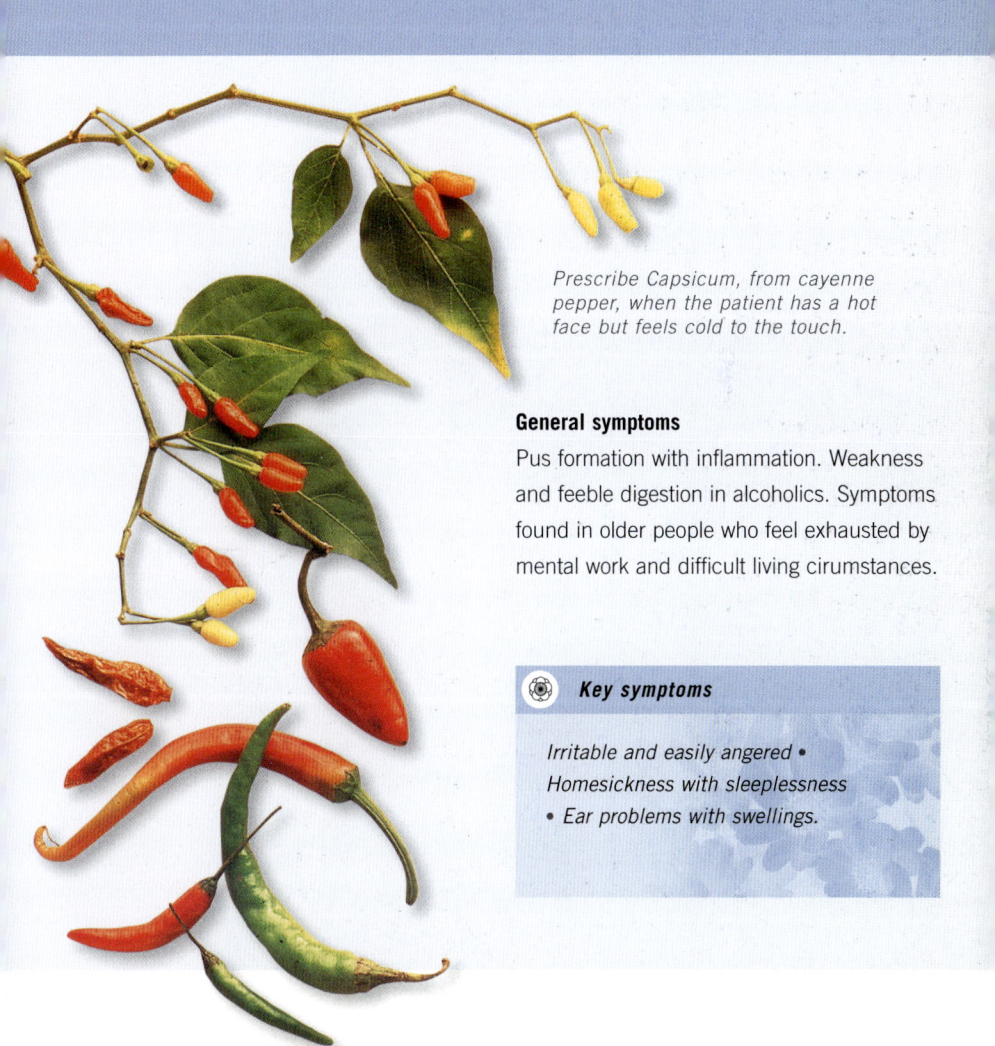

Prescribe Capsicum, from cayenne pepper, when the patient has a hot face but feels cold to the touch.

General symptoms

Pus formation with inflammation. Weakness and feeble digestion in alcoholics. Symptoms found in older people who feel exhausted by mental work and difficult living cirumstances.

Key symptoms

Irritable and easily angered • Homesickness with sleeplessness • Ear problems with swellings.

CARBO ANIMALIS

(+FA, CB, M, GR) animal charcoal

This is a good remedy for old people after a debilitating illness, where they experience a weak constitution and low energy. Carbo animalis helps to revive the system after illness.

Mind and emotions

The patient prefers to be alone; they are sad, reflective and want to avoid society. They experience anxiety at night.

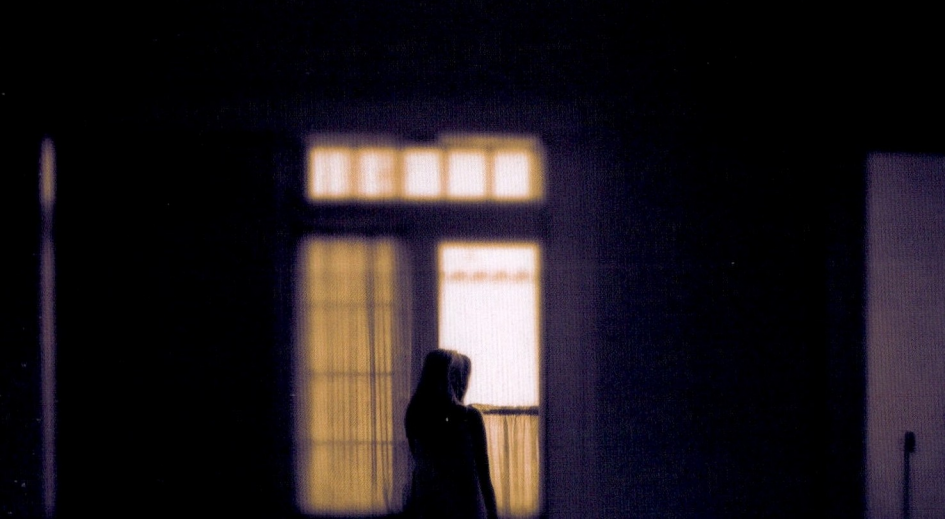

Physical complaints

- Headaches are so intense that the head feels as if it will burst into several pieces, so sharp is the pain.
- The patient has blueish lips and their hearing is confused.
- Patients suffer from weak digestion with flatulence. It is a good remedy to use after food poisoning when the system is weak.
- It is also used for nausea in pregnancy and exhaustion after menstrual periods.
- Use Carbo animalis as a support remedy for cancer of the uterus that is accompanied by burning pains.
- A remedy for coughs with green sputum.
- It is also useful for rosacea (enlarged blood vessels on the face) and when the glands are hard, swollen and painful.

A patient who is reflective and prefers to be alone might benefit from taking the remedy Carbo animalis.

Key symptoms

Anxiety at night, sad and wanting to be alone • Weak digestion • Weakness after a digestive illness • Nausea in pregnancy.

General symptoms

Good for ulceration and where tissues have broken down and begun to decompose. All secretions are offensive. All symptoms are characterized by weakness.

CARBO VEGETABILIS

(+FA, CR, F, GR, Ma) wood charcoal*

A major first-aid remedy, Carbo vegetabilis is used for fainting and collapse. The remedy is to be taken after loss of fluids, from too much medication, or after disease. Also useful as a remedy for scabies.

Mind and emotions

The patient has an aversion to being in the dark, suffers from loss of memory and is frightened of ghosts.

Physical complaints
- The patient can suffer from nosebleeds, bleeding after straining on the toilet, or blood oozing from the gums.
- Complaints of vertigo, nausea and tinnitus.
- Hair can fall out and scalp feels sore.
- The face is puffy, pale and sweaty.
- There are many stomach symptoms as well as becoming emotional after eating. Their digestion is slow and food putrefies before it digests, causing flatulence. The simplest foods distress them.
- They have bloated abdomens and burning in the anus; also old people will have painful diarrhoea.
- Female symptoms include premature and copious periods.

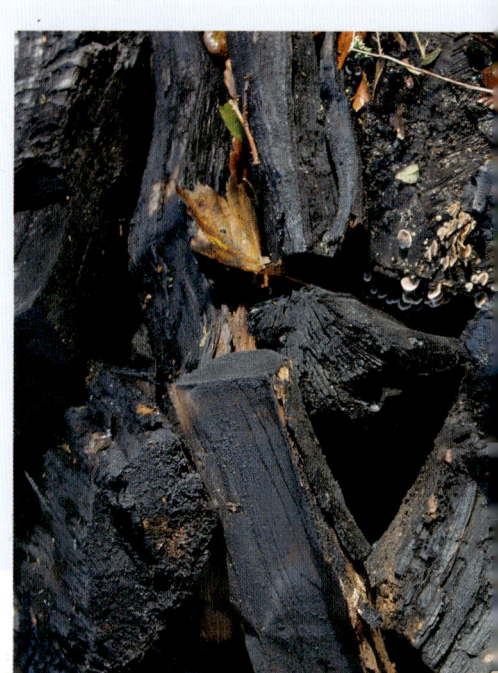

carbo vegetabilis

- This is also a remedy for whooping cough and for hoarseness and where the voice fails easily.
- Other symptoms include coughing with burning in the chest, where the limbs also feel heavy. There is no muscular energy, only exhaustion.

Key symptoms

Bad flatulence • Stomach and digestive problems • A bloated abdomen causing clothes to feel tight around the waist.

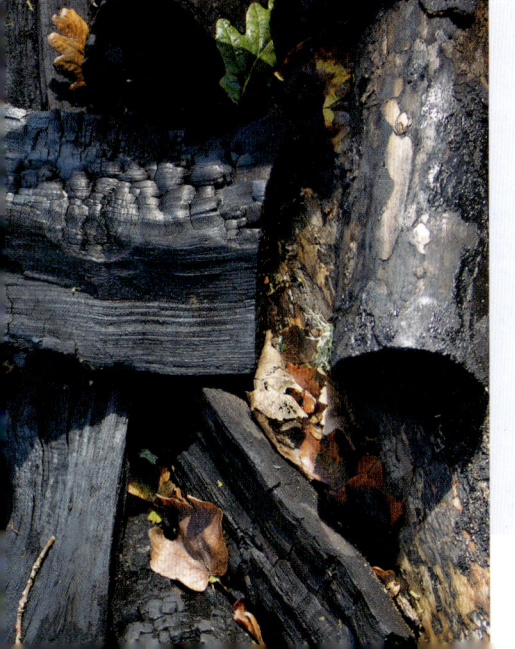

General symptoms

The skin has a blue tinge from lack of oxygen. The patient craves fresh air but this makes them feel worse; also worse in cold weather, and from drinking coffee and eating fatty foods such as butter and milk. They are better for being cold, and from fanning. This is a remedy for states of collapse with utter exhaustion where the body is broken down. Also for food poisoning from tainted fish.

Wood charcoal is the source of the remedy Carbo vegetabilis, which is an essential first-aid remedy for fainting and collapse.

CAULOPHYLLUM

(CB, F) root of blue cohosh plant

The remedy Caulophyllum is used for women who suffer from nervous disorders, negativity and problems relating to the female organs. It is a useful remedy for helping to bring on labour in childbirth and for other ailments relating to pregnancy, birth and lactation.

> **Key symptoms**
>
> *Ailments during pregnancy • Erratic labour pains • Tendency to miscarry.*

Mind and emotions

The patient is nervous and excitable. They are weakened, hysterical and exhausted from labour in childbirth.

Physical complaints

- This is a remedy for ailments that relate to pregnancy, childbirth and lactation.
- The patient has erratic labour pains, with sensations of cramping and shooting pains during pregnancy.
- Also used for labour that does not progress, or to bring on labour in the last stages of pregnancy.
- It is used for unbearable pains during labour due to a rigid cervix.
- Use this remedy for rheumatism of the small joints during menstrual periods.
- It might also be considered when there has been repeated miscarriage.

General symptoms

It is used to treat nausea and vomiting during menstrual periods and severe dysmenorrhoea (painful menstruation with abdominal cramps).

The root of the blue cohosh plant is used in a remedy for many female disorders.

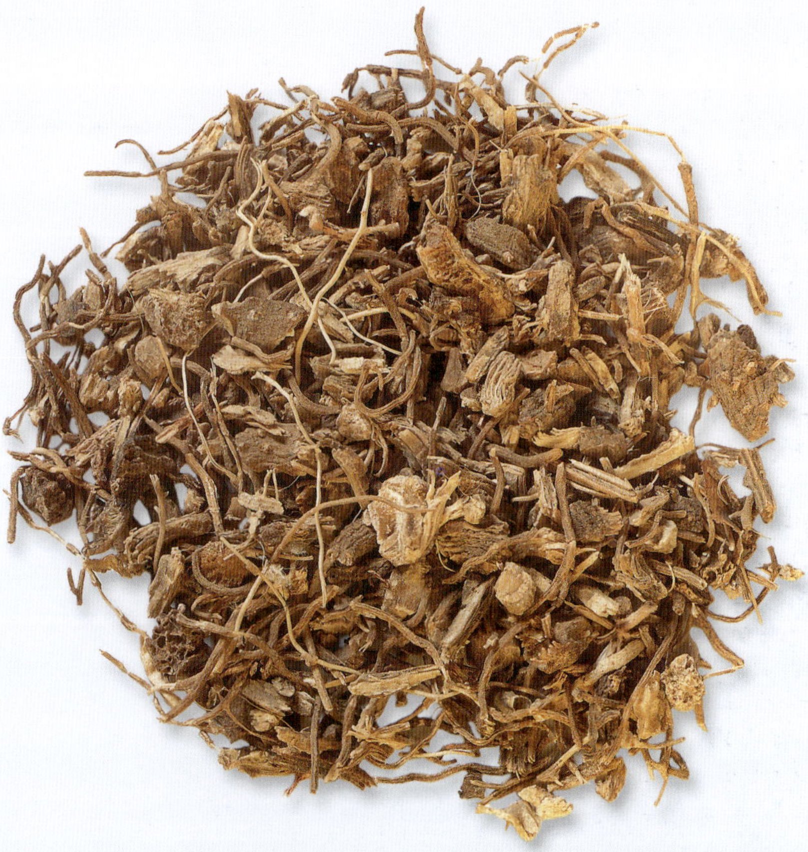

CAUSTICUM

(GR, M) potash

The remedy Causticum is for those who give too much to others, and it is useful for incontinence, blisters and burns.

Mind and emotions

The patient suffers from ailments caused by grief and sorrow over problems in the world. Social injustices affect their emotions and they fight for a better world. It is a remedy for those who feel oppressed; for those who are over-religious and who wish to see drastic social change.

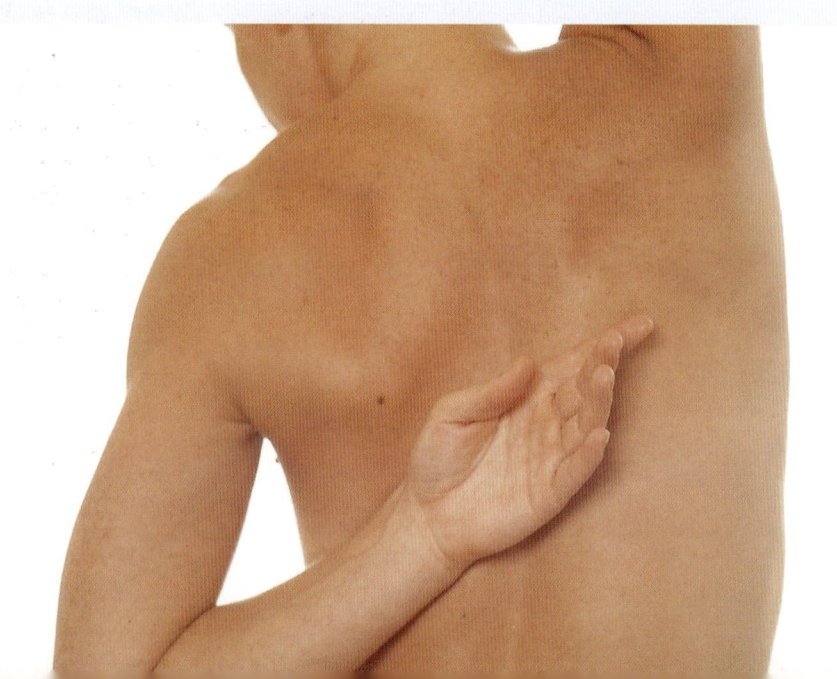

The Causticum patient is inclined to have strong views and ideas. However, they have a weak memory, often feeling as if they have forgotten something. They worry about their relatives, and are inclined to weep with jealousy, with drunkenness and out of sympathy for others. They are also inclined to stammer when angry.

Physical complaints
- The patient suffers from burns, warts, ulcers and blisters.
- They feel burning pains as if the flesh is raw, on the scalp, in the throat, in the anus and vagina, and when breathing.
- It is good for all burns on the skin.
- Other symptoms include muscular pains that feel as if the muscles are too short.
- Also for a dry cough, aversion to sex and for constipation.

One of the complaints suffered by the Causticum patient is muscular pains, where the muscles feel tight and short.

Key symptoms

Burns and blisters • Illness brought on by grief • Muscular pains.

General symptoms
The patient shakes during dry weather, and suffers weakness from grief. They can suffer physical breakdown causing back pain. They might become ambivalent about getting too involved with another person because they have given so much of themselves in the past, which has weakened their spirit. This causes a kind of 'paralysis' on the physical, emotional and mental levels; it starts with irritation and sets into the body, mind and spirit.

CHAMOMILLA

(CR, GR, M) German chamomile plant

This is a specific remedy for teething babies and for children who throw temper tantrums. It works well on very irritable people.

Mind and emotions
The patient is angry, cross and uncivil. They are quarrelsome and vexed. They are oversensitive about all their pains. A child wants to be carried and has an aversion to being spoken to. They can cry in their sleep, without waking. Their strong emotions give them stomach pains and they can scream, yell and throw tantrums.

Physical complaints
- The patient experiences hot perspiration on the scalp, flickering before their eyes, and are extremely thirsty.
- Children who have difficulties when teething, often accompanied by diarrhoea, will benefit from this remedy, which is also used for the relief of asthma that is made worse by cold air.

General symptoms
A change of position makes symptoms better. The patient loves to be carried or rocked. Useful for children who become extremely upset when corrected or punished.

Key symptoms
Excessively irritable • Hot perspiration and a great thirst • Babies who are teething and have diarrhoea.

A useful remedy for teething babies is derived from the chamomile flower and can be taken in granular form.

chamomilla

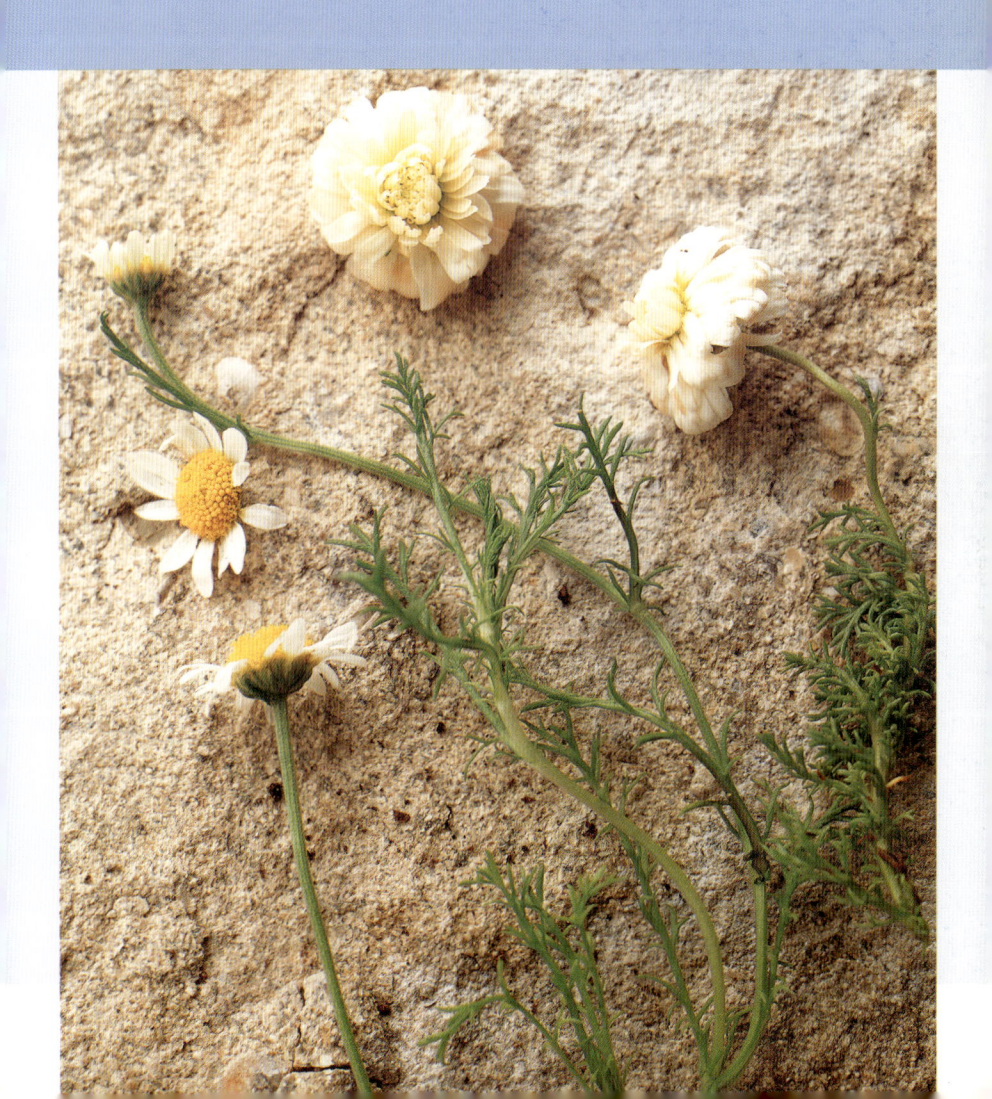

CHELIDONIUM MAJUS

(D, GR, M) celandine

This remedy is excellent for liver dysfunction and gallbladder problems.

Mind and emotions

The patient is a no-nonsense, down-to-earth, strong-minded person who is not impressed by any authority. They have a strong sense of morality and they are not emotional. They are convinced that they are ill and will not recover.

Physical complaints

- Complaints occur on the right side.
- Pains and cramping in the stomach, pain in area of the gallbladder and liver.
- Nausea and perspiration from pain.
- Patient has liver pains that move towards the back or upwards, and pains in the gallbladder. The patient can have gallstones and pain under their right shoulder blade.
- They can also suffer migraine headaches and vomit bile.
- Infants might suffer from pneumonia that begins as bronchitis with a deep but strained cough.

General symptoms

The patient craves very hot drinks. Pain is worse at 4.00 a.m. or 4.00 p.m., and better at noon after eating. The patient has an aversion or desire to eat cheese.

Key symptoms

Practical, sceptical, strong-minded people • Complaints are on the right side of the body • Symptoms are better for hot drinks • Ailments and pain found under right shoulder blade • Pain with nausea and perspiration.

chelidonium majus

A typical Chelidonium majus patient craves very hot drinks, is strong-minded and suffers with liver and gallbladder problems.

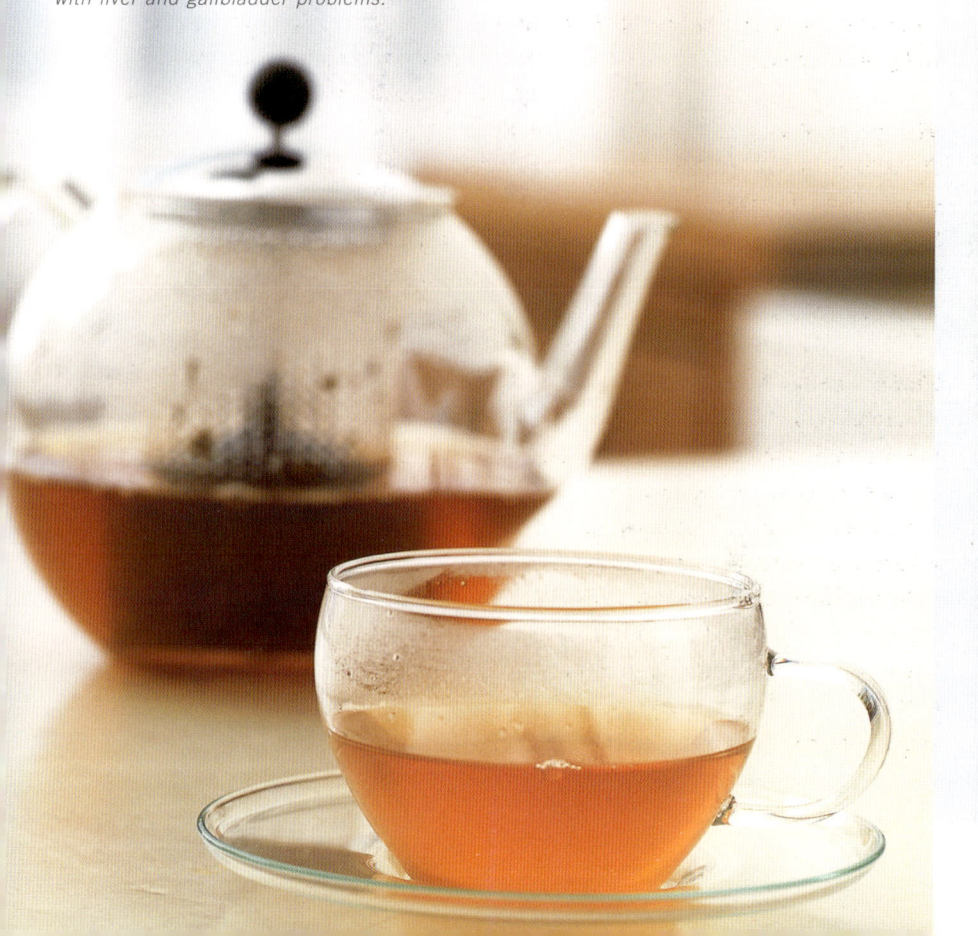

CHINA OFFICINALIS

(CR, D, GR, M)
Peruvian bark, also *Cinchona officinalis*

This is a remedy for highly sensitive, artistic people with a strong sense of beauty. It is for those who suffer from digestive and circulatory problems, and from flatulence. Also good for faintness after the loss of blood.

Mind and emotions

The patient expresses themselves only to close friends, as they are averse to superficial contact. They want only deep, meaningful contacts and friendships. They also want the best of things in life. They have a strong imagination, thinking of wonderful and imaginative things, and are full of plans and ideas. Everything that is experienced externally by this patient leaves a deep impression on them.

Because they are intense by nature this can lead to exhaustion, where they become irritable, insulting and abusive. When in a negative frame of mind they can feel unfortunate and that the world is hostile towards them. They can experience apathy following a severe illness.

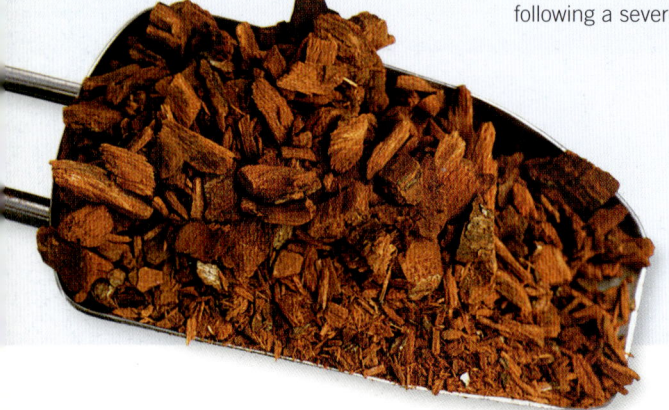

Peruvian bark is potentized to make a remedy for creative, imaginative people.

Physical complaints

- This is a remedy for ailments due to loss of fluids and heavy discharges including flu, perspiration, vomiting, diarrhoea, lactation and masturbation.
- It is a remedy for nervous and overly sensitive people who are worse for being touched, and even the least noise can irritate them.
- China officinalis people are also susceptible to cold winds.
- They can suffer from a bloated belly, which is full of gas.
- They may experience circulatory problems and have gallstone colic (when the patient passes small stones).
- They can also have headaches that feel as if the head is bursting, accompanied by a red face and a throbbing head.
- They may perspire continuously.

Key symptoms

Patient is imaginative and inventive • Ailments from loss of fluid make the patient tired and weak with headaches and stomach problems • Bloating of the belly, which belching does not relieve • Symptoms worse for the slightest touch and better for hard pressure.

General symptoms

The patient is reserved unless they feel that another person is receptive and genuine. Their dislike of superficial contact makes them appear aloof and distant. They can be extremely hungry at night and suffer from drinking too much tea, which causes a nervous stomach, sweating and diarrhoea.

CIMACIFUGA

(F, M, GR)
black cohosh plant (also *Actaea racemosa*)

This is a woman's remedy used for suppressed menstruation (which occurs when using the birth pill) and for labour that is controlled using drugs; Cimacifuga is also used for emotions.

Mind and emotions
The patient is talkative and jumps from one topic to another. She may feel gloomy and sad, as if enveloped in a black cloud. She weeps for others and fears both insanity and death, especially during the menopause. She can suffer from post-natal depression, and feel she is imprisoned, and might have fears and delusions about creatures. The patient can feel insecure and uncertain and is inclined to be restless and nervous, often sighing, especially during her periods and the menopause. She might feel confused and hysterical before her period.

Key symptoms

All complaints that relate to menstrual periods, labour in childbirth or the menopause • Sighing, depression and sadness accompanying physical symptoms • Problems with the nape of the neck, tension and stiffness • Symptoms are worse when periods are late.

Physical complaints
- The patient is chilly, and might suffer weakness from nursing the sick, or have ailments associated with her periods and the menopause.
- She might also suffer with problems connected to the nape of the neck, as well as nausea and vomiting caused by

Cimacifuga is used for ailments that are caused by a lack of menstrual periods.

pressure on the spine, pain in the hips, heaviness in her head, and aching in the thyroid area during her period.
- This is a remedy for those women who suffer from repeated miscarriage. They feel sore and bruised, and are sleepless.
- It is also a good remedy for rheumatic problems during the menopause as well as ailments during pregnancy such as nausea, vomiting, sleeplessness, shooting pains, sadness and nervousness.
- To be used for severe dysmenorrhoea (painful menstruation with abdominal cramps) where the pains extend into the legs, and in labour when the delivery is slow due to a rigid cervix, or with false labour pains in a particularly sensitive patient.

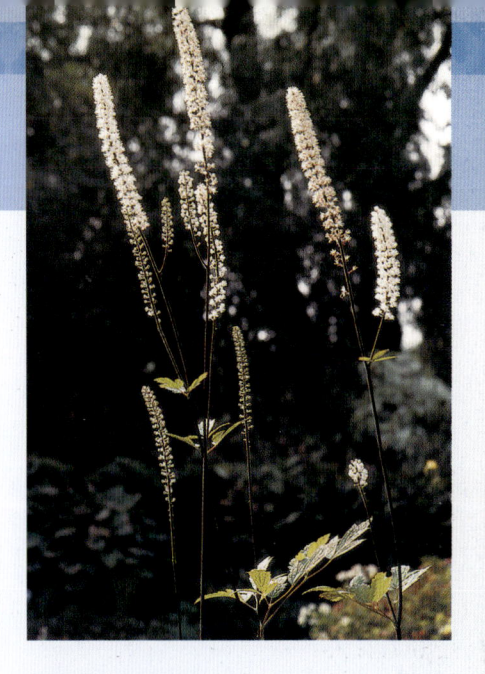

General symptoms

The patient is worse when periods are late, and during a delayed onset of labour; also when emotional, and during damp cold weather. She feels better when wrapped up warm, in the fresh air, with pressure from clothing or a strong, firm touch, gentle continuous motion, eating and rest. Pains in the breast during menopause are alleviated by Cimacifuga. The keynote symptom is depression with physical symptoms.

CINA

(D, CR, GR, M) wormwood

The remedy Cina is useful for children who are ill-humoured and suffer from worms. It is also used for digestive problems.

Mind and emotions

The patient is often a touchy and difficult child, who is inclined to be overexcited and weak – often screaming and hitting, cross and unpleasant. The child is constantly ill-humoured and doesn't want to be touched, caressed or looked at. They scream at night, grind their teeth, and can only lie on their belly; they also chew and swallow during sleep. The child refuses anything that is given to him or her, and will throw it away and try to hit you.

Physical complaints

- This is a remedy for worms, where the patient is also excessively hungry after eating or if they vomit.
- It is also used to treat ailments in nursing children who refuse breast milk, or are allergic to cow's milk.
- It is used to support the treatment of epilepsy where the child awakes and screams without apparent cause and cannot be consoled.
- The child stiffens up before coughing, rubs their nose and complains of stomach ache. They have blue rings under their eyes.

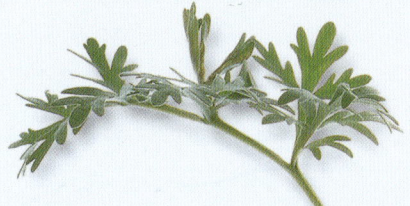

Wormwood is the source for this remedy suitable for pale and sickly children who suffer from worms.

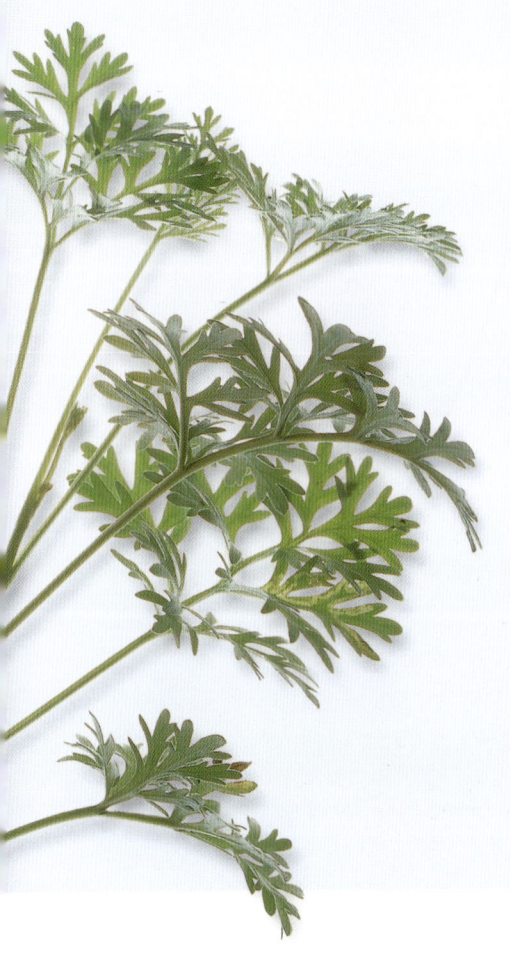

> ### Key symptoms
>
> *A touchy and difficult child who easily becomes overexcited • Intestinal worms • Babies who refuse breast milk or are allergic to cow's milk • Stomach ache.*

General symptoms

The patient may suffer from convulsions while teeth grow, from worms, during heat and when shuddering; also during drinking or while swallowing. The remedy can help while you wait for medical assistance.

COCA

(M, GR) cocaine

This remedy works on the nerves. It is especially good for altitude sickness and substance abusers who have previously used cocaine. A remedy for sleeplessness at altitude.

Mind and emotions

This is a remedy for shy and bashful people who choose to withdraw from the world and who love solitude. They fear heights and falling. They also feel isolated. People who have experienced cocaine substance abuse might hold the energy from that drug in their body and can be helped with this remedy.

Physical complaints

- Vertigo. The patient is worse when ascending stairs, has head pains at altitude and sleeplessness at altitude, feeling very euphoric.
- Also a good remedy for coughing in athletes and old people.

Key symptoms

Vertigo • Coughs in athletes and old people • Suited to shy people who prefer solitude to company.

General symptoms

Worse for ascending heights. Mental tiredness alternating with brightness. It is a mountaineer's remedy; useful in a variety of mountain-climbing complaints, such as palpitations, laboured breathing, anxiety, insomnia and all altitude-sickness symptoms. Generally for people who are weary because of the physical and mental strain of a busy life, and who suffer from exhausted nerves and mind. Also for ailments in old people and inflammation of the nerves. They might feel a sensation of a worm under their skin.

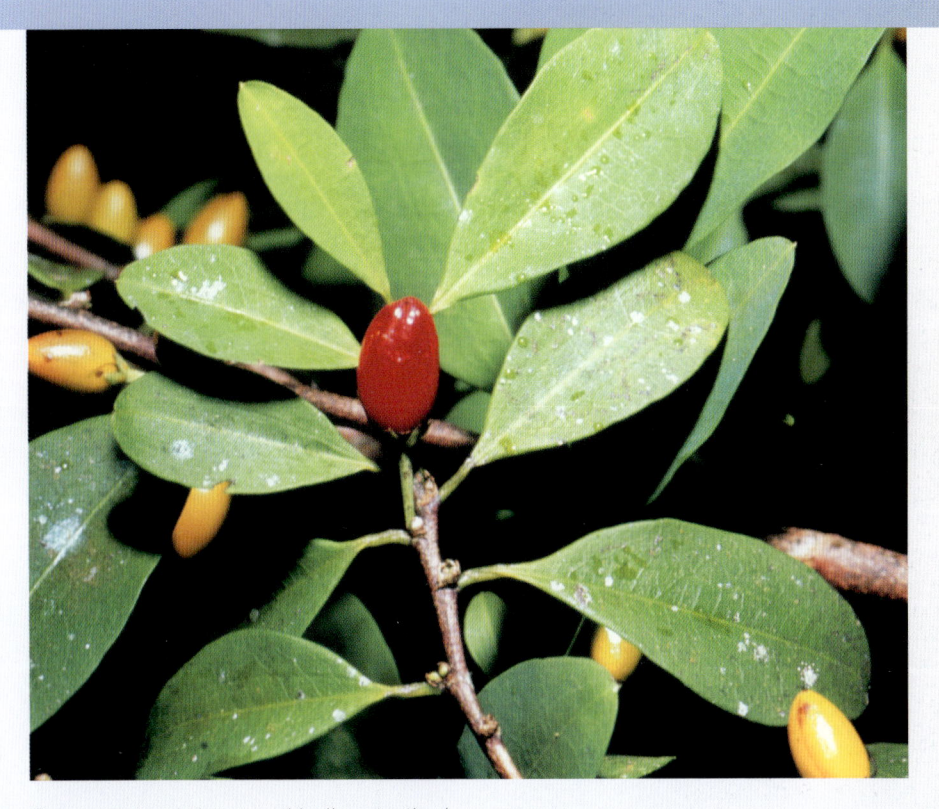

The coca plant is homeopathically potentized to create a remedy suitable for nervous complaints and altitude sickness.

COCCULUS INDICUS

(M, D, CB, GR) Indian cockle tree

The remedy Cocculus indicus affects the senses. It is used for motion sickness, anxiety and nausea.

Mind and emotions

The patient dislikes being disturbed and becomes angry when interrupted, saying they need time to answer and respond. This is a remedy for ailments that relate to a combination of physical and mental stress, such as nursing the sick, loss of sleep, or anxiety about the health of others. It works well with ailments caused by cares and worries combined with physical exertion. The patient feels as if time passes too slowly. They are sensitive to everything that happens to them, and are greatly affected by events.

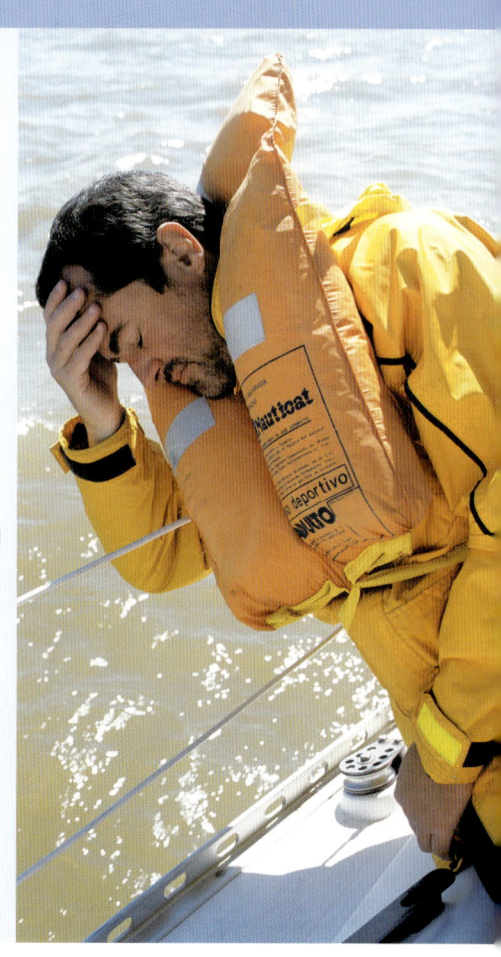

Physical complaints

- This is a remedy for travel sickness, car sickness and seasickness.
- The patient is oversensitive in all ways, such as being worse for noise, odours, excitement and cold.
- They are averse to food – feeling nauseous at the sight of it.
- It is a good remedy for morning sickness.
- Women might be extremely weak during and after their periods, where they can scarcely speak or stand.
- Other symptoms include copious saliva and a raging thirst, numb hands when grasping something, trembling hands and a sensation of a stone in their bellies.

Key symptoms

Travel sickness • Morning sickness • Copious saliva and a raging thirst • Tiredness due to loss of sleep, nursing the sick or anxiety over others.

General symptoms

A sense of faintness, pain in the belly, loss of sleep, trembling from the slightest emotions or from noise, pains or being touched.

Cocculus indicus is a useful remedy for travel sickness and seasickness, especially in sensitive people who are also carers.

COFFEA CRUDA

(M, CB, GR) raw coffee bean

This is a remedy for severe pain and excessive emotions, including joy that is so great that they can become ill. It is used in childbirth to relieve the pain of labour.

Mind and emotions

The patient suffers from conditions that are linked to anger, excitement, fright and also excessive joy and happy surprises. It is also a remedy for disappointed love where the emotions run high. The mind can become overstimulated and the thoughts wander. Ideas gush out and the patient answers incoherently. This is a remedy for overactive minds. The patient loves to theorize and is often sleepless. Despair from physical pain is a prominent symptom.

Physical complaints

- The patient is oversensitive to pain and all their senses are acutely heightened. The eyes will be dilated and shining; there is a marked redness in both cheeks and the patient is very talkative, with an active memory and heightened feelings.
- In childbirth the mother will be sleepless after delivery. This is an excellent pain remedy for childbirth.
- Coffea cruda is also excellent for toothache that feels better when there is cold water in the mouth.
- It works with ailments suffered during the menopause combined with overexcitement, sleeplessness and palpitations.

General symptoms

Aversion to the fresh air, where all symptoms get worse. A remedy for joy with weeping, sleeplessness from excitement or mental activity, congestion in the head, inflammation in the uterus, asthma and palpitations.

coffea cruda 141

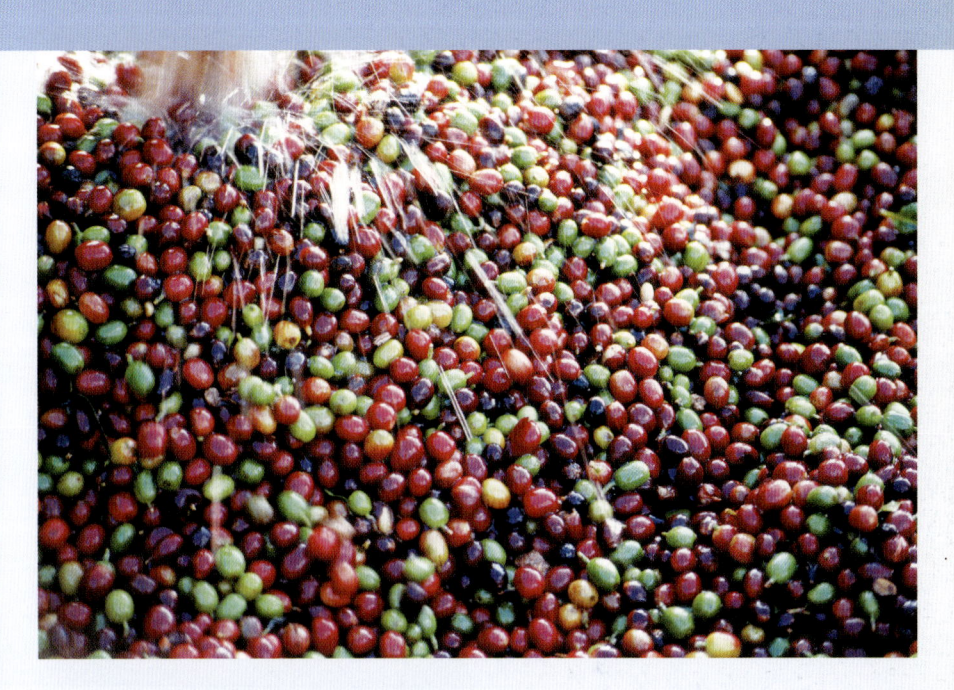

Key symptoms

Excitement, fright or excessive joy in an overactive mind • Menopausal ailments.

The ground raw coffee bean is used to make a remedy for severe pain and can be used for labour in childbirth.

COLCHICUM AUTUMNALE

(D, F, GR, M) meadow saffron

The remedy Colchicum affects the mind and body, working on muscles, joints and alleviating gout.

Mind and emotions

The patient suffers from ailments caused by studying and watching the sick during the night. It is suited to sensitive people who tend to be unable to cope with the day-to-day problems of life. They suffer conditions caused by their sensitivity to the rudeness they encounter in other people. Colchicum is also for people who suffer from gout and who are irritable and unpleasant. The patient is forgetful, dull and has a weak memory.

Physical complaints

- A remedy for gout, pains in the heel and inflammation of the big toe, where the patient cannot bear to be touched or to move the affected area.

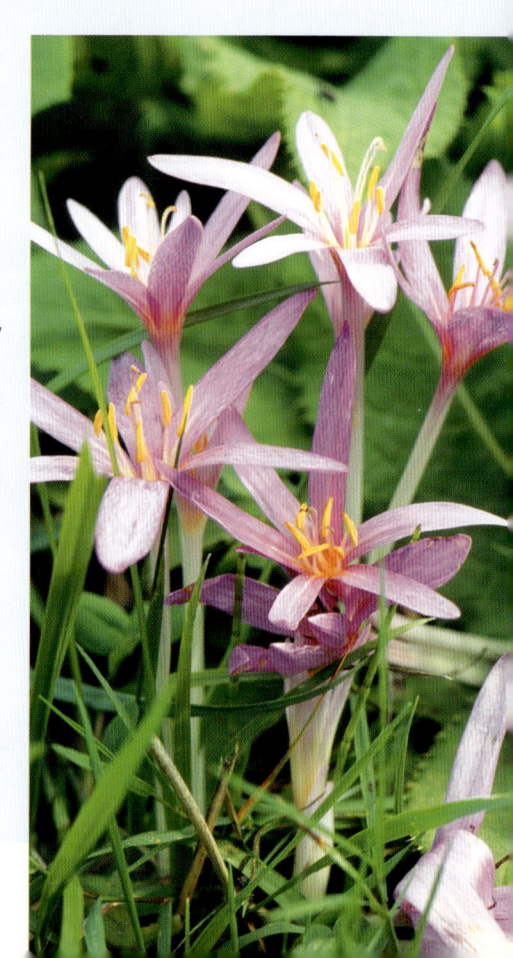

Used for rheumatic problems and gout, the remedy Colchicum autumnale is derived from the bulb of the meadow saffron plant.

- The remedy works well to relieve swelling of the legs and feet, as well as aches in the lumbar area and lower backache. Symptoms are better for rest and pressure.
- Colchicum is also a headache remedy where there is pain above the eyes and in the temples.
- The smell of food creates nausea and fainting, with vomiting of mucus and bile.
- Other physical symptoms include a stomach bloated with gas, where the patient is unable to stretch out their legs because of the discomfort.
- Also used in the treatment of liver ailments and rheumatism.

Key symptoms

Sensitivity to the behaviour of others • Rheumatic and gouty problems, especially of the small joints with swelling and inflammation • Bloated stomach • Liver ailments.

General symptoms

Extreme physical weakness. Tearing pains in warm weather; stinging pains in cold weather. Pins and needles in hands and fingers. Pains worse in the evening and during warm weather.

COLOCYNTHIS

(D, F, GR, M) bitter cucumber

A remedy used to treat trigeminal neuralgia, sciatic pains, digestive ailments and disturbed emotions.

Mind and emotions

The patient suffers from pent-up emotions, especially anger. Where there is anger with silent grief this leads to physical complaints, especially cramps. The patient is restless with pain and does not like others to know they are suffering. Their emotions are expressed with physical pain.

Physical complaints

- The patient is always better when doubled over with hard pressure on the abdomen. Violent cramps make them twist and cry out in pain.
- They suffer from cutting, pinching, gnawing, clutching and boring pains, often with nausea.

Key symptoms

Colic and neuralgia caused by pent-up emotions, especially from anger and irritation • Pains make the patient cry out and become upset • Diarrhoea and other digestive problems.

- Other symptoms include abdominal colic from anger, indigestion and diarrhoea; sciatica that is worse when moving; digestive problems after eating unripe fruit; constipation caused by medication.

General symptoms

Always worse from anger and indignation. This is an acute remedy for very painful conditions.

The bitter cucumber plant is dried and powdered to form a major colic remedy.

colocynthis 145

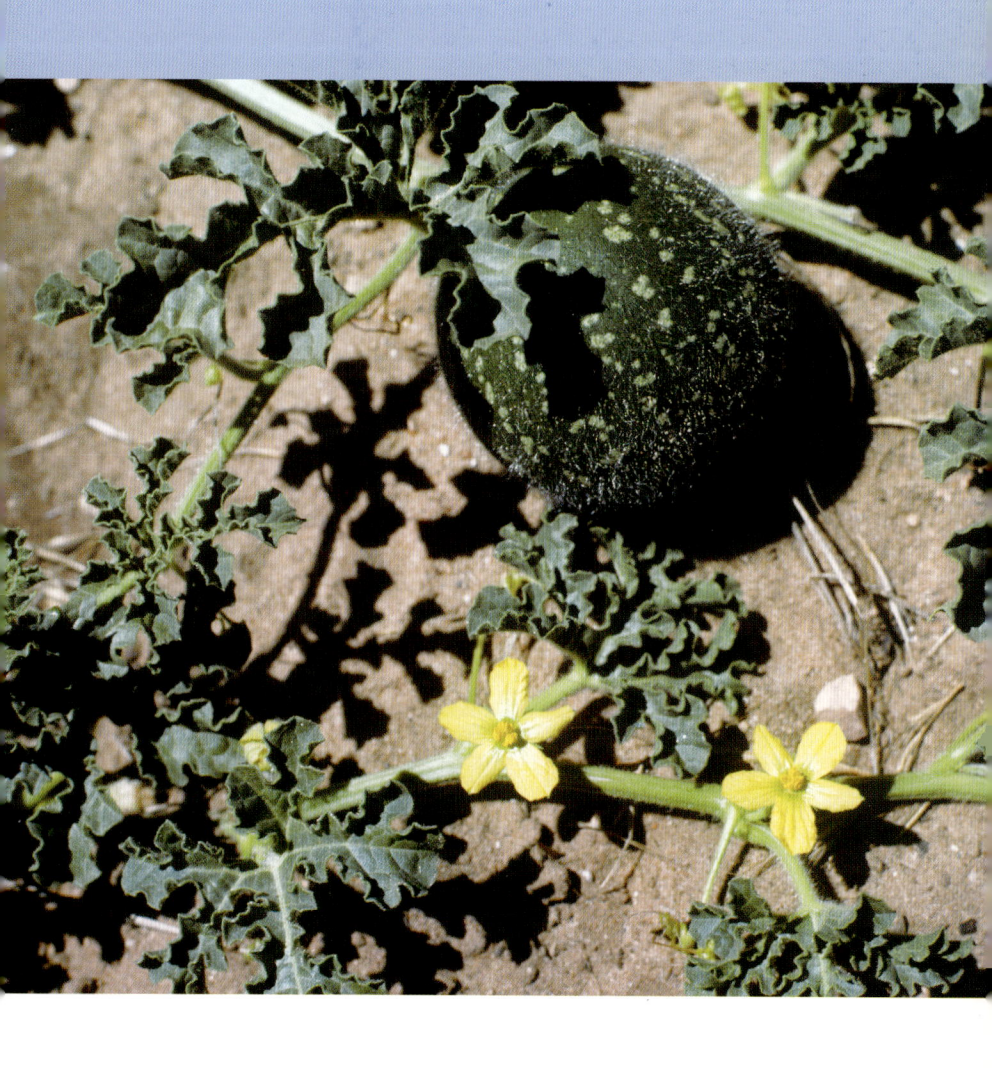

CONIUM MACULATUM

(C-C-F, F, GR, M, Ma) poison hemlock

This is a remedy for paralysis, known since Plato described its use in the death of Socrates. When a person starts to withdraw from life they can stop moving physically, mentally and emotionally and it is at these times that Conium is useful. It is good for trembling, difficulty in walking and loss of strength. It is a remedy for weakness of all kinds, including dizziness, exhaustion and injuries. It can be used with conventional medicine as a cancer remedy for hard tumour formation in the breast and other parts of body.

Mind and emotions
The patient is timid and shy, and wants to be left alone. There is little desire to study or work, or there will be little interest in life. The patient suffers from a weakened memory and mental depression. The 'paralysis' is gradual and goes unnoticed.

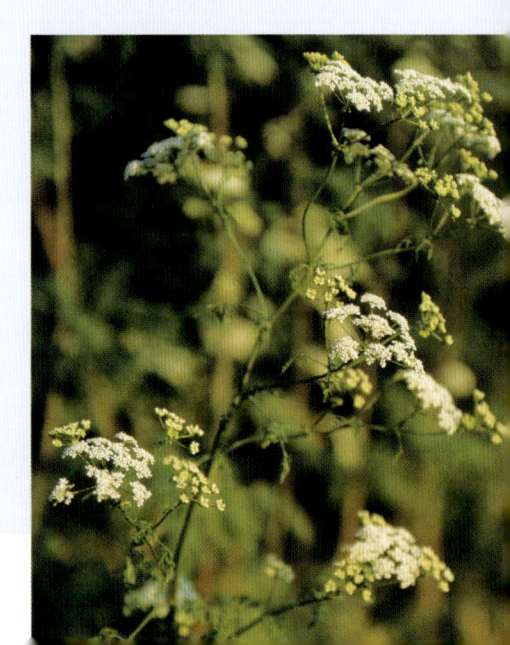

The patient becomes more introverted, and won't discuss their symptoms because they become unwilling to express themselves emotionally. However, there was more emotional suffering in past, but it has now lessened. Although having often had a wild past, the patient has gradually calmed down. Now, he or she gradually withdraws and becomes isolated and dislikes company. This shutting down can lead to ritualistic and compulsive behaviour, especially about diet and health issues.

They may show a lack of anxiety when faced with an uncertain future. The patient cares for little. They lack sexual desire and are materialistic, but this changes into indifference.

Physical complaints

- Sexuality is suppressed; this might be the result of the loss or sickness of a partner, fear of AIDs, fixed ideas about sex, or spiritual reasons.
- There might also be clear signs of premature ageing.
- There can be glandular problems that could lead to cancer.

The poison hemlock plant is potentized to form a remedy for glandular problems.

Key symptoms

Ailments due to sexual suppression
- *Glandular problems.*

- Females experience menopausal problems, dizziness and perspiration that prevent sleep.
- Male symptoms are inflammation of the prostate gland, weak or failed erections.
- Coughing constantly at night and dryness are also indications. This is a remedy to support conventional medicine for cancer of the breast and is also good for hard tumour formations. Always consult your doctor first.

General symptoms

A remedy for injuries to soft tissue. The patient suffers weakness, both physical and mental.

CUPRUM METALLICUM

(C-C-F, GR, M) copper

This is a remedy for spasms, cramps and congestion. It is good for mental as well as physical problems.

This remedy from copper is for cramps, twitching and asthma, and is also suited to behavioural problems in children.

Mind and emotions

This is a remedy for serious people, who are emotionally cramped in their lives or in their work. Good for adolescents who are worried about how they will be accepted in the world and for extremely self-critical people who are afraid of their emotions or have negative thoughts. This is a good remedy to use when the expression of love comes out in a cramped way.

Cuprum metallicum is also used for children with behavioural problems, such as those who are destructive and who hit, bite and spit. Also applicable for those children who will hold their breath until they are blue in the face.

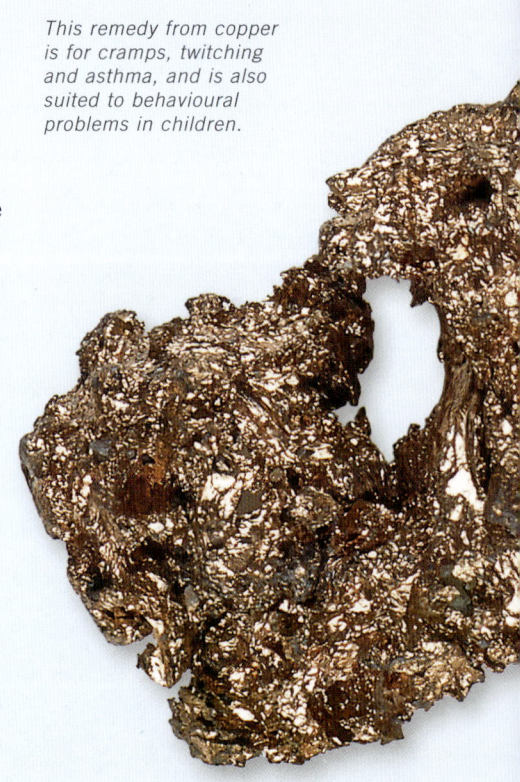

cuprum metallicum

A remedy for dictatorial people, who avoid company or even seeing people.

Physical complaints
- Symptoms include convulsions, spasms, cramps, twitching and jerking: convulsions start in the fingers and toes and work inwards.

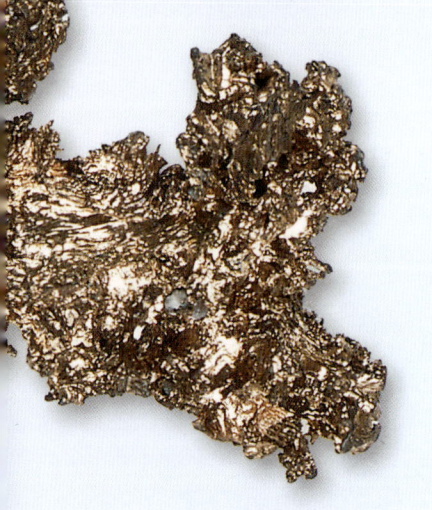

> **Key symptoms**
>
> Symptoms appear in people who are emotionally and physically cramped
> - Behavioural problems in children
> - Convulsions that begin in the fingers and toes, spasms, cramps, twitching and jerking • Asthma.

- Asthma that is spasmodic with nausea and vomiting, cough and respiratory problems where breathing can cease altogether.

General symptoms
Convulsions from becoming wet, or from loss of sleep. Shaking and vertigo can accompany the symptoms.

DIOSCOREA VILLOSA

(CR, D, GR) wild yam

This is a remedy for pain and is especially suited for colic in children and severe abdominal pains in adults.

Mind and emotions

The patient has an aversion to certain people. They make written and spoken mistakes, such as calling things by the wrong name, and using wrong words in a sentence. There is acute restlessness.

Physical complaints

- A remedy for the weak, old or the young with poor digestive systems.
- The pains radiate to distant parts of the body and are unbearably sharp, cutting, twisting, griping and grinding. Pains come in bursts; a baby might have colicky pains where it has to stretch or bend backwards or forwards for relief. There are cutting pains as well as sciatica shooting down the thighs.
- This is a remedy to accompany conventional medicine for gallstone colic (when the patient passes small stones) with radiating pains as well as severe gastric distress, and cramping pains extending along the sternum into both arms.
- Also a remedy for renal colic.

> **Key symptoms**
>
> *Cramping, griping, grinding and twisting pains in the abdomen that radiate in all directions • Strong pains that suddenly shift direction • Symptoms are worse for drinking tea.*

dioscorea villosa

General symptoms

Burping relieves all the pains. Pains are worse for drinking tea, which causes a nervous stomach, sweating and diarrhoea.

Wild yam, shown here dried, is used to prepare the remedy Dioscorea villosa that can be prescribed for colic in children.

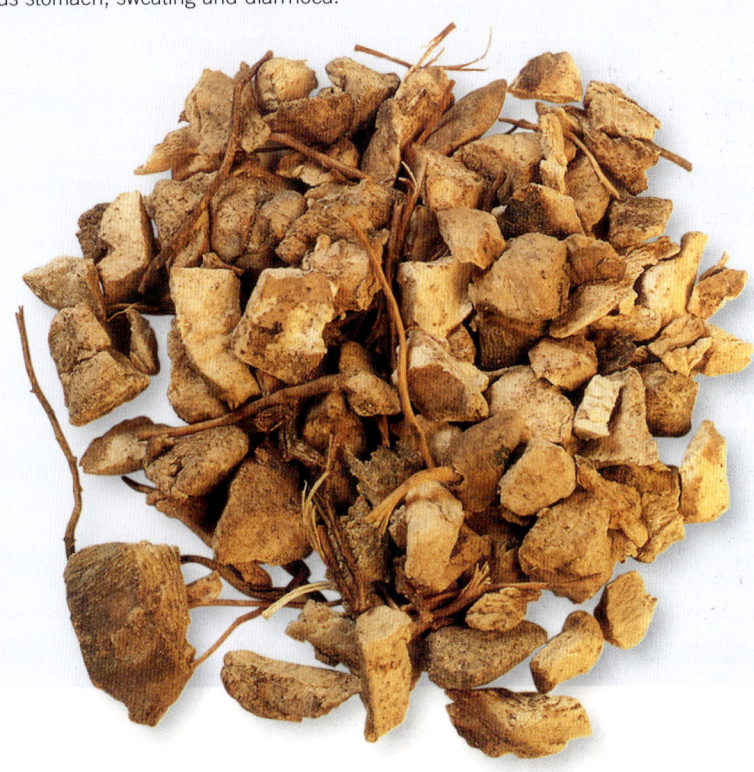

DROSERA ROTUNDIFOLIA

(C-C-F, CR) sundew plant

This is a first-rate cough remedy, good for colds, flu and whooping cough.

Mind and emotions

A remedy for peevish children who are anxious and mistrustful of others. The patient has great restlessness and difficulty with concentration. Full of mistrust, the patient is concerned that they are being deceived and will be anxious about being alone, as they have a fear of the paranormal. Obstinacy is a marked characteristic of someone who would benefit from Drosera rotundifolia.

Physical complaints

- A good remedy for growing pains in children and adolescents.
- It is also a scar-tissue remedy, as well as working for pains in the joints, hips, shoulders and ankles. It is especially suited to stiffness and inflexibility of the ankle.

Key symptoms

For restless people who are mistrustful of others • Symptoms, such as coughing, pain and difficult respiration, are worse after midnight • Growing pains in children.

- Use Drosera rotundifolia for asthma and a violent spasmodic cough.

General symptoms

Coughing is worse after midnight. Symptoms are worse for warmth and better for fresh air.

An effective cough remedy, suitable for restless and mistrustful people, is derived from Drosera rotundifolia, *the sundew plant.*

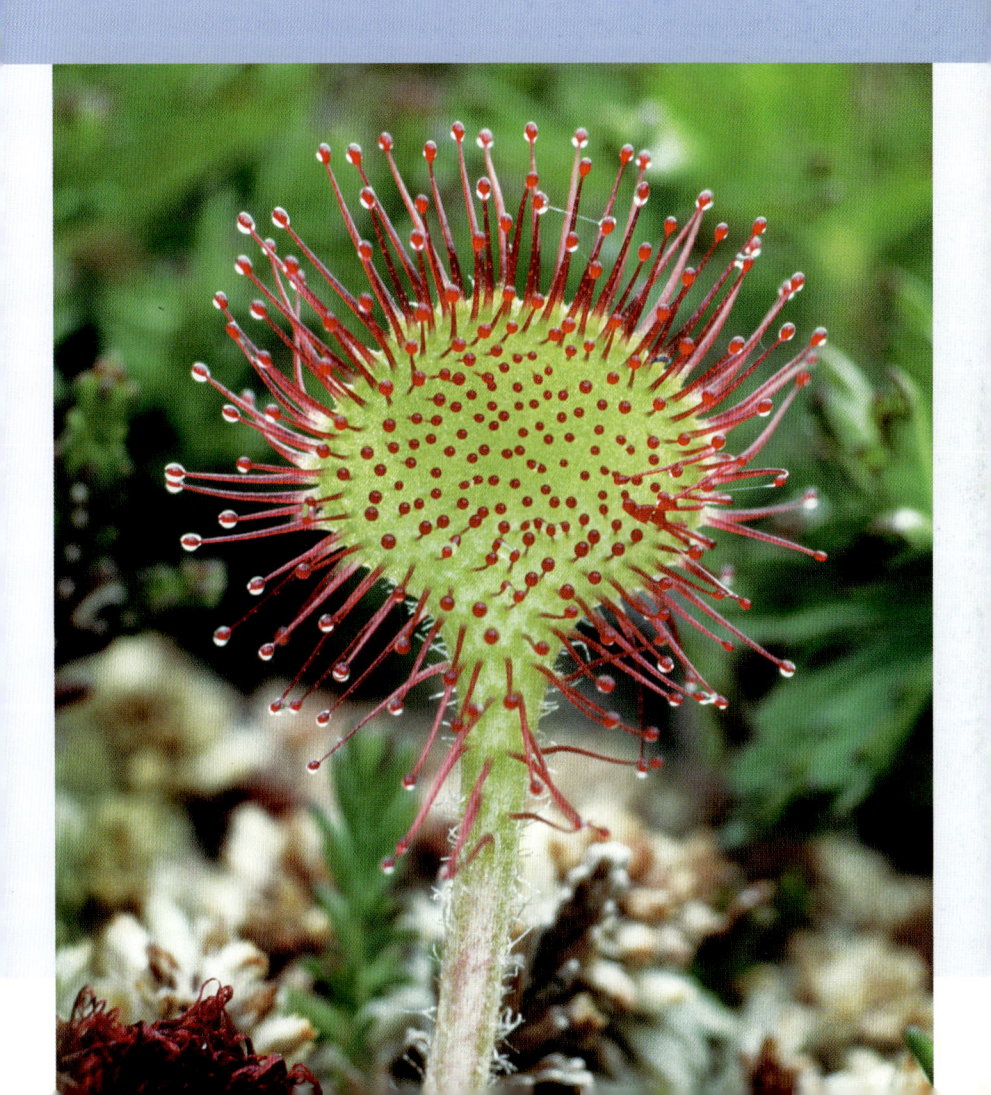

drosera rotundifolia 153

EUPATORIUM PERFOLIATUM

(C-C-F, CR, D) thoroughwort

The remedy Eupatorium perfoliatum is excellent for the aches and pains that accompany flu.

Mind and emotions
The patient will be miserable from suffering with flu and might be moaning with discomfort.

Physical complaints
- The patient's head will feel so heavy that they feel they cannot raise it off the pillow without use their hands.
- They will have pains while in bed in the morning, which are accompanied by nausea, and also during a fever.
- The patient will vomit, and will be chilled and perspiring.
- They will feel pains in the chest caused by coughing, and will hold their hands up to the chest during a coughing fit.

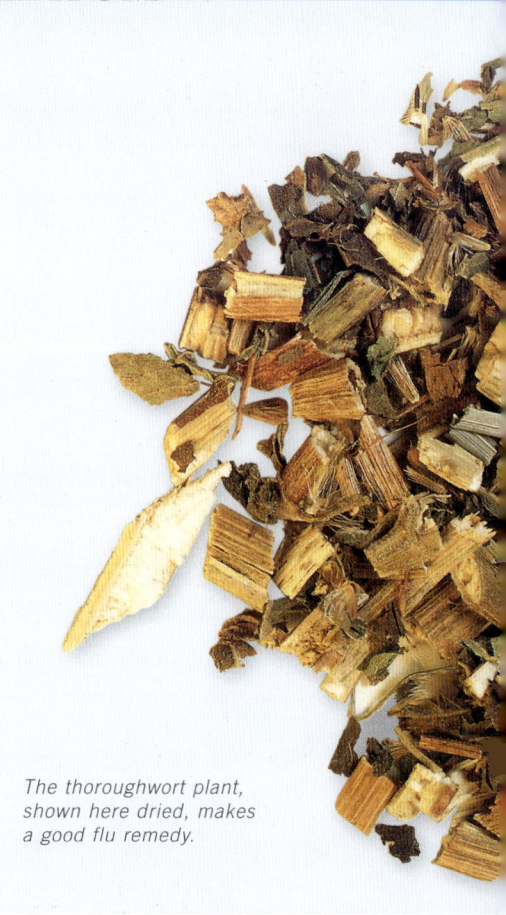

The thoroughwort plant, shown here dried, makes a good flu remedy.

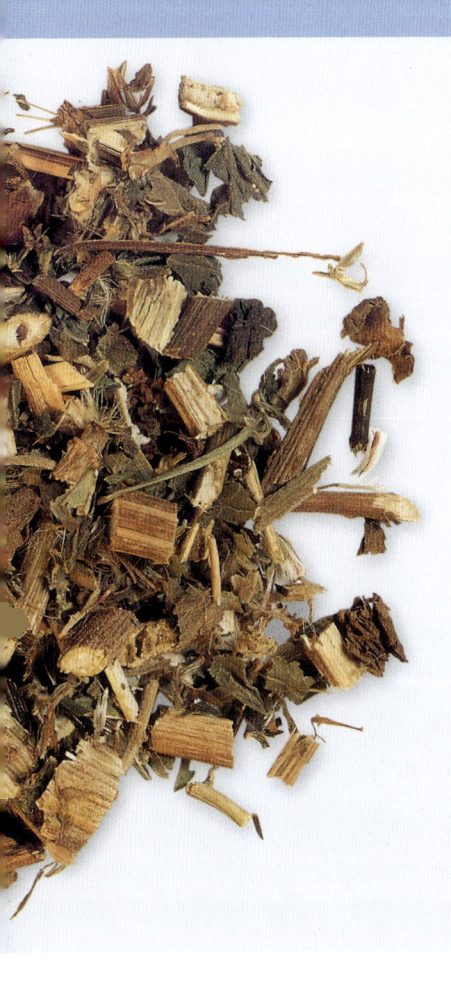

- Pains will be felt in the back, from flu, and there will be growing pains in the legs, which might feel as if the bones were broken.
- The patient will tremble during a fever.
- The patient will be very thirsty for cold drinks and cooling foods, such as ice cream.

General symptoms

The fever changes frequently. The patient is very thirsty, desiring cold drinks and ice cream. The chill begins in the small of the back.

> **Key symptoms**
>
> Aching bones and back, which are worse during flu and fevers • Great restlessness and discomfort • Patient desires cold drinks and foods.

EUPHRASIA

(+FA, CR) eyebright plant

A specific remedy for ailments of the eye and mucous membranes.

Mind and emotions
No symptoms.

Physical complaints
- Thick and yellow pus or acrid mucus from the eyes.
- Itching, tearing; wounds to the cornea; pain in the eyes.
- Fear of light, redness in the eyes after injury and spots around the eyes.
- Other symptoms include swollen or thickening eyelids, ulceration of the cornea and dim vision.
- Symptoms are worse after contracting a fever or measles.
- There is discharge from the nose with coughing and phlegm; also sneezing with hay fever.

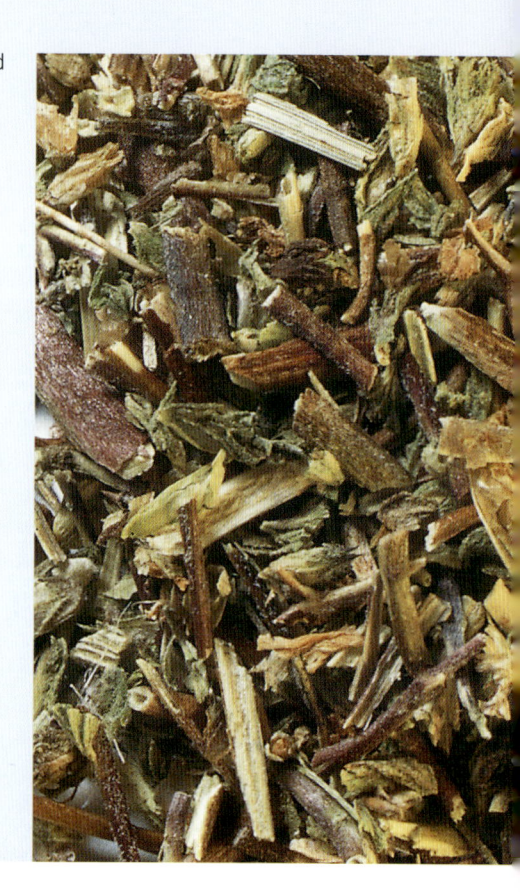

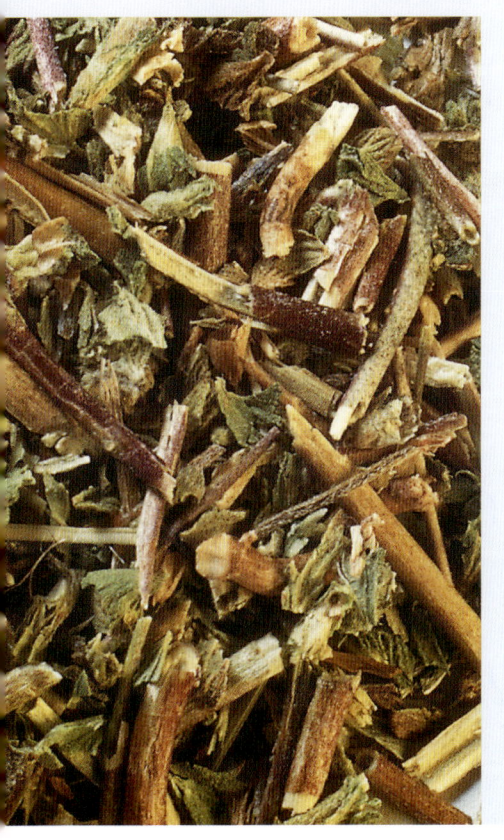

Key symptoms

Tearing and mucus from the eyes • Burning and stinging eyes, and an aversion to light • Coughing with large quantities of mucus during the day but better at night.

General symptoms

Smoke aggravates all symptoms. Vision is worse in dim light. This remedy is good for tired and strained eyes, worse from excessive reading or looking at a computer for long periods of time.

The Euphrasia *plant is used to make a useful remedy for all kinds of ailments affecting the eyes.*

FERRUM METALLICUM

(CB, CR, D, GR, M) iron

The remedy Ferrum metallicum is for young, weak people, who are anaemic and oversensitive, with all symptoms worsening after any effort. Weakness characterizes all symptoms. This is a remedy to use in times of change: from childhood to puberty, at the beginning of periods and the onset of the menopause later in life.

Mind and emotions
The patient is extremely irritated by even the slightest noise. They can be abusive and insulting. This is a remedy for someone with changeable moods, where they flit about from one subject to the other. They can weep and laugh at the same time, and get overexcited by trivial things. They prefer to

Iron, extracted from the ore, is the source of a remedy suited to weak people who are anaemic and oversensitive.

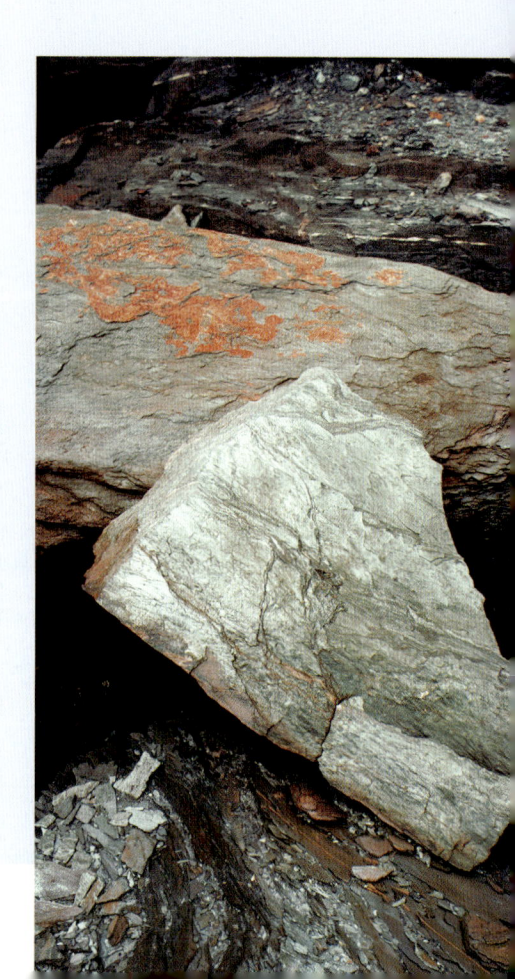

be alone, and they avoid company; their symptoms are worse from conversations. Motion also aggravates their symptoms; they prefer to sit or stay in bed but their pains force them to move. The patient is restless because of the pain.

Physical complaints

- The patient's face becomes flushed from the least excitement or exertion.
- Other symptoms include a hammering headache, which is worse after eating or drinking.
- Diarrhoea during and immediately after eating; nightly diarrhoea around midnight, which is painless.
- The patient might vomit after midnight, without any preceding nausea, as well as having urinary incontinence during the day.
- Varicose veins during pregnancy as well as a prolapsed vagina during pregnancy.

Key symptoms

Patient wishes to be alone and is irritable, with changeable moods • Flushed face from the least excitement or exertion • Diarrhoea during and immediately after eating.

General symptoms

The patient dislikes eggs and the symptoms will be aggravated by them. Although wishing to eat tomatoes and fat, these will also aggravate the condition.

GELSEMIUM

(+FA, CB, C-C-F, CR, GR, M)
yellow jasmine

A first-aid remedy for flu when all the symptoms are worse from anticipation and strong emotion.

Mind and emotions

The patient experiences anticipatory anxiety, great apprehension, and timidity. They dread ordeals such as exams and suffer with stage fright. They are always worse in new or unusual situations. They lack willpower and also suffer from muscular coordination problems. There is weakness at the mental, emotional and physical levels. The patient has a fear of losing control and a fear of falling. They desire to be quiet and dislike being disturbed. They can tremble in their hands and legs, often before a big event, and suffer from fatigue and generally weak limbs. The onset of symptoms is slow and they may follow an emotional upset or shock.

Key symptoms

Muscular coordination problems • Anxiety and timidity • Extreme exam nerves or stage fright • No thirst with a fever • Symptoms are worse for hot, sultry weather.

Physical complaints

- Acute ailments with slow onset accompanied by mental weakness and trembling characterize Gelsemium's physical portrait.
- This is a remedy for trembling during labour; diarrhoea from anticipation.
- Also for people who have never been well since contracting flu.
- The patient has heavy, droopy eyelids; while ill with flu they cannot keep their eyes open.

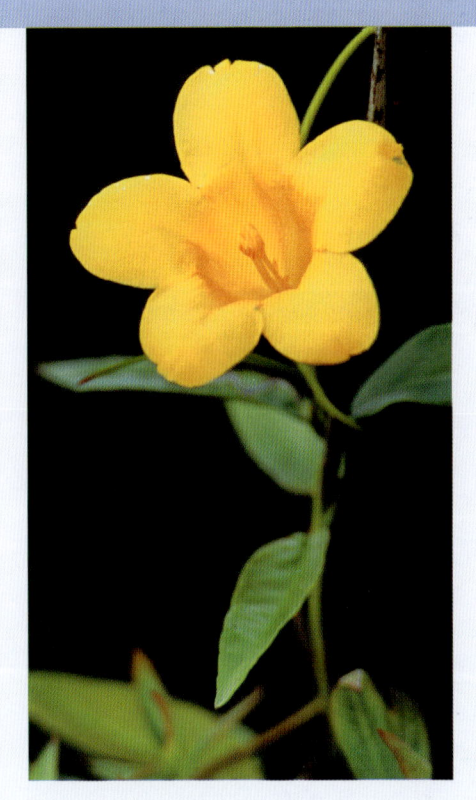

The root of Gelsemium sempervirens *is used to prepare a remedy for ailments connected to anxiety, such as exam nerves.*

- Useful to overcome fear in childbirth.
- It is accompanied by weakness, drowsiness and trembling, and for a headache that is caused by sickness or exhaustion.
- Their knees tremble when they walk downhill or down stairs.
- Use Gelsemium for miscarriage that was caused by emotions, fright or influenza.

General symptoms

All conditions are worse in hot, sultry weather, summer heat and before thunderstorms. The patient suffers from weariness in spring and weakness in summer because of the sun's heat. There is no thirst during the heat. The patient's head feels congested during the heat, and they can feel dull minded, although they feel better if they urinate copiously. This is a remedy for convulsions before thunderstorms, with faintness and fright afterwards.

GRAPHITES

(M, D, GR) black lead

This is a remedy for skin conditions and where a person is unable to absorb and digest nutrients in the body.

Mind and emotions

The patient is hesitant and timid with a pronounced lack of confidence and is full of doubts. Their thinking is unclear and they are unable to plan or analyse. The patient anticipates problems that might lead to anxiety. They suffer from overexcitability with sadness and despair, and are upset over minor issues. They weep when expressing their feelings, and can be compulsive about trivial situations.

Physical complaints

- Their glands, eyelids and nails can be lumpy and hard, and they can have hard, thick skin or scars.
- Female symptoms include dryness of the vagina, with pain in the uterus.
- The patient is often inclined to either obesity or emaciation.
- There are cracks in the skin of their hands, eyes, nostrils, mouth, nipples or anus.
- They might have offensive foot odour, and the soles of their feet can be raw from excess sweating.
- Often they have the accompanying symptoms of chronic constipation, where their stools are hard with mucus.

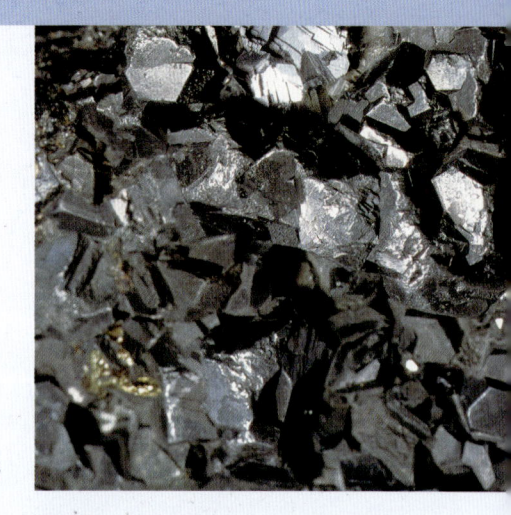

graphites 163

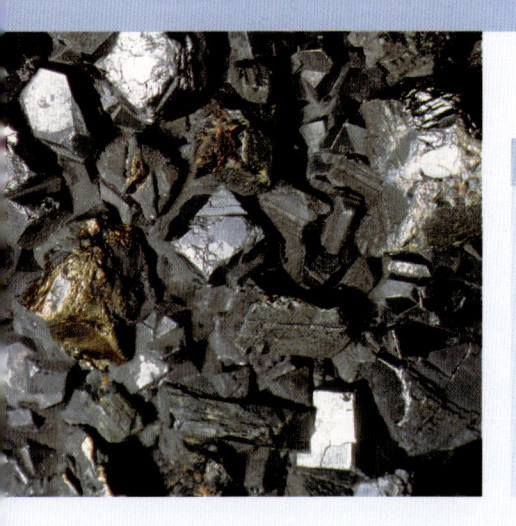

Key symptoms

Difficulty in concentrating • Patient anticipates difficulties and is easily upset by them • Symptoms are worse for the cold weather and the patient is generally chilly • Cracks in the skin, such as the hands, eyes, nostrils and mouth.

Graphites *makes a remedy that is good for skin conditions.*

- The patient can be asthmatic, where eating improves their symptoms.

General symptoms

Weariness and trembling during menstrual periods. The patient is chilly and worse for cold weather, for becoming cold and when entering a cold place. Pains shift to the body part that was lain on; obesity, lumpy, hard skin on the glands, eyelids and scars; crusts on the face, back or chest; cracks in the corners of the eyes, nostrils and mouth, on the fingertips and nipples. There is a sense of burning and numbness, and the brain feels numb. A very small appetite, where the patient only nibbles and has to take frequent small bites. Symptoms are worse for hunger.

HAMAMELIS VIRGINIANA

(+FA, D, F, GR, M) witch hazel plant

A major remedy for congestion, haemorrhages, varicose veins and haemorrhoids (piles), Hamamelis virginiana is also excellent for open, painful wounds and for weakness from loss of blood. A useful remedy to use after operations.

Mind and emotions

The patient feels numbness over the frontal bones of the head. They feel a need to be respected by others.

Physical complaints

- Hamamelis virginiana is a remedy for haemorrhages and varicose veins.
- The patient experiences soreness in all parts of the body; sore pain, swelling of veins, varicose veins and haemorrhoids.
- Use this remedy for haemorrhages that result from injury, such as nosebleeds or a blow to the face, or for long-lasting bleeding from tooth extraction.
- It is a remedy to accompany conventional medicine for phlebitis (inflammation to the walls of a vein), and varicose veins in the lower extremities.
- Think of Hamamelis virginiana to treat a black eye and other injuries to the eyes, as well as varicose veins during pregnancy, injury to the testicles and bleeding from haemorrhoids.

General symptoms

Colds from exposure to warm, moist weather.

A remedy for haemorrhages is derived from the pounded fresh bark of Hamamelis virginiana, *witch hazel.*

Key symptoms

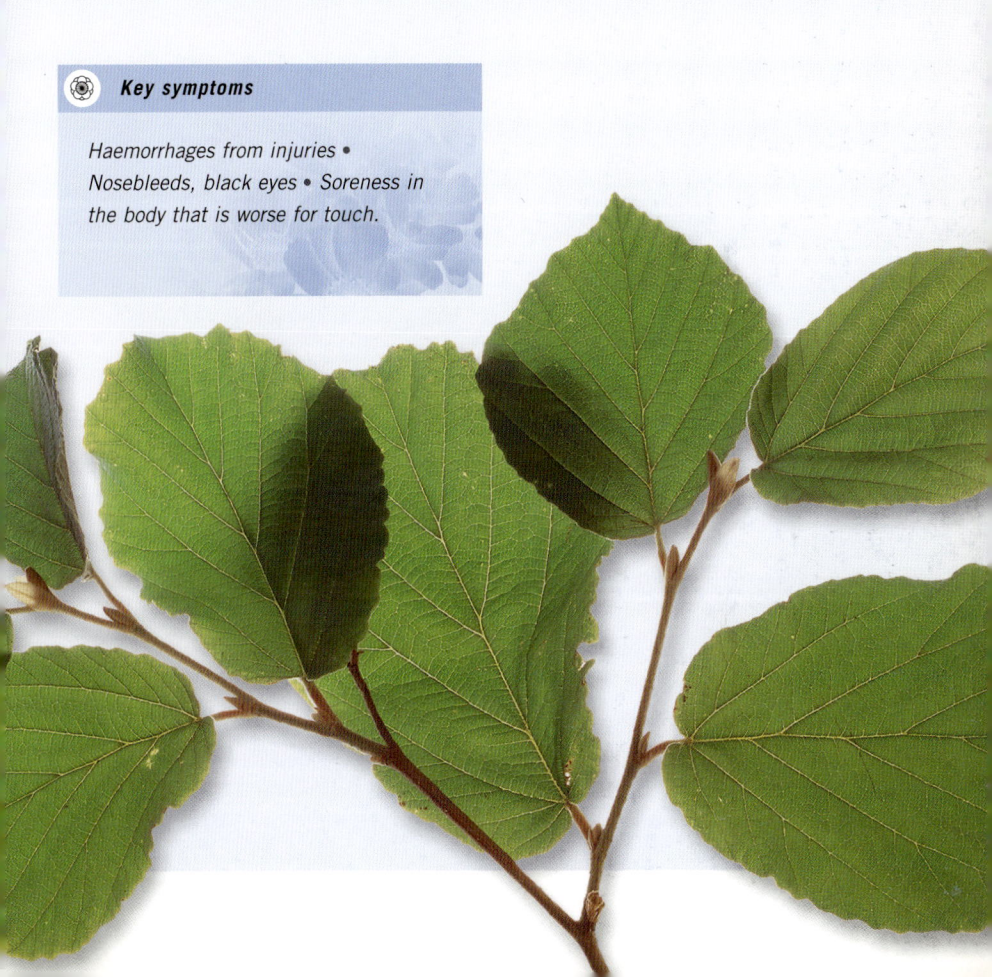

Haemorrhages from injuries • Nosebleeds, black eyes • Soreness in the body that is worse for touch.

HEPAR SULPHURICUM

(+FA, C-C-F, D, GR, M)
impure calcium sulphate

A remedy for skin eruptions, glandular swellings and mental anguish. Suited to chilly, hypersensitive people with splinter-like pains. The patient is worse for draughts.

Mind and emotions

The patient is anxious at night, is deeply depressed and will speak, eat and drink rapidly. The symptoms are intense. Pains create extreme emotional reactions with anger and violence. The patient feels vulnerable and insecure with a great need to be protected, finding solace in money, security, position and comfort. They are sensitive to emotional stress and deeply affected by sad stories.

Physical complaints

- There are stitching and stabbing pains, the scalp is sensitive and sore, and there are boring pains in the temple every morning.
- This is a remedy for ulceration of the cornea, and conjunctivitis with profuse discharge, where the eyes and lids are inflamed and the eyeballs are sore to the touch.
- Also suitable for discharges of pus, especially from the ear, with whizzing and throbbing and hardness of hearing.
- Also use for wet coughs with yellow mucus, and for sore throats with colds.

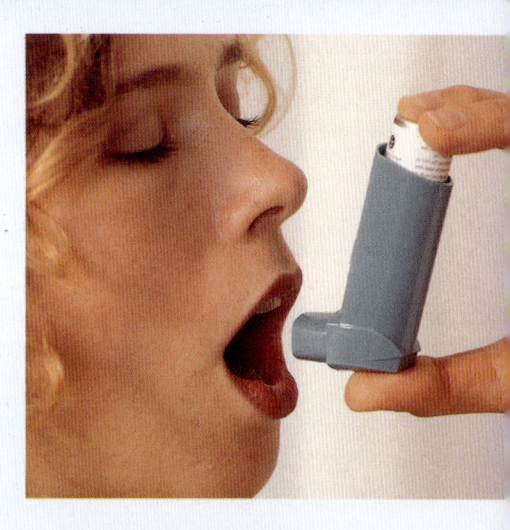

Where a patient suffers from asthma that is worse from dry, cold air, the remedy Hepar sulphuricum might be appropriate.

- Also for deafness caused by scarlet fever.
- There can be ulceration of the nose with sneezing in cold draughts.
- It is good remedy for hay fever.
- A key symptom is unhealthy skin where every injury festers; use for chapped skin, ulcers and cold sores.

Key symptoms

Pains cause irritability and anger • Unhealthy skin where every injury festers • Stabbing pains • Extreme sensitivity to pain; soreness to the touch • Patients are chilly, symptoms are worse for draughts.

- Consider this remedy for bleeding gums and quinsy (inflammation of the throat) with pus.
- Other symptoms include burning in the stomach and constipation.
- Female symptoms are spotting between periods; sensitive abscesses on the labia; profuse perspiration at menopause.
- Also for hoarseness and troublesome coughs, loss of voice from colds. It is used for anxious wheezing, croup and asthma that is worse from dry, cold air.
- Also use Hepar sulphuricum for abscesses on the skin and acne in young people.

General symptoms

Worse in dry, cold winds; the slightest draughts irritate. Heavy perspiration during a fever. The patient is better when wrapping their head up in a hat, from warmth, and improves after eating.

HYDRASTIS

(+FA, C-C-F, D, GR) golden seal plant

The remedy Hydrastis is important for drainage, especially useful after surgery and to accompany conventional medicine during cancer treatment. Used for goitre, smallpox and digestive problems.

Mind and emotions

The patient feels depressed, feeling that they wish to die or are going to die.

Physical complaints

- The symptoms are degenerative conditions, with weakness and emaciation.
- Patients may be suffering from cancer of the skin, breasts, cervix, uterus or liver – Hydrastis can be used as a suitable support therapy.
- It is also useful for liver problems caused by alcohol abuse.
- Other symptoms include chronic catarrhal problems with thick, yellow discharges from the nose, throat and lungs as well as purulent sinusitis, especially with post-nasal drip and a headache. There is often a large quantity of mucus, which might also be found elsewhere in the body – in the urinary tract and vagina.

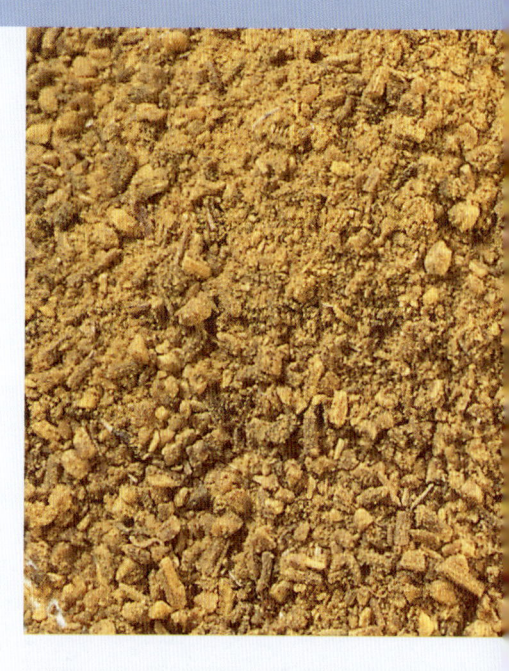

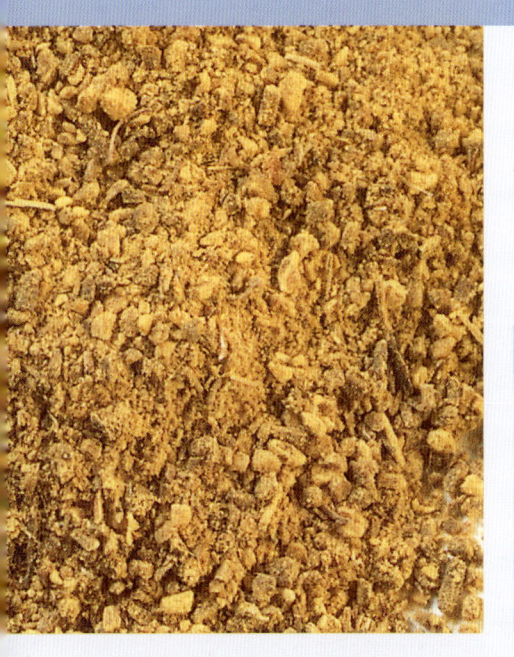

The golden seal plant, shown here dried, is a remedy for degenerative conditions where there is a thick, yellow discharge.

Key symptoms

Thick, yellow discharges • Constipation without urging • Degenerative conditions • Use for drainage after surgery or dentistry.

- The patient's digestion is slow and sluggish. There is constipation with no desire to pass a stool. Useful for children and old people who are constipated.
- Use also alongside conventional medicine for goitre during puberty and pregnancy.

General symptoms

Intolerance of bread or vegetables. Patient is weak and very thin.

HYOSCYAMUS NIGER

(M, CR, GR) henbane

The remedy Hyoscyamus niger is used for mental and nervous disorders.

Mind and emotions

The patient is jealous and suspicious, and may have delusions that they will be injured, poisoned or murdered, or that they are being watched. They also feel that others are favoured whereas they are not and that they are being deceived, cheated or tricked by the people around them. The patient also believes, unreasonably, that their partner is unfaithful, and they try obsessively to control everything around them.

Feeling like an outsider, the patient can be silent for hours, sitting and staring into space or, alternatively, very talkative, mocking, slandering and maligning others. Because the patient wants to harm those who create their pain, they can be violent in outbursts due to disappointed love.

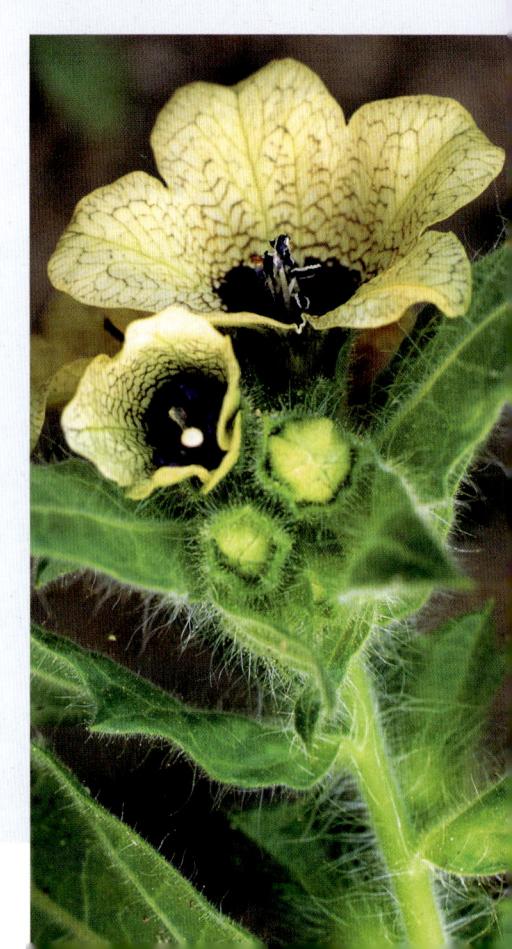

Hyoscyamus niger is used to treat nervous disorders in jealous and suspicious people.

There may be a strong sexual element of exhibitionism, with the patient sometimes acting defiantly. Hyoscyamus niger is also a remedy for children who use foul language and laugh foolishly or who feel shameful and have a strong aversion to exposing themselves by taking their clothes off.

Physical complaints
- The patient fumbles with their hands or wants to wring them constantly. They are worse for being touched.
- Hyoscyamus niger will benefit early masturbation in children.
- Can be used alongside conventional medicine for epilepsy that is preceded by ringing in the ears, restlessness or vertigo.
- Other symptoms include sleeplessness in irritable, excitable people, accompanied by spasms, twitching, and jerking, involuntary stool or urination after excitement.
- A dry, spasmodic cough that is worse for lying down.

General symptoms
The patient can experience a ravenous appetite before a seizure or catalepsy from jealousy. All convulsions begin in the face during grief.

Key symptoms

The patient is jealous and suspicious and has violent outbursts • They can also be either shameless or shameful about their body • Constantly moving their hands or wringing them; worse for being touched • Dry, spasmodic cough.

HYPERICUM PERFORATUM

(+FA, CR, GR) St John's wort plant

A major remedy for injury to the spine and nerve endings, such as the fingers and toes. To be used for the effects of shock and all injuries as an emergency remedy while waiting for medical treatment.

Key symptoms

Injuries to nerves • Shooting pains from injury • Head and spinal injuries • Injuries to toes, fingers or coccyx.

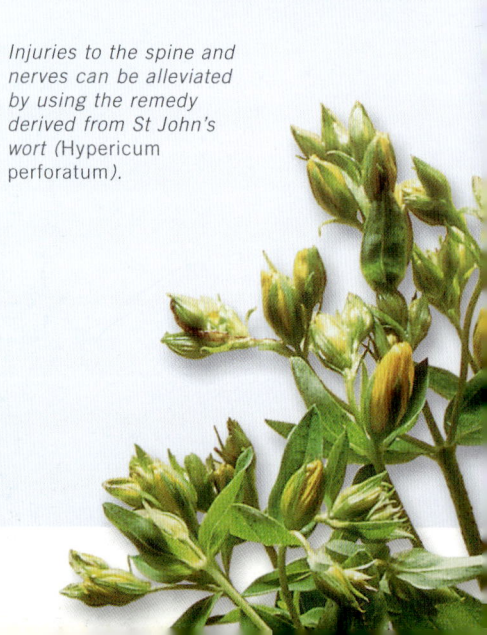

Mind and emotions

The patient feels as if they are floating and has anxiety with a fear of falling. They may make mistakes when writing.

Physical complaints

- To be used for injuries to all parts of the body that are rich in nerve endings, especially the fingers, toes and coccyx.
- Use also for injuries to the head or spine, for penetrating wounds, especially to the palms of the hands or the soles of the feet, where the patient feels pain shooting up the nerve.
- Use Hypericum perforatum as an emergency remedy after a penetrating

Injuries to the spine and nerves can be alleviated by using the remedy derived from St John's wort (Hypericum perforatum).

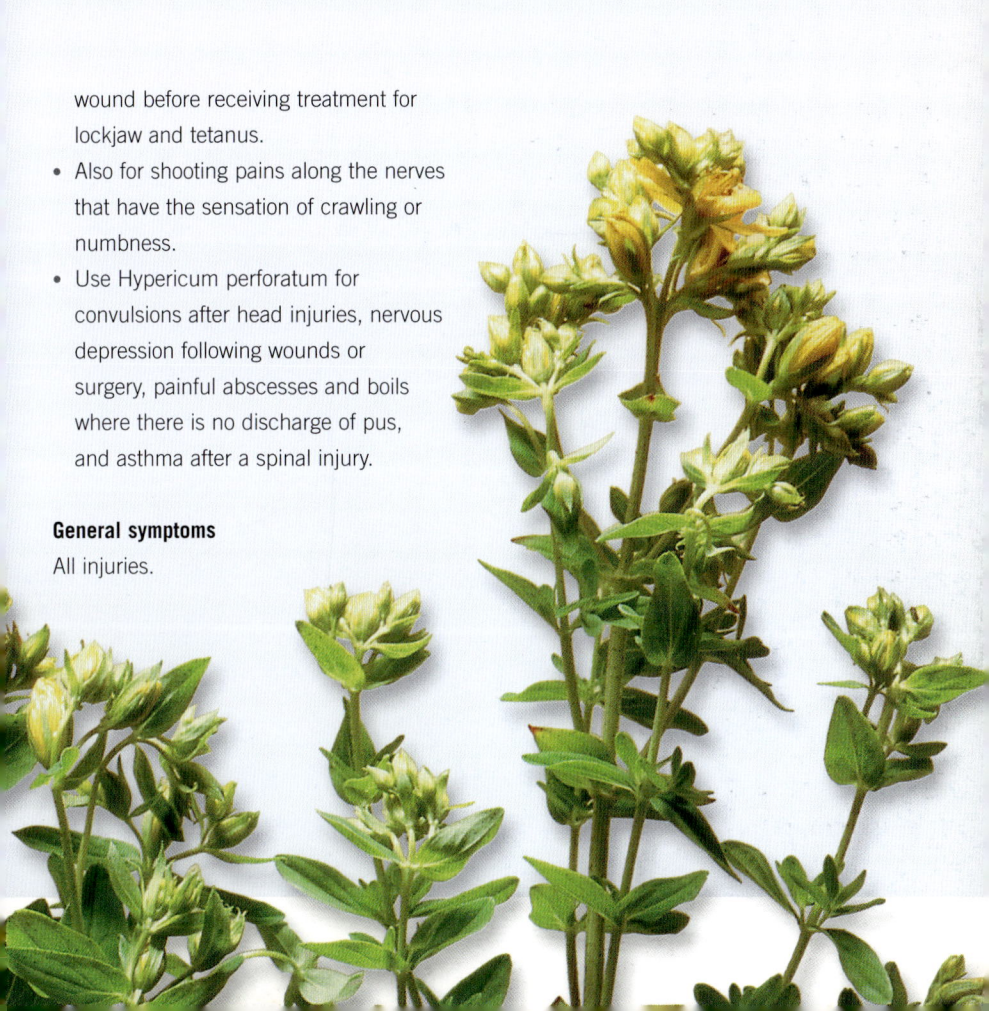

wound before receiving treatment for lockjaw and tetanus.
- Also for shooting pains along the nerves that have the sensation of crawling or numbness.
- Use Hypericum perforatum for convulsions after head injuries, nervous depression following wounds or surgery, painful abscesses and boils where there is no discharge of pus, and asthma after a spinal injury.

General symptoms
All injuries.

IGNATIA

(+FA, C-C-F, GR, M) St Ignatius bean*

A major remedy for grief, Ignatia is also used whenever the structure of a person's life breaks down, emotionally or physically. It is excellent for back injury, a croup-like cough accompanied by fright and for a sore throat caused by grief.

Mind and emotions

A remedy for all the ailments that relate to silent grief: bad news, disappointed love and disappointments of all kinds, as well as for fright, reproaches and shame. The patient has high ideals and expectations, with a strong drive to make them true, and they expect others to be perfect. They have a strong sense of duty; women who benefit from Ignatia may be very competent working in a man's world.

Patients can suffer from self-reproach and inner conflicts where they believe they have neglected their duty, or have done wrong or committed a crime. After disappointment or grief the patient may develop ailments that arise through contradictions: wanting one thing but choosing another. The patient might have emotional, even hysterical, outbursts but controls them too quickly, with short sobs, a few tears and swallowing to hide their feelings. It is also suitable for

The powdered bean of Ignatia is the source of a useful remedy to ease illnesses caused by grief and disappointment.

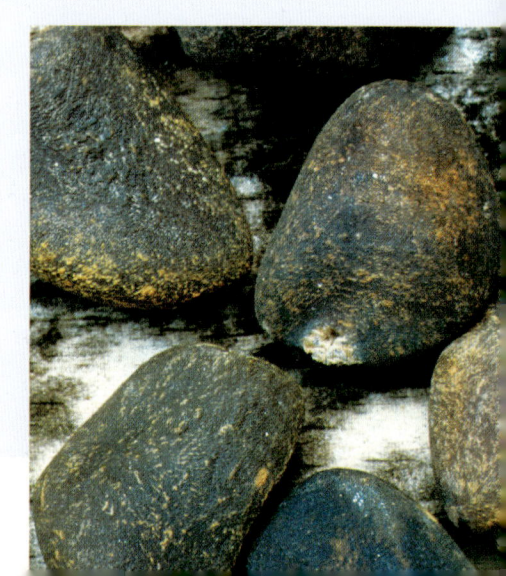

people who eat to comfort their stress and have a sinking feeling in the pit of their stomach that is relieved by eating food. Conversely, the Ignatia character may have an aversion to food.

Physical complaints
- The patient has a strong loathing of tobacco smoke. They often experience a sensation of a lump in their throat.

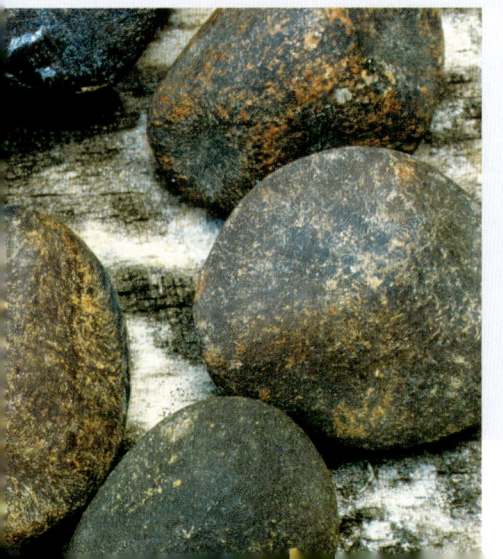

> **Key symptoms**
>
> *Grief, inner conflict, disappointment • Brooding • Dislike of tobacco smoke.*

- They can suffer from backaches when the structure of their life breaks down after a loss, shock or disappointment.
- They can develop a nervous twitch or a dry, constant cough, as if they have dust in their throat.

General symptoms
The patient can experience pains in small areas. Sleeplessness, nausea and faintness. They can have an aversion to fresh air and are better when close to a source of warmth. They may also be better for physical exertion, such as running or walking fast.

IODUM

(M, C-C-F, GR) iodine

This is a remedy for degenerating glands, emaciation and breakdown of a person's general health. Iodum arouses the body's natural defences and kick-starts immunity.

Mind and emotions

The patient will be anxious when they are quiet. They can be forgetful and often disorganized, but try to stay busy. They may have bad thoughts and be very depressed. Having a fear of people the Iodum patient is inclined to shun society, and can also have a strong impulse to be violent, so they prefer to be busy and keep in constant motion until they are exhausted. They tend to suffer from restlessness that can become intolerable and can be very discontented.

Physical complaints

- The patient suffers from weakness that is worse from hunger.

Key symptoms

Patient can suffer extreme restlessness and prefers to be busy • Swollen glands.

- Also swollen glands followed by degeneration of the thyroid, ovaries, breasts, uterus, prostate, lymph or tonsils.
- Other symptoms include pains with constricting sensations, bone pains, constipation, croup caused by damp weather, an external goitre that is painful.

General symptoms

Lead poisoning and swollen testicles – use Iodum as an emergency remedy while waiting for medical treatment.

A person who is restless and prefers to be alone might benefit from Iodum.

iodum 177

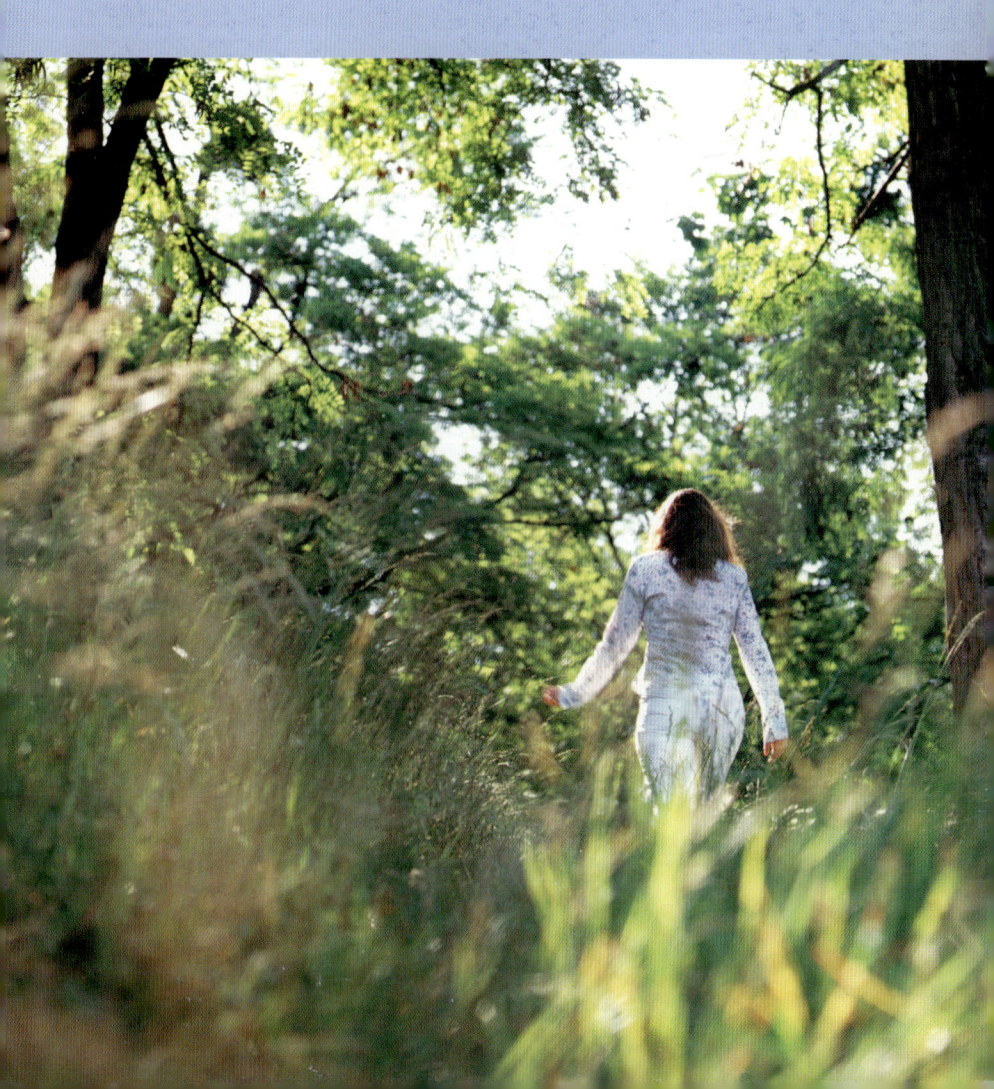

IPECACUANHA (IPECAC)

(C-C-F, D) root of ipecac plant

A remedy for nausea, vomiting and pain; also used as an emergency remedy to stop bleeding.

Mind and emotions

The patient is difficult to please. They are irritable and hold everything in contempt. They have a sense of longing, but they are not sure what for.

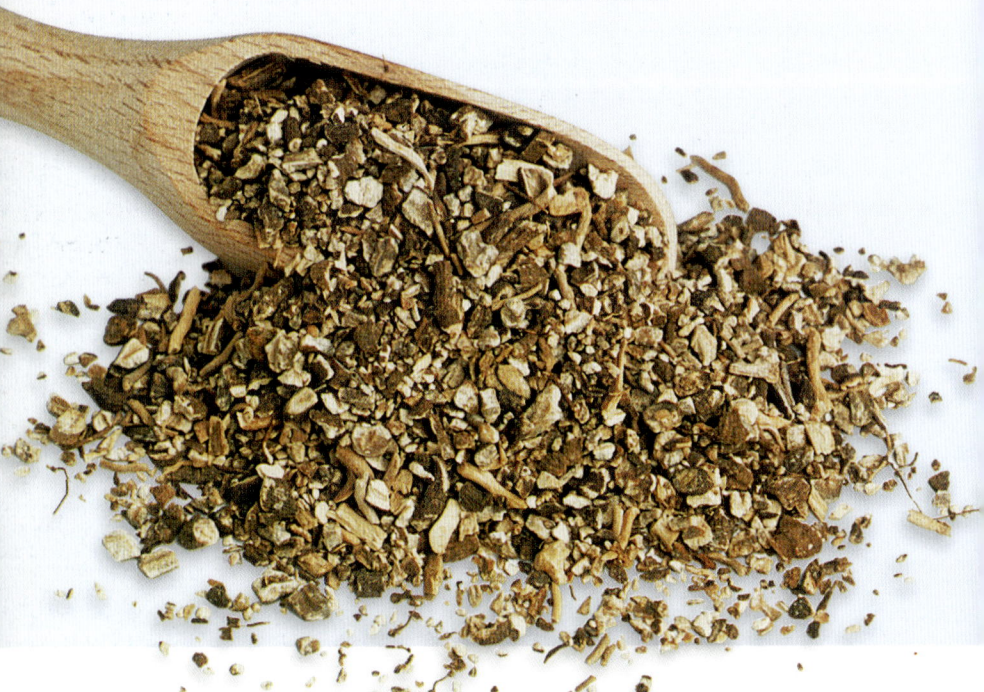

Physical complaints

- A remedy for stomach and gastrointestinal tract ailments with nausea.
- Also use this remedy for respiratory ailments such as asthma that are accompanied by nausea.
- Ipecac is a remedy to accompany conventional medical treatment for uterine haemorrhage with bright red blood accompanied by nausea.
- To be used for convulsions from indigestion, bronchitis or asthma with a suffocating cough accompanied by retching and vomiting.
- Ipecac is also for nausea, vomiting in pregnancy and a support remedy in the treatment of dysentery.

The powdered dried root of Ipecac makes a treatment for nausea as well as an emergency remedy to slow bleeding.

Key symptoms

Patient is irritable • Nausea accompanied by other ailments • Lack of thirst • Asthma.

General symptoms

Summer heat aggravates the symptoms. Nausea and faintness in warm rooms. Patient has no thirst. Symptoms are worse for any kind of movement.

IRIS VERSICOLOR

(GR, D) blue flag iris plant

This is a remedy for headache and indigestion. It increases the flow of bile.

Mind and emotions
Iris versicolor is suited to delicate and nervous people.

Physical complaints
The patient can feel bilious, with sour or acrid vomiting, and will have burning feelings that accompany a headache.
- This is a remedy for headache with visual disturbances. To be used for migraine headache with vomiting and copious urination after a headache.
- Saliva from the mouth is profuse. It may be thick and drip.
- An excellent remedy for indigestion accompanied by headache.

Key symptoms

Headaches with vomiting and bile • Patient craves sweets, but these make the symptoms worse • Profuse saliva that drips • Burning feelings along the digestive tract.

General symptoms
People who get overly tired, and who feel a headache coming on when they are run down. This is usually accompanied by nausea, vomiting and eye disturbances. The patient may develop pain in the pancreas (which is located behind the stomach) and be sensitive to sugar, which they indulge in when they are tired.

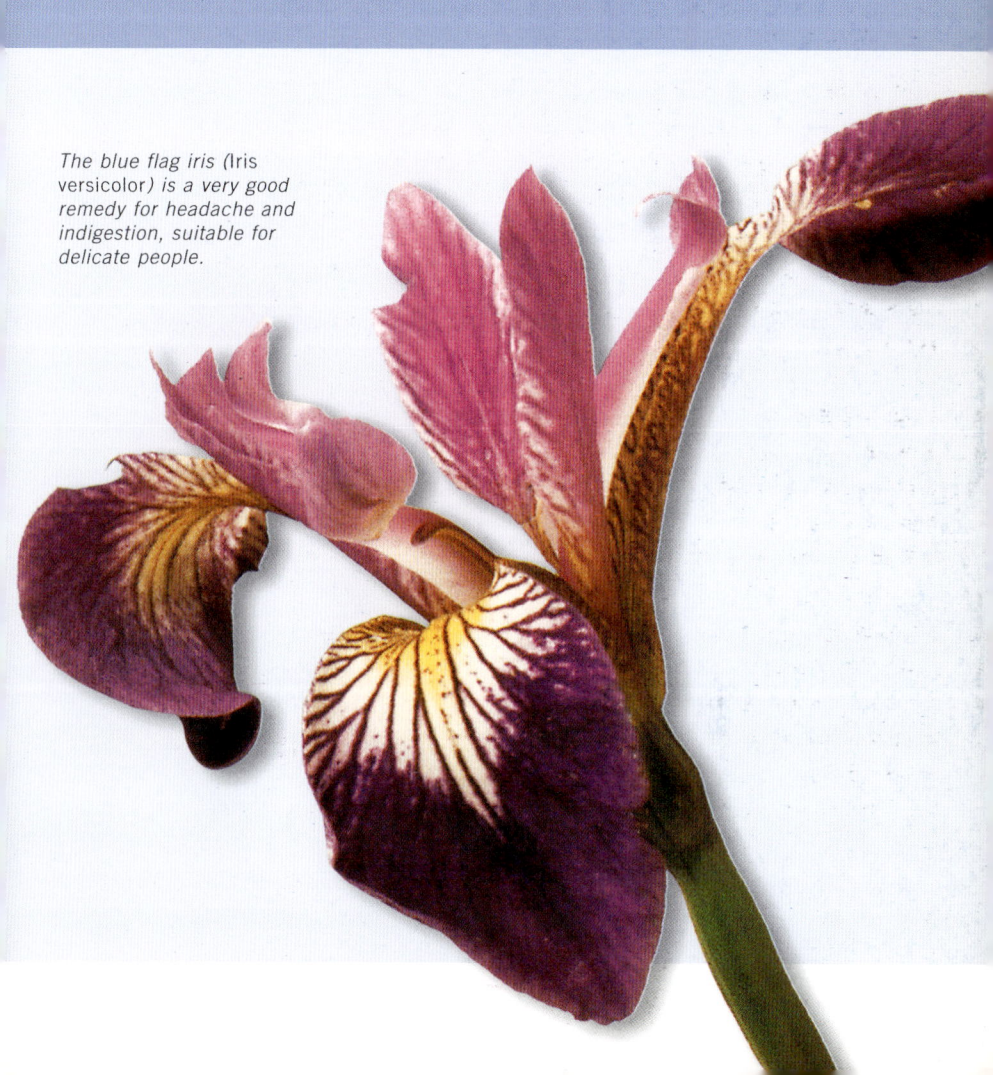

The blue flag iris (Iris versicolor) is a very good remedy for headache and indigestion, suitable for delicate people.

KALI BICHROMICUM

(C-C-F, D, F, GR, M) potassium bichromate, bichromate of potash

A remedy for pain, congestion and digestion.

Mind and emotions

The patient is very consistent and rule abiding. They can be narrow-minded and have an aversion to getting into trouble. They will also be someone who is self-occupied and who likes to be with the family.

Physical complaints

- The patient experiences thick, stringy, yellow and white discharges.
- Kali bichromicum is a useful remedy for colds with congested mucus.
- It is also used for pains that shoot rapidly from one part of the body to another, such as rheumatism that appears every day at the same hour.
- Also appropriate for migraine where there are pains in small spots, preceded by

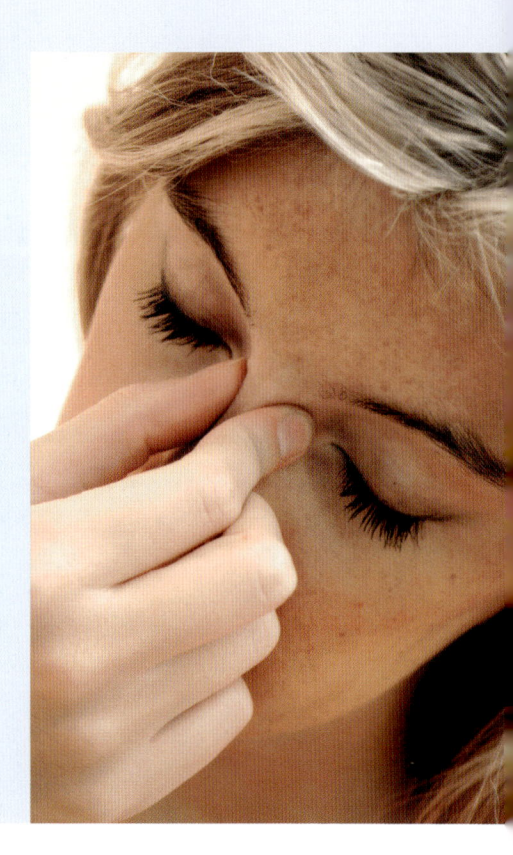

visual disturbances, such as blurred vision and blindness.
- This is also an important remedy for sinusitis where there is pressure and fullness at the top of the nose, accompanied by stringy yellow discharge when acute; it can be used for colds that move into the sinuses.
- Good also for rheumatic disturbances that alternate with digestive disorders.

General symptoms
Diarrhoea that occurs in warm weather; skin eruptions in summer; serious burns.

> ### Key symptoms
>
> The patient is a conformist who is rule abiding • Thick, stringy, yellow and white discharges • Skin and rheumatic problems that are worse in summer • Respiratory and digestive problems that are worse in the spring and autumn.

The remedy Kali bichromicum is useful for relieving sinusitis, especially in people who are rule abiding and conformists.

KALI CARBONICUM

(C-C-F, CB, D, GR, M)
potassium carbonate

This is a remedy for backaches, headaches and mental conditions.

Mind and emotions

The characteristic portrait of this remedy is a person whose mind rules their emotions. They tend to be conservative, regular, proper, down-to-earth people with a strong emphasis on morality. They fear losing control, and can be dogmatic with a strong sense of duty. People who are suited to Kali carbonicum experience their emotions, such as fear and fright, in the stomach and stomach area of the abdomen. They can make life difficult for those around them who have a will of their own. During menstrual periods women can experience emotional instability with strong mood swings. Good for those who develop symptoms such as headaches and lower backache from working too hard for too long.

Key symptoms

Backaches, especially in the lumbar region after childbirth or abortion • Sharp and cutting pains • Symptoms are worse between 2.00 and 4.00 a.m.

Physical complaints

- The patient craves sweets.
- They can have flatulence and stitching pains in the area around the liver.
- They perspire easily with little exertion.
- They can be exhausted from coughing.
- A keynote symptom is backache in the lumbar region that is worse after childbirth and abortion. All the patient's emotions affect the small of their back, and so their pains originate in the lower back.

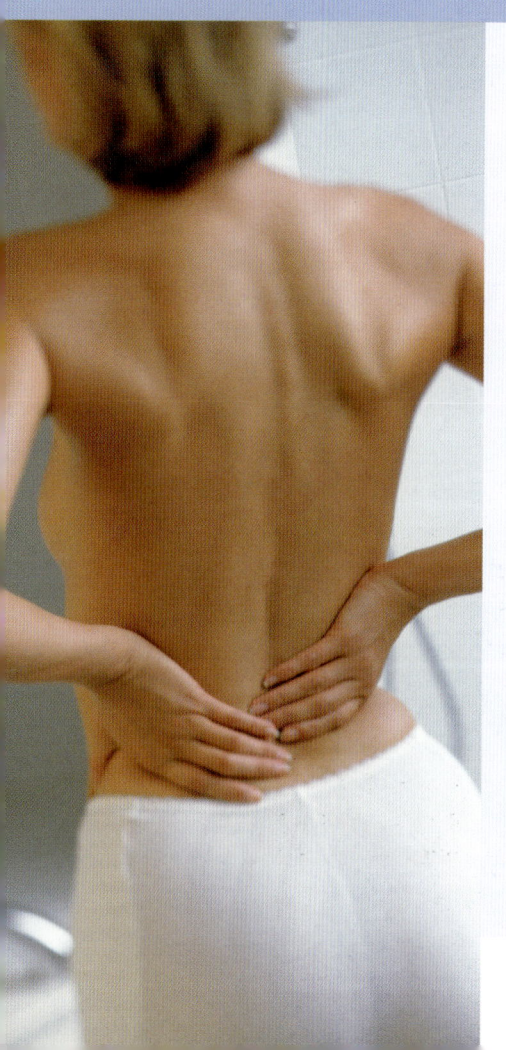

Consider Kali carbonicum for backache.

- During childbirth it appears that labour is delayed because of violent backache.
- Patient suffers from palpitations and burning in the heart region.
- They can have a weak, rapid pulse owing to digestive disturbances.
- Other symptoms are swollen upper eyelids, coughing with breathing difficulties; recurrent colic.
- Symptoms are worse between 2.00 and 4.00 a.m.

General symptoms

A soft pulse that can hardly be felt, coldness, general depression and stitching pains felt in all parts of the body. All pains are sharp and cutting. The patient is sensitive to any atmospheric change.

KALI MURIATICUM

(C-C-F, D, GR) potassium chloride

This is a remedy for excess catarrh, subacute inflammations and glandular swellings.

Mind and emotions
The patient is exhausted and tired of taking care of others. They have done too much mothering of others and feel deprived of attention and affection.

Physical complaints
- Sticky, white, thick secretions from the ears, nose, base of tongue, the vagina, and from lumps on the tonsils; also coughing with phlegm.
- There are tough, fibrous discharges and hard swellings.
- Other symptoms include coughs that affect the eyes (which feel as if they are protruding from the head), skin eruptions after vaccination, deafness from swelling of the Eustachian tubes (which are worse

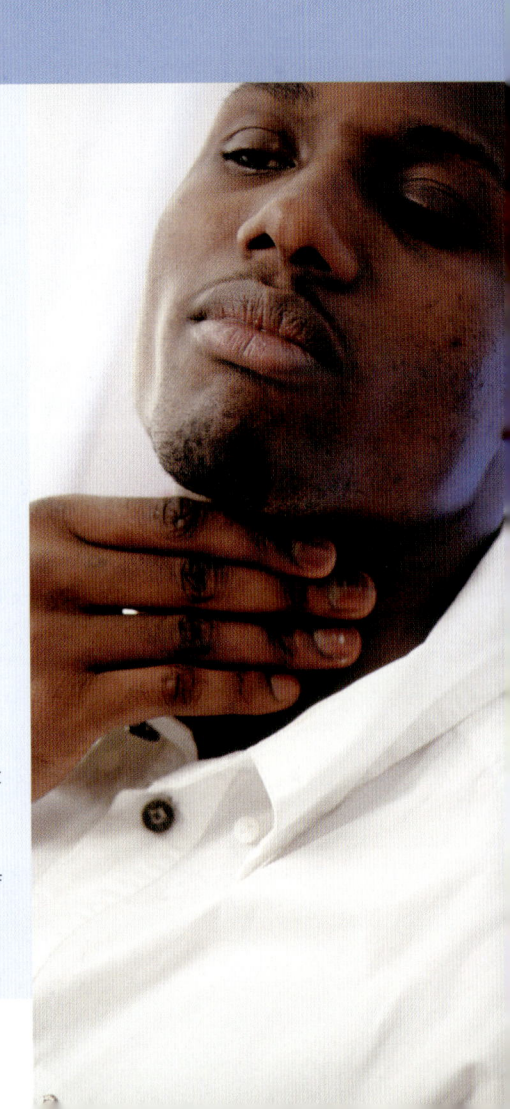

kali muriaticum

Kali muriaticum is a treatment for swollen glands and tonsillitis, especially suited to someone who is exhausted.

after flying), swollen glands, glue ear, tonsillitis when the patient can swallow only by twisting the neck, and asthma with gastric symptoms.
- Especially suitable for eczema and other skin diseases, such as warts.
- Useful for rheumatic fever with swelling around the joints, nightly rheumatic pains that are worse from the warmth of the bed and bursitis (inflammation of the sac-like cavity in a joint). Acute symptoms should be referred to a doctor immediately.

Key symptoms

The patient is exhausted from taking care of others (remedy is especially suitable for mothers) • White, sticky discharges • Painful ear problems that are worse for flying • Tonsillitis.

General symptoms

A remedy for loss of voice and inflamed tonsils. Mouth ulcers in the mouth also respond to Kali muriaticum.

KALI PHOSPHORICUM

(CB, C-C-F, F, GR, M, Ma)
potassium phosphate

A remedy for exhaustion, nervous disorders, weakness and fatigue, Kali phosphoricum is also useful when a person wastes away, usually from grief.

Mind and emotions

The remedy is appropriate for times of excitement, overwork and worry. The main mental symptoms are anxiety, nervous dread, exhaustion and fatigue. The patient does not like to meet people and feels very weary and depressed. They are shy and disinclined to talk and socialize. This is a remedy for nervous people who startle easily, for those who are suffering from brain tiredness due to overwork and study, for loss of memory, and despair about business concerns. This is also a remedy suitable for use in the treatment of grief, where the patient shows signs of feeling drained and exhausted.

Physical complaints

- Conditions arising from a lack of nervous energy, causing the patient to be languid without the energy to do the things that they need to, as well as mental and physical depression.
- Where there are suspected malignant tumours this remedy can support conventional medicine. It can also help healing after the removal of a cancer when the skin has become tight over the wound.
- Kali phosphoricum is good for speeding up a delayed labour in childbirth and boosting the mother's energy during a long and difficult labour.
- The patient might have a bitter taste in the mouth in the morning and a loss of appetite.
- Other symptoms include headache with a weary, empty feeling and spongy, receding gums.

kali phoricum

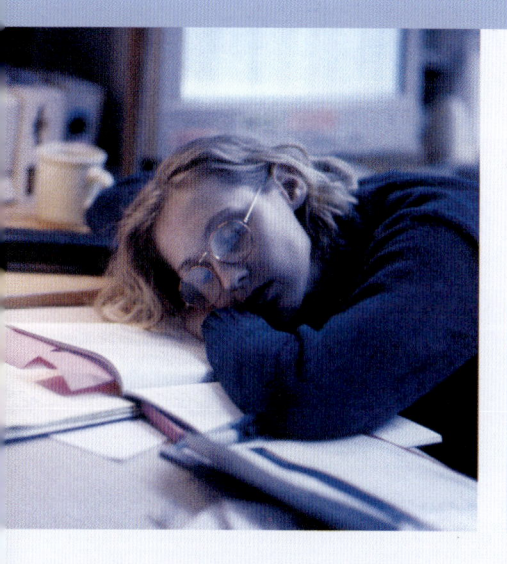

Prescribe Kali phosphoricum for a patient who is exhausted because of overwork and feels weakened by fatigue.

Key symptoms

Mental and physical exhaustion, such as in a delayed labour • Symptoms are better for gentle motion.

- Use for men who experience impotence or the lack of desire and for women where sexual desire increases after their periods.
- Patients have a tendency to perspire, especially after meals or from excitement. Their body odour smells like onions. The patient cannot keep their feet still, and there is weakness and pain centred on the seventh cervical vertebra.

General symptoms
Better for gentle motion. Weakness from pain.

KALI SULPHURICUM

(GR, M) potassium sulphate

A remedy for profuse yellow discharges and complaints caused by cold hands and feet.

Mind and emotions
The patient is lazy and indolent, worse in warm weather and a warm room, and always complains about being tired. They like fresh air and are impatient, and are worse for any form of consolation. They are self-absorbed and worried about themselves, and also feel sorry for themselves.

Physical complaints
- This remedy treats profuse yellow discharges and wandering arthritic pains.
- It is a remedy for cold hands and feet. Kali sulphuricum warms the blood and raises the body temperature.

Key symptoms

The patient is lazy and worse for warm weather or a warm room • Profuse yellow discharges • Wandering arthritic pains • Complaints caused by cold hands and feet.

General symptoms
Coarse, dry, itchy skin, sometimes with a rash. Symptoms occur in people who are generally warm and who dislike warm rooms or other forms of heat. They also tend to perspire a great deal, especially in the middle of the night. and are extremely thirsty with a strong craving for sweets.

Cold hands and feet can cause other complaints, which can be treated with Kali sulphuricum.

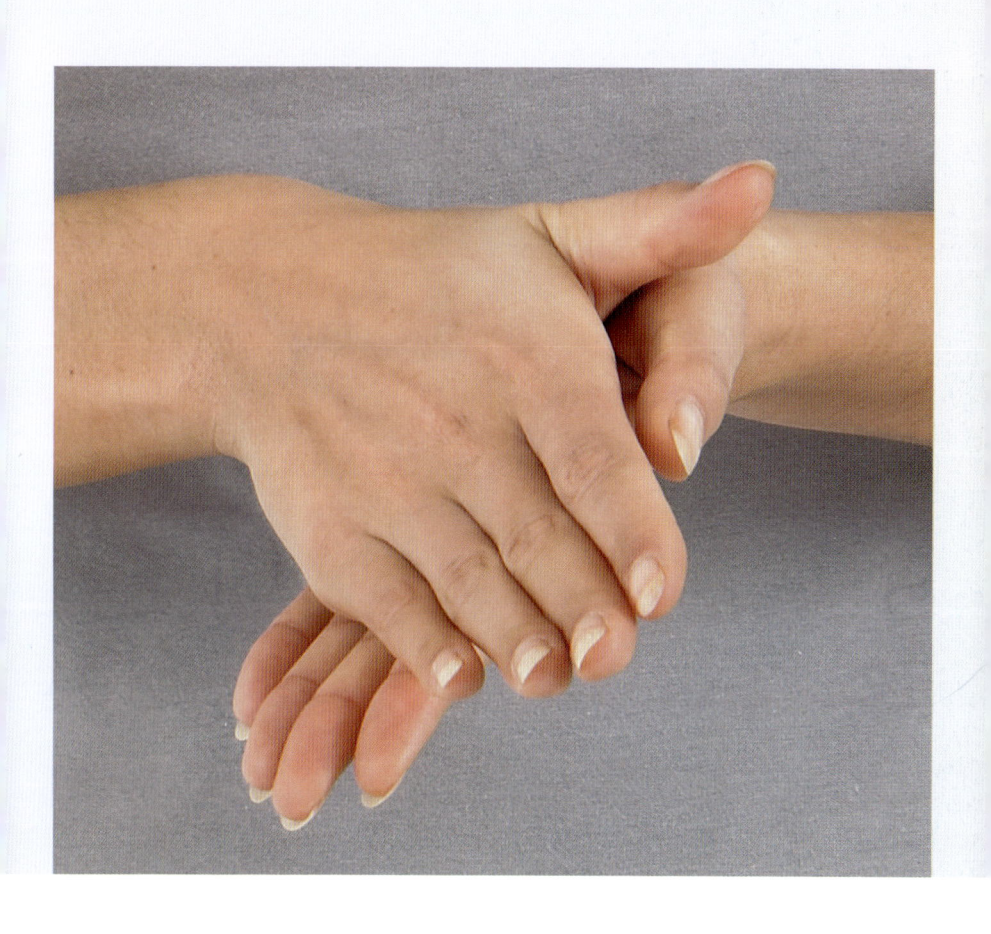

kali sulphuricum

KREOSOTUM

(CR, F, GR, M) beechwood creosote

This is a remedy for anxiety, bedwetting in children and female difficulties. It can also be used in conjunction with conventional medicine to help cancer.

Mind and emotions
The patient has many fears – of sex, rape and all types of interactions with other people. Children are generally irritable, continually asking for things but then throwing them away.

Physical complaints
- A remedy for female problems connected to menstruation.
- The patient may become overexcited and restless.

Women who suffer with headaches, problems connected to menstruation, and abdominal pains might benefit from taking Kreosotum.

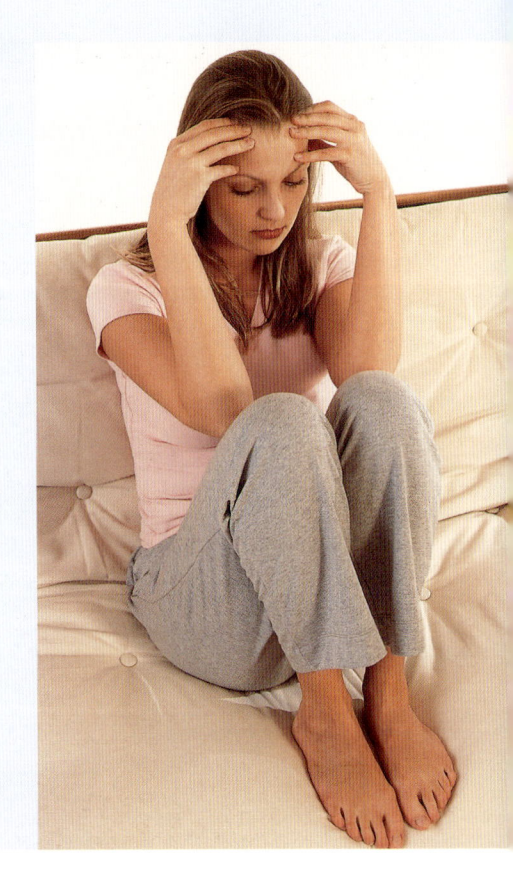

- Common symptoms are headaches and impaired hearing, accompanied by vomiting, abdominal pains, diarrhoea and constant chills.
- Women will also have itching of the vulva and labia. The burning sensation of the labia with inflammation is so intense that it creates rawness and swelling.
- Other symptoms include hot, often foul-smelling discharges.
- This is also used for boys who grow too fast, children who are too tall for their age, and for problems with growing teeth where the gums are painful and swollen and the teeth decay easily. Also for toothache.
- Kreosotum is also a remedy for bedwetting where it is difficult to wake the child.

General symptoms
Wounds bleed freely.

> **Key symptoms**
>
> *The patient avoids and fears sex as well as intimate contact • They are chilly • Menstrual problems • Bad-smelling discharges • Children have problems with growing teeth, also bedwetting.*

LAC CANINUM

(C-C-F, F, GR, M) female dog's milk

This is a remedy for low self-confidence and self-hatred. It is excellent for sore throats and many female problems.

Mind and emotions

For people who have had a difficult childhood, separated from their mothers for periods of time, or who experienced conflicts with their mothers; also for those who stopped breastfeeding too soon, and for any time the mother–child relationship has been disturbed in any way. These problems result in a lack of confidence and a feeling of abandonment, accompanied by low self-esteem and even self-hatred. Especially for young women who suffer from self-loathing and have a disgust for their bodies. The patient feels dirty, and as if they are falling to pieces. They also have a a fear of failure. They are full of fears, hypersensitive and hysterical, as well as forgetful and aggressive.

Physical complaints

- A painful, swollen throat that extends to the ears, and where the symptoms change from one side to the other accompanied by a stiffness of the neck and tongue.
- Menstrual problems include periods that are too early or too frequent, or a heavy flow.
- Breasts that are swollen and painful; mastitis. This remedy can dry up breast milk, so this is suitable for mothers who are bottle-feeding their baby.
- It is also used for sciatica on the right side, where the legs feel numb and stiff and there are cramps in the feet.

General symptoms

Dreams of snakes. Symptoms are better for cold drinks. Glands swell during menstrual periods. The patient desires pungent foods and salt and experiences a sensation as if they are floating.

lac caninum

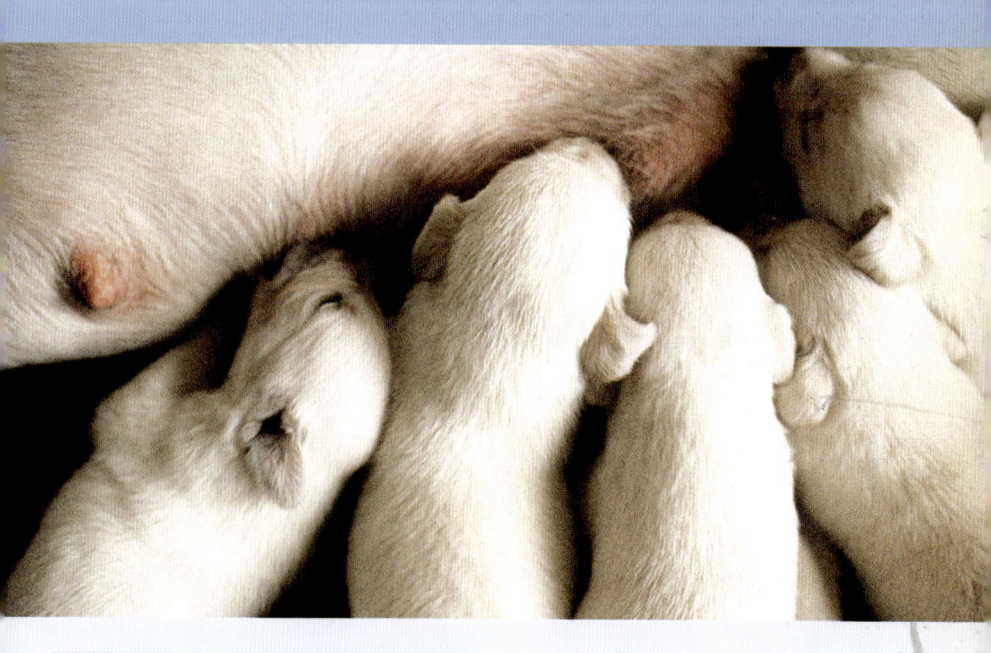

Key symptoms

The patient suffers from low self-confidence and self-hatred • Sore throat that changes from one side to the other • Desire for salt and pungent foods.

The potentized milk of a female dog creates a remedy for people who suffer from low self-confidence.

LACHESIS

(C-C-F, F, GR, M) bushmaster snake

A remedy for jealousy and intense passion.

Mind and emotions
The patient's mind is overactive, they are continually talkative and their conversation jumps from one subject to another. They never listen to others and are bombastic, exaggerated and rambling. The patient will be jealous and suffer ailments that are caused by disappointment in love. They might be very highly sexed or their passions might be transferred to the moral–spiritual plane where they have high moral standards and strong spiritual drives. This is a remedy for people who are passionately over-religious.

People who might benefit from Lachesis are restless and often have difficulty concentrating on their work.

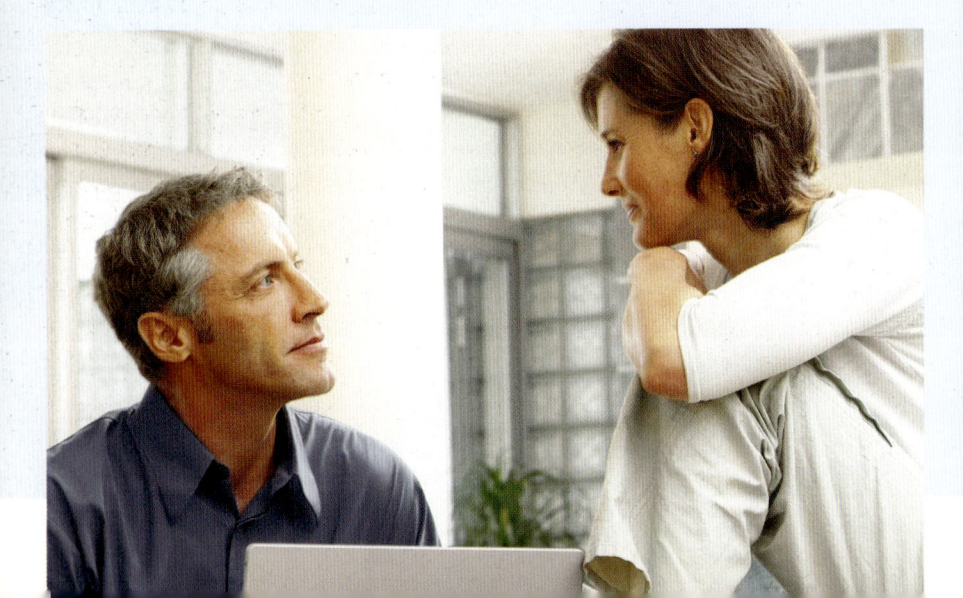

Other symptoms include sadness in the morning and dislike of mixing with others. The patient is restless and loves to travel. They find it difficult to attend to business, although they love mental work late at night and have a vivid imagination. Symptoms are worse on waking.

Physical complaints
- Circulatory problems, with purplish discolouration of skin.
- A sore throat that is worse for wearing tight clothing around the neck or waist, septic throat and a feeling that something is swollen in the throat and can't be swallowed.
- There might also be a sensation of suffocation and strangulation when lying down, a dry fitful cough and heart palpitations with fainting spells that occur especially during the menopause.
- Good for many menopausal symptoms.

Key symptoms

The patient has an overactive mind. Continually talkative and inclined to be jealous • Illnesses are felt on the left side of the body • Sore throat • Menopausal symptoms • Symptoms are worse after sleeping.

General symptoms
The patient awakes unrefreshed and often with a headache. Symptoms are better for losing a lot of fluid during their menstrual period. Complaints are generally felt on the left side of the body.

LEDUM PALUSTRE

(M, +FA, GR) marsh tea plant

The remedy Ledum palustre is appropriate for puncture wounds, bites, stings and a black eye.

Mind and emotions

The patient is a loner who likes seclusion and the female Ledum palustre character will dread men – they can appear to be misanthropic and hateful. It is a good remedy for constitutions that are broken down from taking drugs and too much alcohol; the patient craves whisky.

Physical complaints

- A remedy for eye injuries, stings and bites.
- This is a first-aid remedy for all puncture wounds. Use Ledum palustre as an emergency remedy for tetanus where there is twitching near the wound, before receiving medical treatment.
- Good for back and spine injuries, stiffness on waking or rising from a seat, and for all forms of rheumatism, particularly when it starts in the feet and rises upward.
- Patient is chilly, lacks vitality and warmth.
- Other symptoms include anal cracks, bleeding haemorrhoids (piles), cramps, gouty pains and swelling pains in the joints.

General symptoms

Cold, but finds heat intolerable.

> **Key symptoms**
>
> *The patient is a loner • Rheumatism and gout • Puncture wounds.*

The marsh tea plant makes a remedy for puncture wounds and rheumatism, especially for those who prefer to be alone.

ledum palustre 199

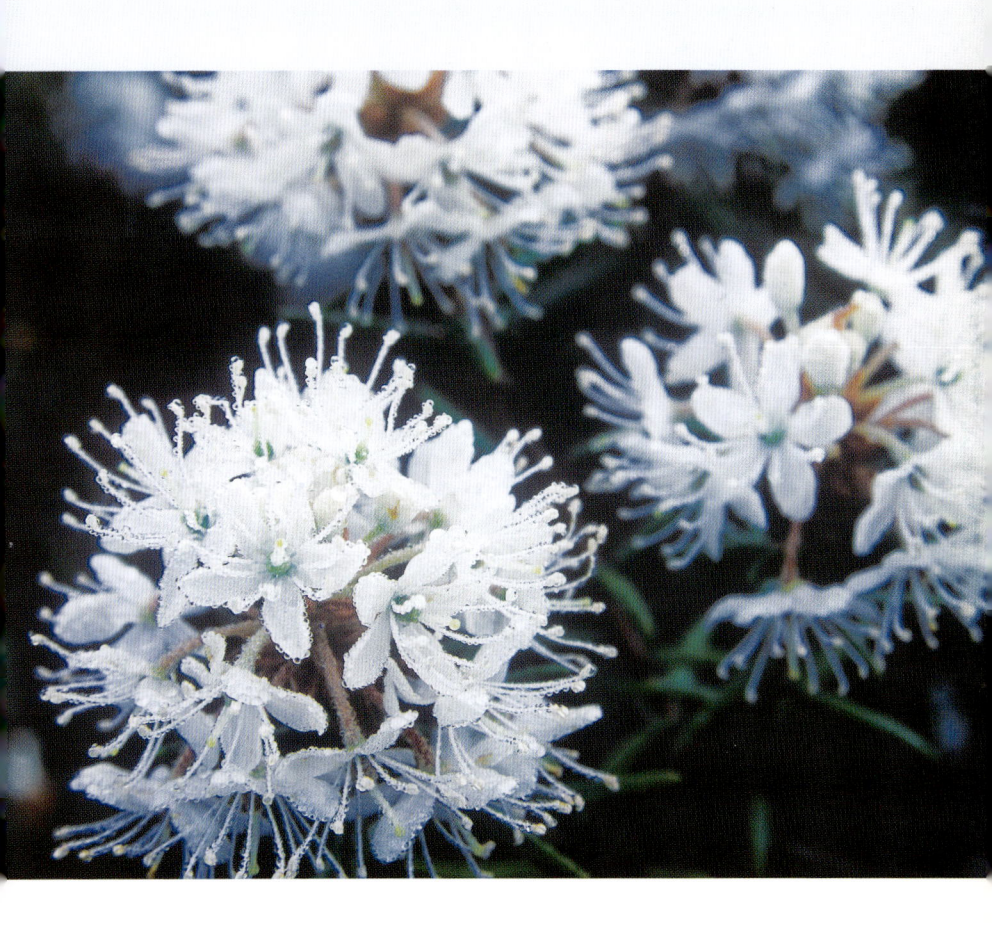

LYCOPODIUM

(D, F, GR, M) club moss plant

This remedy assists the body to absorb and digest nutrients and it works on the liver, gallbladder and digestive tract. Lycopodium is useful to treat infected styes, body lice and impetigo and is good for mental conditions such as fear and a lack of confidence.

Mind and emotions

The patient is extremely lacking in confidence. They also dislike new things and can appear sophisticated and haughty. They can also be dictatorial and presumptuous; although pleasant while in company they can be a tyrant when at home. They also suffer from an inflated ego. The patient is irritable on waking, shuns responsibilities, is afraid to be alone and is melancholy. They fear that stress will cause them to break down. Known as 'the teacher's remedy', it can be useful when timidity and fear block a patient's ability to express themselves personally.

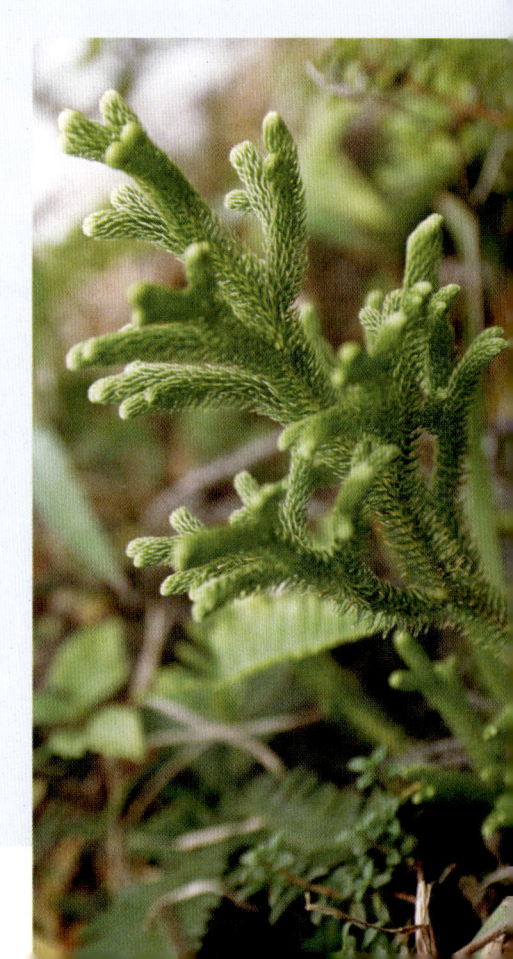

The club moss plant makes a remedy for scabies, impetigo and itching in those who lack confidence but can appear haughty.

Physical complaints

- The patient is easily satisfied with food and becomes bloated after eating, often accompanied by flatulence; all food gives them gas. They might also be constipated.
- They have a strong mind but a weak body.
- Other symptoms include pain in the right ovary, bearing-down pains in the uterus when bending over, anxiety felt in the stomach, depression with a menstrual period, cystitis, coldness in one foot while the other is hot, early greying of hair and premature ageing.
- Good for feeilngs of pressure on the bladder, where the patient has an urge to urinate, often at night.
- Lycopodium is a remedy that supports the liver and tonifies the gallbladder.

Key symptoms

The patient lacks confidence • Gastro-intestinal problems with flatulence • Desires sweets and hot food • Symptoms are worse between 3.00 and 4.00 a.m. and between 4.00 and 8.00 p.m.

General symptoms

Scabies with unbearable itching. The patient always feels better after midnight. Although chilly, the patient has a strong craving for fresh air; they are sensitive to draughts, worse in a warm room but better in a warm bed; full of gas with an inflated feeling, which is worse for flatulent foods; desires sweets and hot food; worse between 3.00 and 4.00 a.m. and between 4.00 and 8.00 p.m.; a keen intellect but with weak muscular power.

MAGNESIA CARBONICA

(CR, D, F, M) magnesium carbonate

This is a remedy for those who feel forsaken and unloved – it is often referred to as the 'orphan's remedy'. It is appropriate for both children and adults.

Mind and emotions
The patient feels neglected; it is a remedy for those who witnessed fights and quarrels between their parents, and for children of divorced parents. It is also a remedy to give to someone who has been deceived by a friend.

Other symptoms include despair from pains, disgust with everything, kleptomania, children who are behind in their work at school, and for problems with writing and reading. Use Magnesia carbonica for people

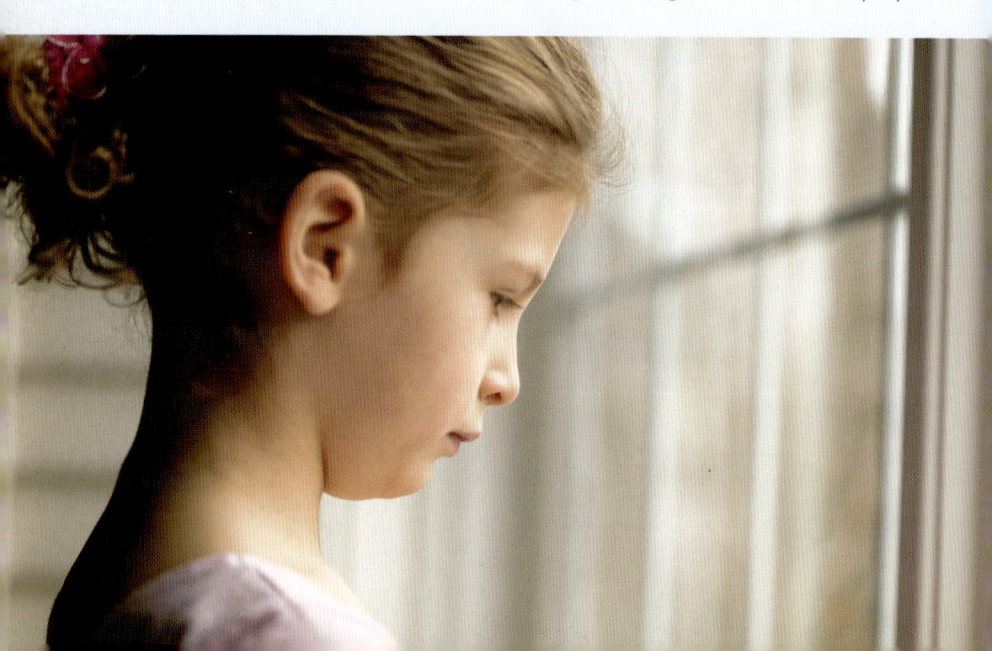

Key symptoms

Patient feels neglected, abandoned and deserted • Sour temper with a sour taste in the mouth and sour-smelling perspiration • Whole body feels exhausted and painful • Symptoms improve when walking in the fresh air.

who are sensitive to conflict – they are the natural peacemakers whose world feels threatened. Also for people who are insecure, which can lead to hyperactivity, especially in children, and for problem children who are bad-tempered and oversensitive.

Consider Magenesia carbonica (often called the 'orphan's remedy') to treat someone who feels neglected, forsaken and unloved.

Physical complaints

- Nervous exhaustion is relieved by Magnesia carbonica.
- All the patient's pains are at night when they are restless. They therefore feel worse when they wake tired and unrefreshed.
- They have a sour temper, a sour taste in the mouth, sour-smelling perspiration and sour secretions.
- Other symptoms include greenish diarrhoea with cramps which force the patient to double over; vomiting, bloating of the stomach, sores and back pains that feel as if the back is broken.

General symptoms

Walking in the fresh air makes them feel better, even if chilly and cold. Weakness with menstrual periods; their body feels tired and painful, especially the legs and feet. Also colic that is better for heat and pressure.

MAGNESIA MURIATICA

(D, F, M) chloride of magnesium

The remedy Magnesia muriatica is used to relieve depression and anxiety; also for severe menstrual cramps.

Mind and emotions
The patient is peaceful and dislikes confrontation and aggression. They have a strong sense of duty and become anxious about fulfilling their responsibilities. At night they get overwhelmed with fear. Although they dislike aggression they are full of suppressed anger, and so when it does find its way to the surface they can be unstable and be depressed with violent outbursts or might experience manic depression.

Physical complaints
- An excellent remedy for severe menstrual cramps, taken on a monthly basis as needed. Heavy, dark, clotted periods with numbness and tingling in the upper limbs.

> **Key symptoms**
>
> *Patient dislikes confrontation; anxious, especially during the night • Menstrual cramps with flooding during a period.*

- Other complaints include heart palpitations, a bloated belly, burping with headaches and craving water when having headaches.

General Symptoms
The patient is worse for bathing in a lake or the sea, also worse for milk, fats and salt. Gushing of menstrual blood while sitting.

Where there is a heavy menstrual period with severe cramps Magnesia muriatica can be a useful remedy.

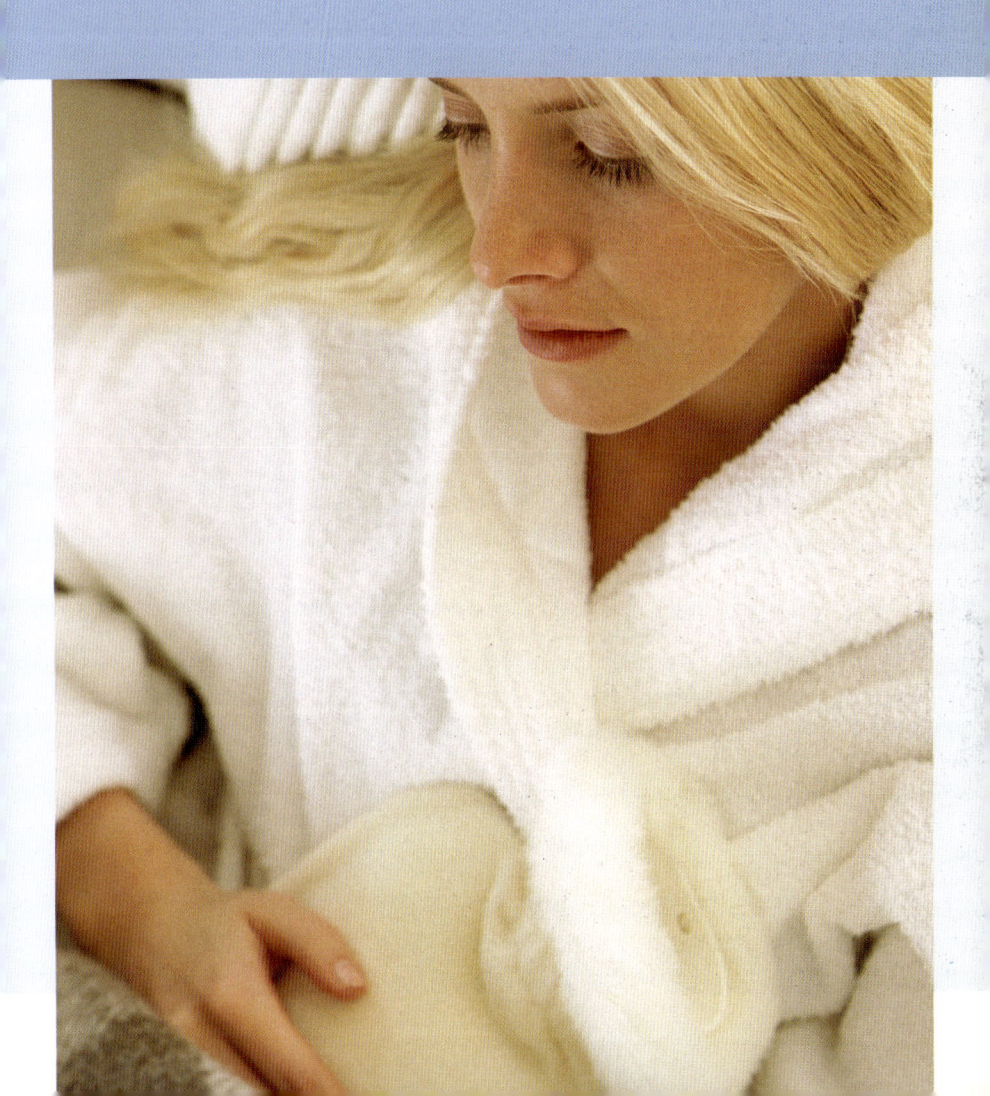

magnesia muriatica

MAGNESIA PHOSPHORICA

(GR, M) magnesium phosphate

Use Magnesia phosphorica as an effective pain-relief remedy for cramps, headaches and general pains.

Mind and emotions
The patient is extremely impulsive, irritable and fearful. This is a remedy for intellectual, sensitive or artistic people, who are nervous, intense, restless and neurotic, and who have cramps and pain. They are always discussing their pains with other people.

Physical complaints
- The patient experiences erratic, wandering pains, radiating pains or cramping, shooting and stitching pains. This remedy is particularly suitable for growing pains in young people.
- Also use for a headache that starts in the nape of the neck then spreads to the whole head.

> **Key symptoms**
>
> *Patient is sensitive, nervous, impulsive and fearful • Cramping, shooting and stitching pains • Headache that starts in the nape of the neck • Better for pressure on the painful area.*

- Use Magnesia phosphorica for pre-menstrual pains that are better when the flow starts.
- Also good for heartburn or indigestion during pregnancy or when caused by medication.

General symptoms
Feeling nauseous with hiccups. Better for hot applications to the affected parts. Better for pressure on the painful area.

Prescribe Magnesia phosphorica for a headache that is better for pressure.

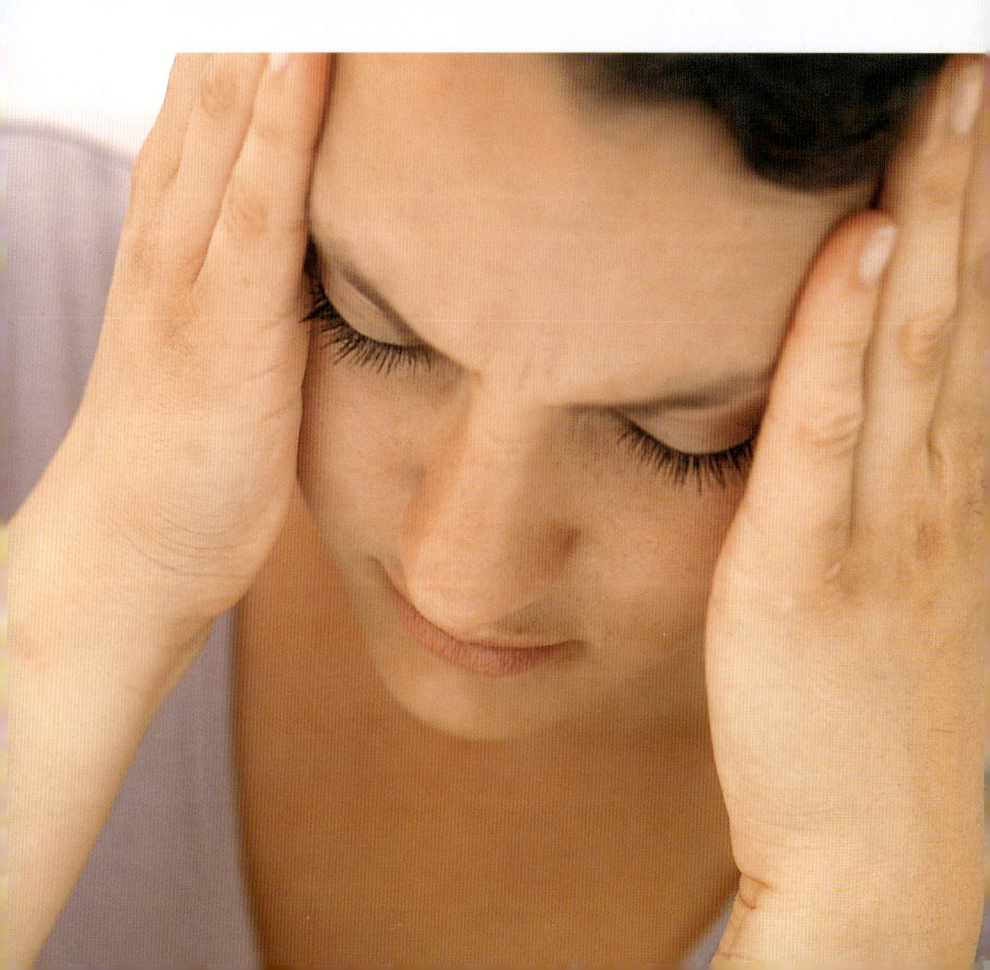

magnesia phosphorica

MERCURIUS VIVUS (MERCURY)

(GR, M) quicksilver

This is a remedy for toothache, enlarged glands and the lymph nodes. It is closely linked to mental states of confusion and fear.

Mind and emotions

Instability is the theme of this remedy. The patient is unsure of him- or herself and experiences instability in many ways. They are slow to answer questions, and have a poor memory and little willpower. They can become lost in familiar streets. Weary of life, the patient's health has begun to be affected. They fear that they are losing their reason, can be very suspicious, cautious and vulnerable, and fear being attacked, as they believe that everyone is their enemy.

Typically, the Mercury patient is emotionally very conservative and wants order in all relationships. Yet they are also discontented, and often have an all-or-nothing attitude. As a result, they can sometimes be revolutionary or an anarchist – they are prepared to fight for the strict moral code that they hold. Because the patient lacks confidence, they tremble inside and become easily embarrassed. They are sensitive to criticism and contradiction, and hate people who have offended them. They are torn between their conservative attitude to law and order and their forceful impulses.

Physical complaints

- The patient is sensitive to heat and cold. They constantly perspire all over their body.
- They also suffer from bad-smelling odours and swollen glands, as well as freely flowing secretions that are thick or thin, slimy, acrid, burning and foul. They have a lot of saliva which dribbles during sleep.
- The patient may suffer from ulcerative colitis and can have diarrhoea or pass hard, slimy stools.

mercurius vivus

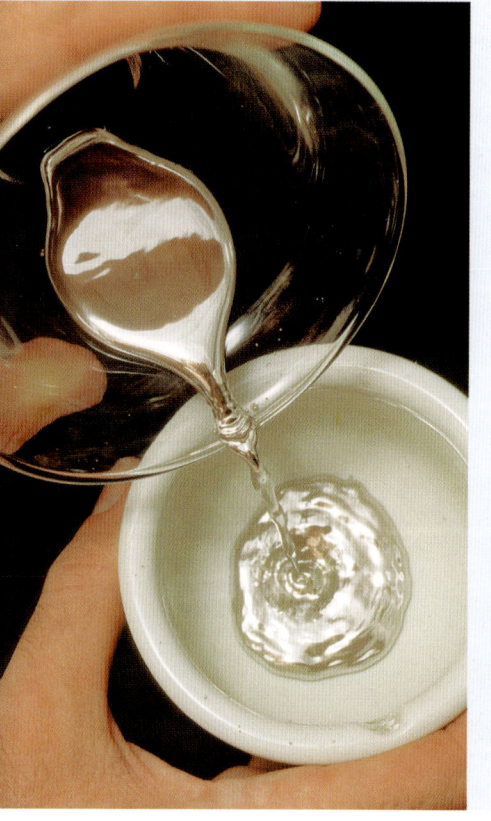

Key symptoms

The patient can behave unpredictably and finds self-control difficult in some situations • Constantly perspiring • Sensitivity to heat and cold • Swollen glands • Symptoms are worse at night or when lying on the right side.

General symptoms

Toothache. Flabby feeling in the chest, legs and the back. Symptoms are worse at night, and when lying on the right side.

The liquid metal mercury is the source of a remedy that is suited to ailments caused by mental instability.

NATRUM CARBONICUM

(D, F, GR, M) sodium carbonate

The remedy Natrum carbonicum is used for weakness caused by summer heat and the chronic effects of sunstroke exhaustion. (Sunstroke can be very dangerous and should be referred to a doctor.)

Mind and emotions

Natrum carbonicum is a remedy for mental exhaustion. The patient is selfless and sweet-natured. They are self-contained, independent, kind and mild, and can be

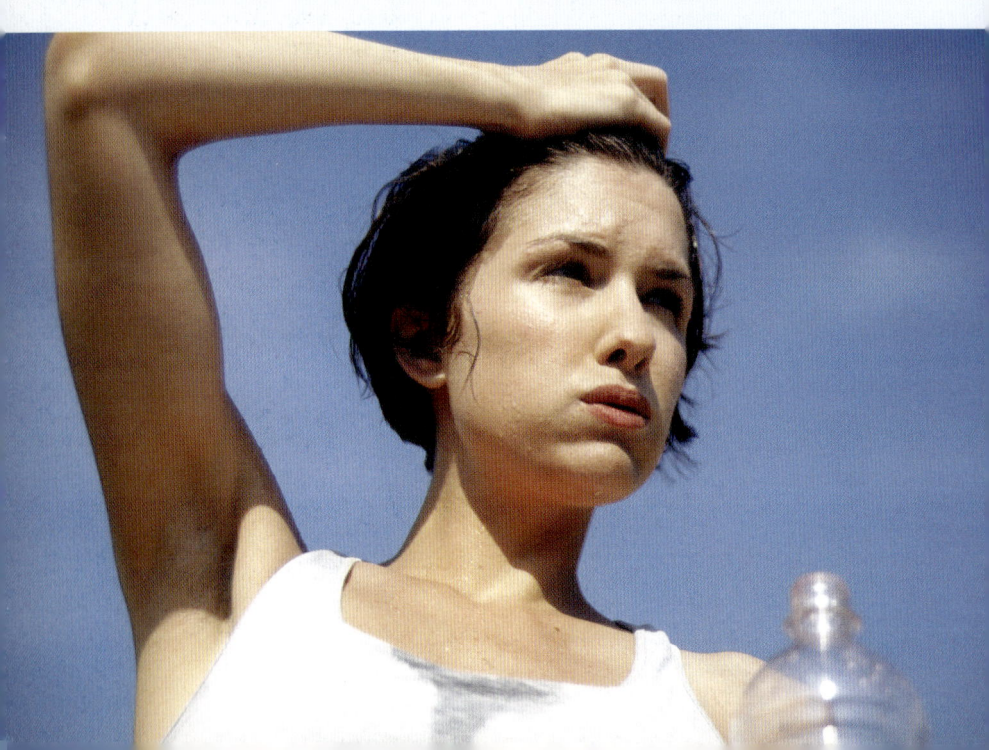

> ### Key symptoms
>
> *Patient is delicate by nature, unselfish and kind • Weak digestion • Weak ankles • Symptoms are worse for extremes of heat and cold.*

unselfish to the point where they will give to others things that they need for themselves. They are devoted, sympathetic and giving to others, and take care of others without asking for anything back. They are cheerful even when sad, sensitive to the ambiance in a place, but sometimes withdrawn. The patient is oversensitive to music and thunderstorms; they dislike certain people, and become estranged from their family.

Prescribe Natrum carbonicum for a gentle-natured person suffering from sunstroke.

Physical complaints

- The patient is weakened by heat and has a weak digestion as well as weak ankles that are easily dislocated and sprained.
- Flatulence and diarrhoea when milk is drunk are also common symptoms.
- Other symptoms include acute hearing, vaginal discharge after sex, and burning perspiration.

General symptoms

Patient gets up at 5.00 a.m. with an empty feeling in the stomach. Better for eating before going to bed at night. Worse for extremes of heat and cold.

NATRUM MURIATICUM

(D, F, GR, M) sea salt, sodium chloride

A major remedy for grief and migraines, Natrum muriaticum is suited to emotionally closed people.

Mind and emotions

This is a remedy for people who are easily hurt and feel rejected. They are exceptionally vulnerable and easily offended. They desire solitude and dwell on the past, recalling negative experiences, which make them become ill or unable to sleep. Although responsible people, they hold feelings of guilt. They can be defensive and cautious and are emotional after sex or drink. If they are given sympathy they only feel worse. They long for love, sympathy and connection with others but cannot seem to create it in their lives. They are torn by inner strife.

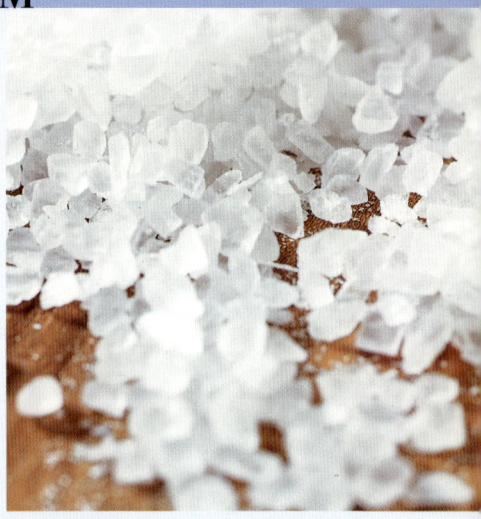

Physical complaints

- The patient has a strong craving for salt and is very thirsty for cold drinks.
- They are always worse for heat and the sun.
- Pains appear and disappear gradually.
- The patient suffers from hammering and bursting headaches that are worse for reading, motion, light, noise, sun and during their menstrual periods.

People who easily feel rejected and suffer from herpes or migraines might benefit from the remedy Natrum muriaticum.

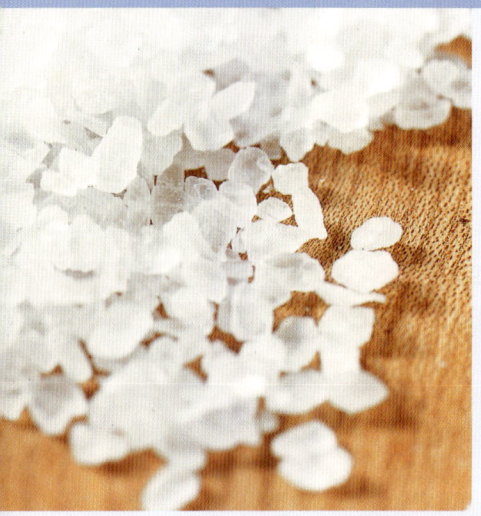

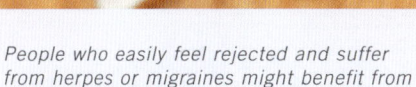

- They may have a thin, watery, profuse nasal discharge.
- Both sexes may suffer from genital herpes.
- Women suffer from a dry vagina and can be sad and irritable before and during their periods.

Key symptoms

The patient is vulnerable and easily offended. They are also inclined to dwell on negative experiences from the past • Craves salt • Severe headaches or migraines • Symptoms are worse for heat, especially the sun.

General symptoms

Sleep is disturbed by anxious dreams, such as of being chased. Skin erupts in spots because it is overheated. Hiccups and warts; faintness in a crowded, hot room. Symptoms might be improved or worsened when the patient is by the sea.

NATRUM PHOSPHORICUM

(C-C-F, CR, D, F, GR, Ma)
sodium phosphate

The remedy Natrum phosphoricum is useful for the initial stages of sore throat and for excessive lactic acid build-up in the body resulting from too much sugar. It is also good for all ailments with excessive acidity caused by eating too much fatty food.

Mind and emotions

The patient can be sad after sex, forgetful after frequent sex and indifferent to loved ones. They might also think that they hear footsteps when there are none.

Physical complaints

- After mental exertion and during thunderstorms the patient's head feels full and the body feels stiff.
- The patient might vomit during a headache.
- The ears are itchy, the nose discharges yellow mucus and the tongue is yellow.
- The stomach feels overly acidic due to eating fatty food.
- Male symptoms are a pain in the spermatic chord after ejaculating and ejaculating every night.
- Female symptoms include vaginal discharge that is like cream, and which smells offensive and sour.
- The patient feels bubbling sensations in the heart area of the chest.
- Other symptoms of note are restless sleep and palpitations that begin during thunderstorms.

General symptoms

Seizures during ejaculation. Flushes of heat during menstrual periods. Weariness in warm weather and during storms. Trembling during thunderstorms. Worse for warm weather. Patient suffers from a sore throat.

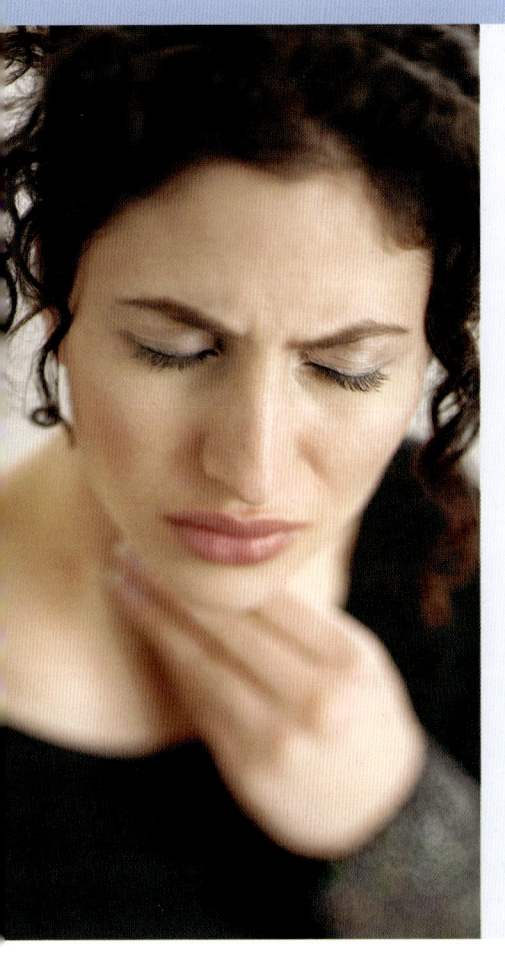

Key symptoms

Craving for fried food and strongly flavoured foods • Reaction to over-rich foods • Yellow discharges • Head that feels full and stiffness in the body after exertion.

Prescribe Natrum phosphoricum for the initial stages of a sore throat as well as for discomfort after eating fatty foods.

NATRUM SULPHURICUM

(C-C-F, D, GR, M) sodium sulphate

A remedy specific for head injuries past or present, Natrum sulphuricum is also suitable to be used as a support remedy in conjunction with conventional medicine for problems relating to head injuries.

Mind and emotions

The patient is a systematic worker who is down-to-earth and has a strong sense of duty and responsibility. They are very grounded, sensible and practical people. They are

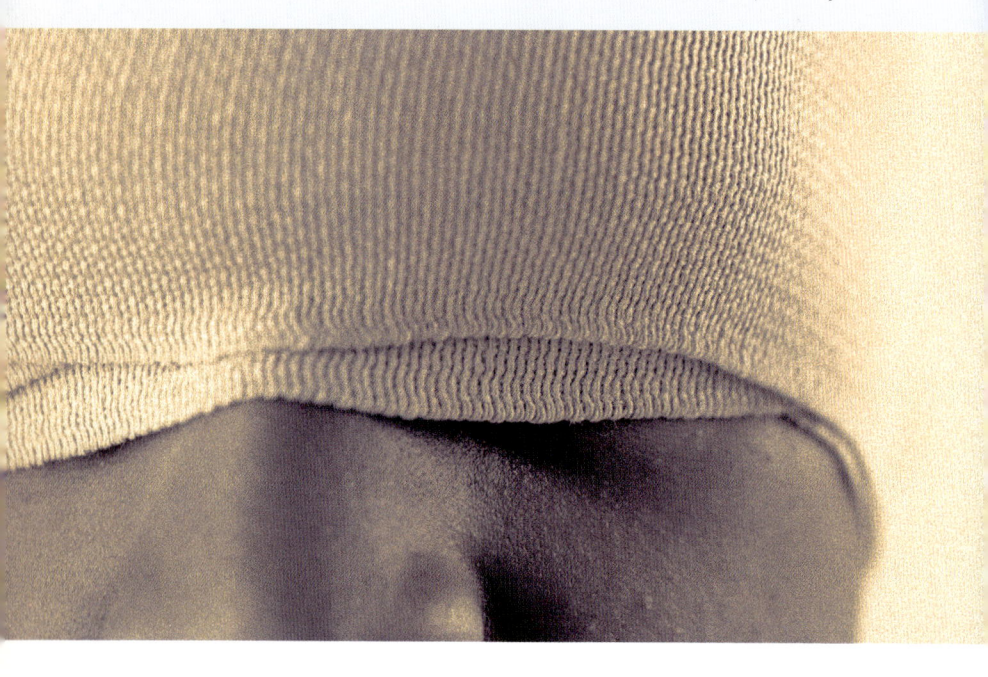

Key symptoms

Patient is a grounded, down-to-earth person. They may have changed emotionally after a head injury • Head injury (past or present) • Yellow and yellow-green mucus • Problems with liver and lungs • Symptoms are worse in the morning after rising, and for changes in the weather.

objective, realistic and always matter-of-fact people, who become emotional only when listening to music. They can be sad and depressed. A keynote symptom is mental change after a head injury.

Use Natrum sulphuricum for people who have suffered a head injury.

Physical complaints

- The patient has profuse yellow, watery discharges or thick yellow-green mucus.
- They will suffer from chronic physical problems that result from old head injuries, including headaches and asthma that are worse from damp, wet weather.
- Natrum sulphuricum is also a liver remedy to support conventional medicine for acute hepatitis, gallstones, colic and jaundice. It is a good remedy for chronic liver pains and inflammation.

General symptoms

Worse for changes in the weather and wet, damp weather; also in the morning after rising. Vertigo from head injuries.

NUX VOMICA

(C-C-F, D, GR, M)
seed of poison nut tree*

A remedy for constipation and sore throat, Nux vomica is also useful for patients who are inclined to be angry and irritable.

Mind and emotions
The patient is a strong, ambitious person who easily becomes angry and irritable. They are often business people who have a sedentary lifestyle, who eat over-rich food and drink too much alcohol. They are cramped and can't relax. They can be very independent and fear marriage and intimacy, as well as being fastidious, fault-finding and reproachful of others. They can also often be irritable and impatient, as well as jealous and abusive, and quarrelsome even to the point of violence.

> **Key symptoms**
>
> *The patient has a sedentary lifestyle and is angry and irritable. They can be jealous and abusive • Constipation • Tension creates symptoms where the patient cannot let go, such as cramps or being unable to urinate or belch.*

Physical complaints
- This is a liver remedy to tonify a lethargic liver caused by irritability and anger.
- It is also a major constipation remedy.
- Also useful when there is gas and colic after eating rich food and drinking alcohol.
- Nux vomica is a remedy for hayfever when the patient wakes sneezing.
- Also for nasal congestion that is worse at night but becomes runny during the day.

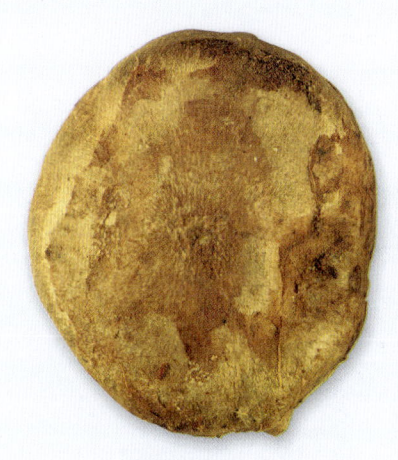

The finely powdered seeds of the poison nut tree are potentized as a remedy for constipation and a sore throat.

- It is also a remedy for loss of sleep.
- Use for sore throats with liver imbalance.
- Other symptoms include trying to pass stool but being unable to, being unable to urinate, to belch, to sneeze, to vomit, as well as cramps, spasms, jerks and feeling very tense.

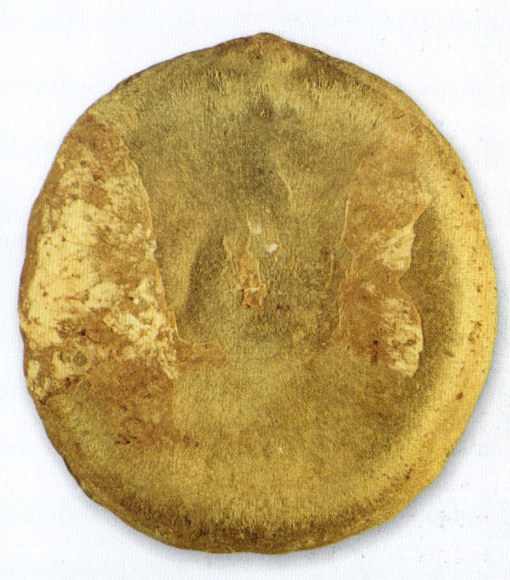

General symptoms

Faintness from the smell of odours or the sight of blood. Nausea, headaches and hangovers that are worse for movement.

OPIUM

(C-C-F, GR, M) opium poppy plant

This is a remedy for fear, fright and joy, and is specifically used to support conventional medicine for head injuries.

Mind and emotions

The patient suffers from ailments caused by disappointment, embarrassment, fear, fright from the sight of an accident, grief, reproaches, shame and shock. Opium is also useful for those who drink excessively.

All these symptoms lead the patient to withdraw into an inner world. They will feel unaffected by pain, with a sense of numbness, and will be unable to react to what is happening around them.

Physical complaints

- The symptoms are vertigo after stress, eyes remaining open during unconsciousness.
- Patient has a face that is pale and discoloured during anger or headaches.
- Constipation is a common ailment, where the stool recedes. However, after a fright the patient might experience diarrhoea (this might also occur after sudden joy), a lost voice or involuntary stool and retention of urine.
- The symptoms will occur after drug abuse, during pregnancy, or in someone with a sedentary lifestyle.
- For women, this remedy can help prevent miscarriage or a prolapsed uterus caused by fright, as well as lessening an overly strong sexual desire.

General symptoms

Patient can suffer convulsions and or twitching caused by fright. Although the patient will perspire, there will be little urination. The patient dreams while awake, breath slows right down or stops intermittently during sleep.

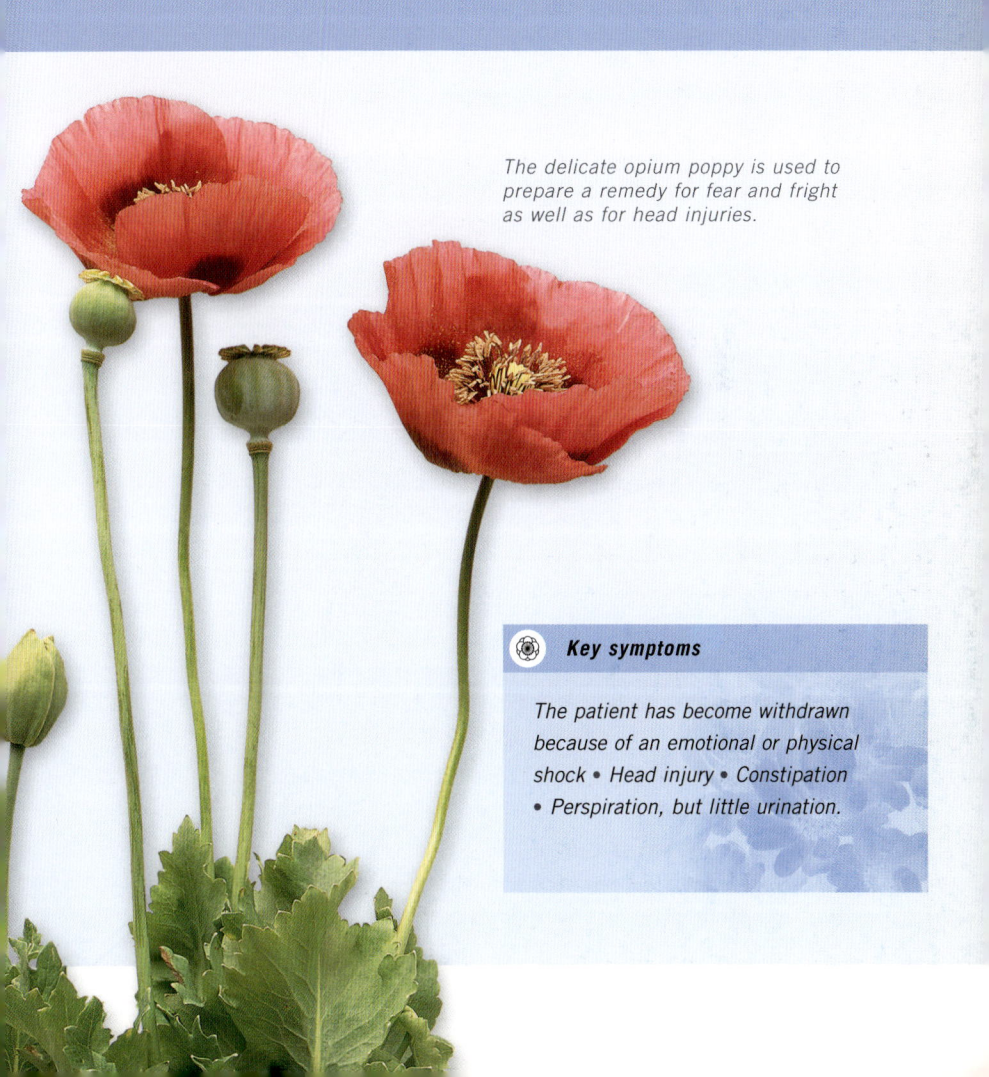

The delicate opium poppy is used to prepare a remedy for fear and fright as well as for head injuries.

Key symptoms

The patient has become withdrawn because of an emotional or physical shock • Head injury • Constipation • Perspiration, but little urination.

PETROLEUM

(+FA, D, F, GR, M, Ma) crude rock oil

This is a remedy for skin eruptions, cuts that are slow to heal and fissures in the skin, as well as asthma and gastric acidity.

Key symptoms

The patient is excitable and easily upset
- *Dry skin with deep bleeding cracks*
- *Asthma • Bloated stomach • Patient is chilly, symptoms are worse in winter.*

Mind and emotions

The patient is excitable and quick-tempered, quarrelsome and worse for drinking alcohol. They feel uncertain and chill easily, dreading the fresh air. The patient also feels as though death is near and that they need to settle their affairs promptly. Feeling low-spirited, irritable and easily offended, they are also easily vexed and sceptical.

Physical complaints

- This is a remedy for moist skin problems found on the scalp that are worse at the back of the head and on the ears.
- The skin around the eyes is dry and itchy, and there will be eczema behind the ears that causes intense itching.
- The skin on other parts of the body might itch and burn, and there might be chilblains, bedsores and eczema. The skin on the tips of fingers will be cracked and there will be other fissures in the heels and hands that will not close.
- The patient's vision is dim and far-sighted.
- There might be a bloated stomach and an empty feeling. Also experiences nausea and vomiting.
- There will be a dry cough and a feeling of tightness in the chest at night; coughing

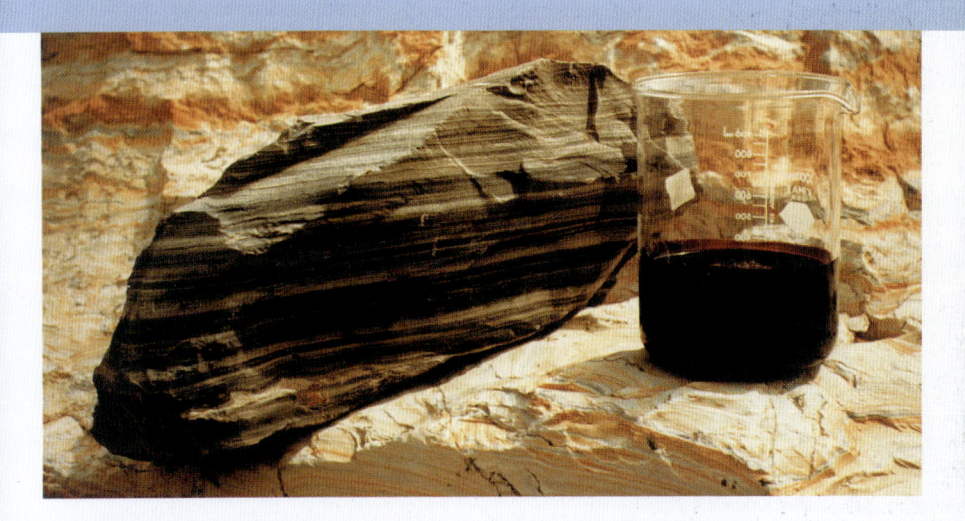

produces a headache or asthma, and is worse indoors.

- Male symptoms may include herpes on the penis, and a painful, inflamed and swollen prostate.
- Female symptoms may include profuse discharge, as well as sore genitals that are also moist.
- Other symptoms include chronic catarrh in the Eustachian tube that affects the hearing, ulcerated nostrils that are cracked and feel burning, and heartburn that is hot and sharp.

Crude rock oil is the source of a remedy for dry skin that cracks.

General symptoms
The patient might have flushes of heat in the daytime and after anger.

PHOSPHORIC ACID

(CB, D, M, GR, Ma)
diluted phosphoric acid

The remedy Phosphoric acid is used for exhaustion caused by overwork, grief and disappointment, as well as in childbirth when labour has exhausted the mother. Alongside conventional medicine, it is useful to relieve the pains of cancer.

Mind and emotions

The patient is a mild, yielding person who is easily overwhelmed by emotions or who is slowly recovering from an acute illness. They are apathetic, burned out and feel weak and indifferent to everything; they are also slow to grasp ideas and have a poor memory. The patient suffers from ailments which are caused by grief, disappointed love and mental shock, as well as being so used to their unhappiness and despair that they make no effort to change and become settled in their despair.

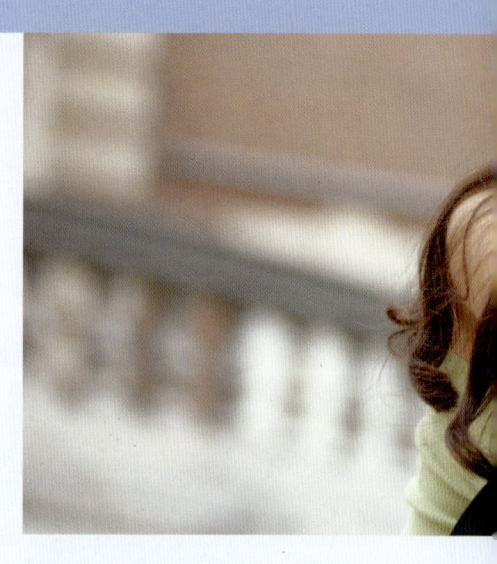

Physical complaints

- The head feels heavy and confused and the patient has a crushing headache.
- The hair becomes grey early and falls out.
- There are blue rings around the eyes, a ravenous appetite at night and a sensation of a lump in the abdomen after eating.
- The patient finds looking at food makes them feel nauseous, and they might suffer

phosphoric acid

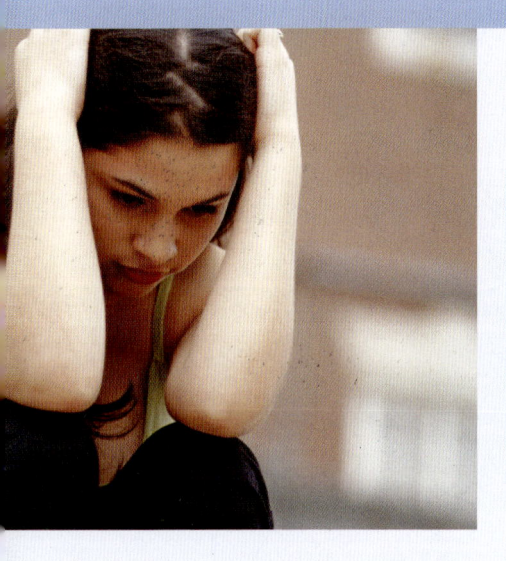

When a person is exhausted due to overwork or grief and feels weak, consider the remedy Phosphoric acid.

Key symptoms

The patient is apathetic, burned out and weak • Ailments caused by grief, disappointment or exhaustion after illness or childbirth • Most food makes them feel nauseous but they crave refreshing foods • Cold hands.

from diarrhoea caused by anticipating something, a change of weather, being cold, or from eating cold food. However, they crave fruit and other refreshing foods.
- Men may suffer from erection problems during sex or seminal discharges after sex.
- The patient has palpitations in bed at night, caused by grief, sexual excitement or disappointed love.

General symptoms

Irritability that has been caused by oversensitivity to too much medicine. Broken bones are slow to repair. Hands are always cold. Weakness occurs as a result of disappointment.

PHOSPHORUS

(+FA, CB, C-C-F, CR, M, Ma, F, GR)
phosphorus

This is a remedy for burning pains, haemorrhage, hypoglycaemia, colds and flu. Phosphorus is also good for recovering from surgery and jet lag.

Mind and emotions
The patient is an extrovert who is very open and affectionate, as well as impressionable and sensitive to things that happen around them. They are also easily distracted and very suggestible.

The typical Phosphorus patient can also be full of fears, such as of supernatural phenomena, what the future might bring, their health, the possibility of disease, and thunderstorms, and will be anxious about being alone. They are unable to cope when they receive bad news and can easily suffer from low spirits. They also have clairvoyant premonitions, and may become egotistical.

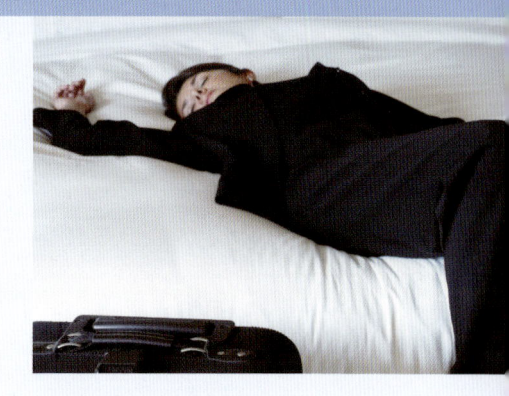

This is a remedy for mental fatigue, excitability and restlessness, suitable for those who are often fidgety.

Physical complaints
- For cataracts, with the sensation that everything is covered with mist.
- Phosphorus is also useful for excessive bleeding following tooth extraction or drilling.
- Stomach symptoms include the patient vomiting warm fluid from the stomach, and unable to hold food down. There might also be exhausting diarrhoea with mucus.

Jet lag can be alleviated by using the remedy Phosphorus.

- Also to treat atrophy of the optic nerve, and glaucoma as a support therapy for conventional treatment. It can be used to treat thrombosis of the retinal vessel and degenerative changes in the retina.
- Throat symptoms: hoarseness (often with laryngitis), sore throat, coughing with a tickling sensation, lung congestion, burning pains and oppression in the chest during flu, pneumonia and tuberculosis.
- Other symptoms include sharp, cutting pains in the stomach, liver congestion, acute hepatitis, jaundice, fatty degeneration of the liver and pancreatic diseases.
- Men may suffer from having no energy for sex or have desire with lascivious dreams.
- Women may have bleeding in between periods or weeping before their period begins, a stitching pain in the breast and profuse discharges.

Key symptoms

The patient is extrovert, affectionate and impressionable but also full of fears • Burning pains • Eye problems • Better for sleep • Craving for ice cream and highly seasoned food.

General symptoms

The patient is worse from touch, mental exertion, warm food and drink, change of weather and thunderstorms. Patient craves highly seasoned food and loves ice cream, feels better in the dark, with cold food, fresh air and from washing in cold water. Sleep, even naps, will improve their symptoms.

PHYTOLACCA DECANDRA

(CR, D, F, GR, M) pokeroot plant

This is a remedy for swollen glands, weakness, soreness and restlessness with illness. It can also be used as a support remedy for cancer and angina.

Mind and emotions
The patient may be very uninhibited and like walking around without clothes or exposing themselves. They act indifferently to life and are indifferent to exposing themselves; they can act shamelessly.

Physical complaints
- The patient experiences wandering and shooting pains that appear and disappear, like electric shocks.
- The patient is restless and wants to move about and keep active.
- Other symptoms include cancer, hard nodules in the breast with enlarged glands, mastitis, breasts that feel like hard stones, heavy and swollen breasts that are worse during breastfeeding. The pains can spread to the entire body.
- Also common are cracked nipples, recurrent or acute tonsillitis, sinusitis and angina pectoris, when the pain moves from the heart and appears in the right arm.

> **Key symptoms**
>
> *Patient may be very uninhibited • Tough, stringy discharges • Symptoms are worse in cold weather • Swollen glands • Wandering and shooting pains.*

phytolacca decandra

Prescribe Phytolacca decandra for swollen glands with weakness and soreness.

General symptoms

Abscess of the breast, where pains suddenly come and go. Unbearable pains anywhere in the body. Symptoms are worse in cold weather.

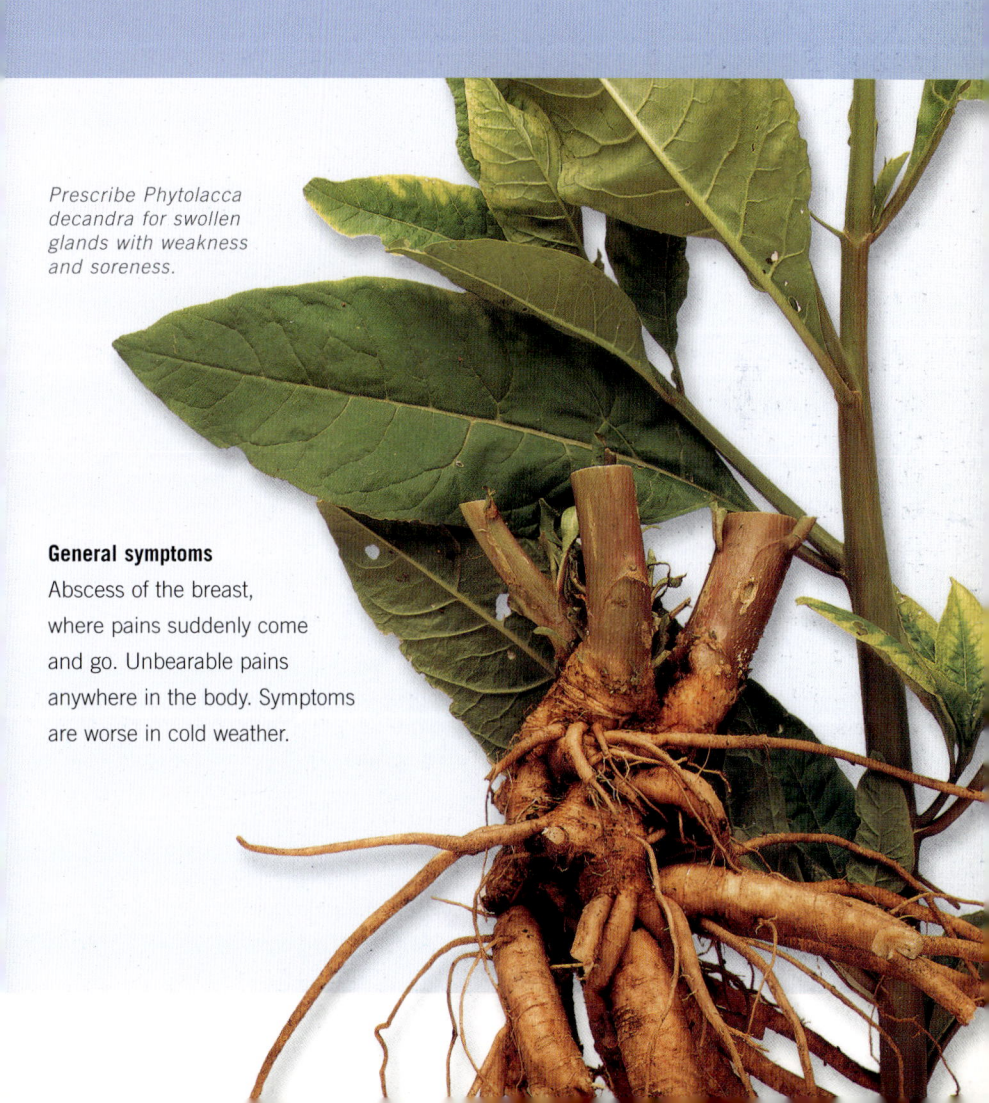

PLATINA

(F, GR, M, Ma) platinum

This is a remedy for female problems relating to emotional and sexual issues.

Mind and emotions

The patient is romantic and idealistic, and suffers from ailments caused by disappointment, sexually related problems, grief and scorn as well as from having been betrayed by others. These can lead to the patient dwelling on the past and feeling abandoned. They may compensate for these feelings by being overconcerned about themselves. The patient has a high sex drive and is easily excited. They also feel superior and can be indifferent to others. This is a remedy for self-love, contempt for others, arrogance and haughtiness.

Physical complaints

- The affected parts might feel numb, stiff and cold, with numbness particularly felt in the coccyx. The pains may appear and disappear gradually.
- Menstrual periods will be short but heavy.
- Other symptoms include violent cramping pains, including vaginismus during sex.

General symptoms

Numbness in spots; pains are worse when pressure is applied. Weakness, which is helped by moving.

Key symptoms

The patient is romantic and idealistic and has experienced sadness caused by relationships or sexually related problems • Numbness and stiffness • Female problems relating to sex and menstruation.

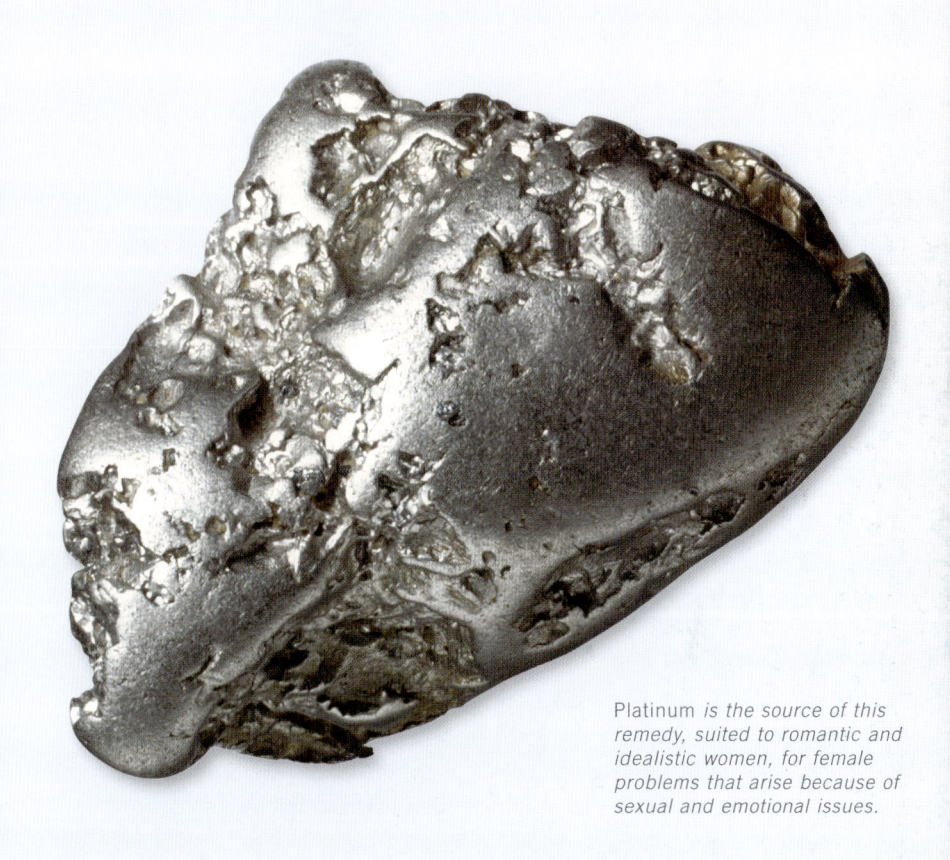

Platinum is the source of this remedy, suited to romantic and idealistic women, for female problems that arise because of sexual and emotional issues.

PLUMBUM

(+FA, CR, F, GR, Ma) lead

This is a remedy that can be used to support conventional treatment for paralysis, multiple sclerosis, infantile paralysis and progressive muscular atrophy.

Mind and emotions
The patient suffers from depression with a fear of being killed. They will be melancholy, apathetic and slow to understand what is happening around them. They may also suffer from a partial or total loss of memory. This is a remedy for mental exhaustion caused by physical exertion, and it is also suitable for inflexible people who are quite selfish, thinking only of themselves, and who are self-destructive and impulsive.

It can be used for children who are oversensitive or have weak memories or those who are experiencing problems at school and who are nervous, emotionally unstable and restless.

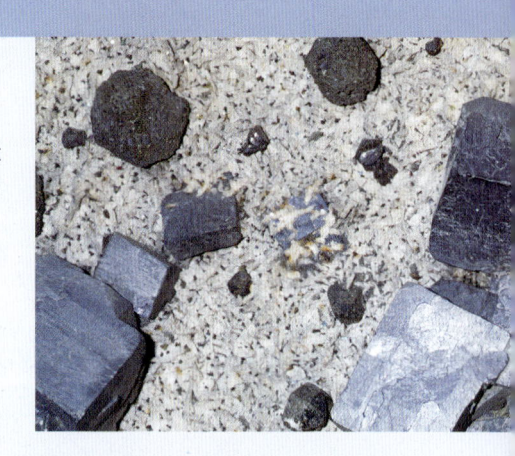

Physical complaints
- The extensor muscles (the muscles that enable a limb to be straightened) are weakened, leading to paralysis.
- Lightning-like pains may be felt in the back with paralysis of a single muscle. This might result in wrist drop and cramps in the calves, or swollen feet and paralysis in the legs.
- The patient has distinct blue lines along the margins of the gums, which can suggest lead poisoning.

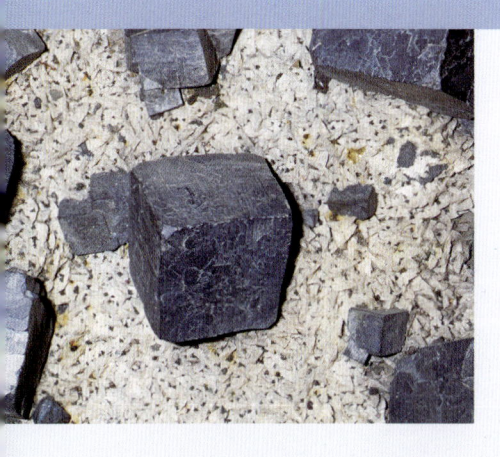

Lead is used to prepare a support remedy for a variety of illnesses.

- Other symptoms include gastralgia (problems with stomach acid), constant vomiting, the inability to swallow food, excessive colic and a strangulated hernia.
- There can be constipation, especially during pregnancy, with hard, lumpy stools and urging that comes in spasms, impacted faeces, chronic interstitial nephritis (inflammation of the kidneys), with great pain in the abdomen.
- Men may experience a lack of libido, with a constricted feeling in the testicles.
- Women may be seriously underweight, constipated and suffer from vaginismus. They may also find that the vulva and vagina are hypersensitive, and that there is a tendency for pregnancies to miscarry.

General symptoms

Worse at night; better for rubbing with hard pressure and for physical exertion.

> **Key symptoms**
>
> *Patient is exhausted and depressed. A child may have a weak memory or experience problems at school. • Pains in the muscles • Paralysis • Upset stomach with vomiting.*

PODOPHYLLUM

(+FA, CB, CR, D, F) May apple plant

This is a remedy for acute diarrhoea and digestive problems to accompany conventional medical treatment.

Mind and emotions
Depression.

Physical complaints
- The patient experiences a headache that alternates with diarrhoea, the face is hot and there is a bitter taste in mouth. The patient will roll his or her head from side to side, moaning and vomiting.
- Also to be used for infants who are having difficulties with teething that is accompanied by diarrhoea, and for babies who vomit milk.
- Podophyllum is also useful for nausea and vomiting, as well as heartburn that is accompanied by gagging or retching.

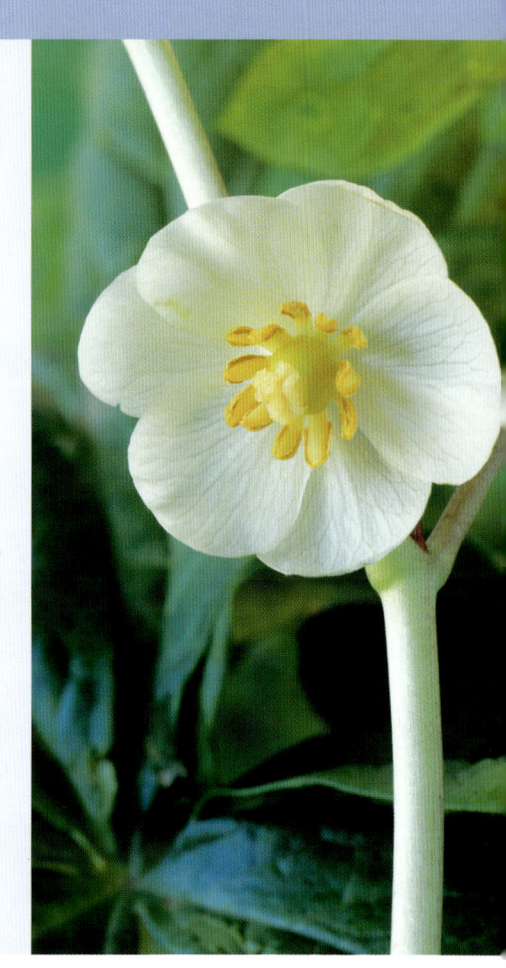

- The abdomen is bloated, hot and empty, and there is a sensation of weakness and pain in the area of the liver.
- Use this remedy also for long periods of diarrhoea that is green, watery, fetid, profuse and gushing.
- Another symptom is constipation alternating with diarrhoea.
- Women may suffer from pain in the uterus and the right ovary, lack of periods that are accompanied by painful spasms in the pelvic area, or haemorrhoids (piles) during pregnancy and after childbirth.

Key symptoms

The patient is depressed • Headaches with diarrhoea • Teething problems in infants • Diarrhoea that is slow to improve • Symptoms are worse in the morning, in hot weather and during teething.

General symptoms

Worse in the morning, in hot weather and during teething.

The May apple plant is used to create a remedy for diarrhoea and digestive problems accompanied by depression.

PULSATILLA

(C-C-F, CR, CB, F, GR, M) wind flower

The remedy Pulsatilla is suited to clinging and dependent people, who are worse for being alone. It is also for heart congestion or non-specific pains in the chest, and colds where there is a yellow discharge, which can come from the eyes or nose.

Mind and emotions

The patient weeps easily and is timid, clingy and uncertain. They fear being alone, and love sympathy and the attention of others. Children love to fuss and be caressed. They have a yielding disposition, are submissive, and cannot say no. They long to please others and can be manipulative to get attention. They are better for consolation and the attention of others.

Physical complaints

- The patient has suffered ailments and not been well since puberty.
- Their symptoms are always changeable, shifting from side to side.
- They are chilly but dislike the heat. They long for air, and are better out of doors or with the windows open. They have a dry mouth but no thirst.
- Pulsatilla patients suffer from digestive problems, and love fat, butter and cream.
- This is a useful remedy in pregnancy for food and air cravings.
- It is also good for colds with a yellow discharge, and for children with running noses and loose coughs.

Key symptoms

Patient is mild, affectionate and weepy • Although chilly the patient dislikes the heat • Digestive and heart problems.

- Men may have swollen testes after they have contracted mumps.
- Women may suffer from profuse vaginal discharge, and extremely painful periods accompanied by painful breasts. They may suffer with headaches because of delayed periods. This is a good remedy for bringing on a menstrual period if it is slow or delayed.

General symptoms

Pulsatilla is a remedy for contradictory and alternating conditions: many of the symptoms are contradictory in nature and can alternate from side to side, or the patient might want to eat, for example, but they are not hungry, or they might love rich food although it makes them ill. Also appropriate for recurrent styes, faintness when in a closed room and for hiccups caused by cold drinks. Also for vomiting when a menstrual period is late.

Pulsatilla is a useful remedy for clingy people who have yellow mucus, and is especially suitable for children.

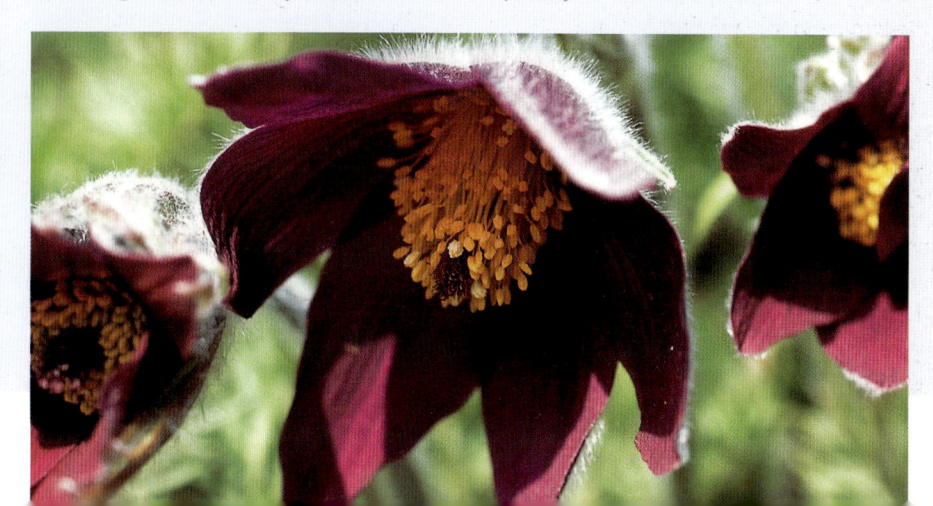

PYROGEN

(C-C-F, CR, GR) artificial sepsis

The remedy Pyrogen is used for serious infections that do not respond to drugs or remedies. This is a homeopathic antiseptic. Use it with conventional medical treatment when there is a septic condition accompanied by restlessness.

Mind and emotions

The patient is full of anxiety and unrealistic thoughts, and they can't stop chattering. They have delusions about wealth and cannot distinguish between a dream and things that happen while they are awake.

Physical complaints

- The patient's head throbs with pain, they suffer bursting headaches and are very restless, and may have septic fevers.
- They have chills that begin in the back and a temperature that rises rapidly. They become overheated and sweat profusely,

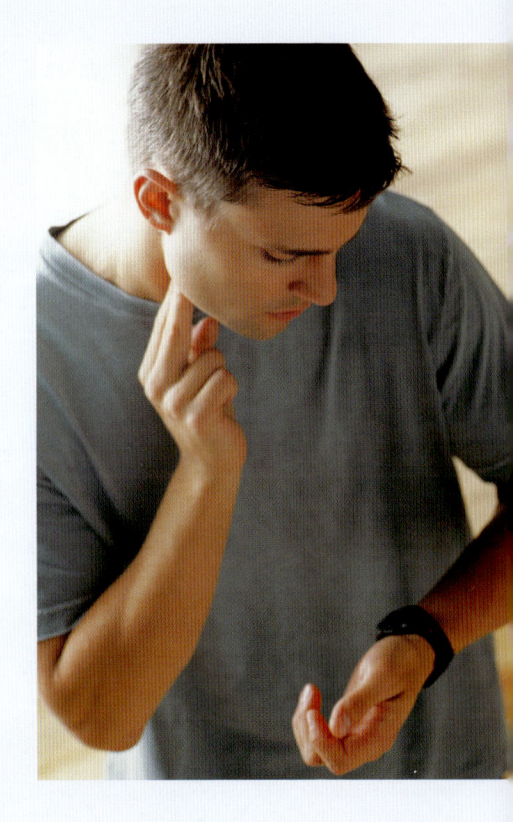

but this does not lower their temperature.
- There is a tired feeling in their heart accompanied by palpitations; their pulse is overly rapid.
- The patient might vomit water when it becomes warm in their stomach.
- Women might have septicaemia following a miscarriage or abortion, offensive-smelling periods and uterine haemorrhage. They can also suffer from a fever every time they have a menstrual period, creating pelvic inflammation.
- This is a good post-operative support remedy for cases where there has been an infection.

> **Key symptoms**
>
> *The patient feels bruised and sore and feels the need to move for relief • Fever and pain • Infections • Heart feels weak from the stress of illness.*

General symptoms

Abscesses that are recurrent and burn. Pain feels as if the bones are broken. Patient is better when moving. Good for cuts that become infected and wounds that do not heal.

The homeopathic antiseptic, Pyrogen, is useful for patients with a rapid pulse who tend to be anxious and unrealistic.

RADIUM BROMATUM

(C-C-F, D, F, GR) radium bromide

This is a remedy for rheumatism and gout, as well as severe aches and pains all over body that are accompanied by extreme restlessness. It is also used as a support remedy to complement conventional medicine for relieving the pains caused by radiation treatment for cancer.

Mind and emotions
The patient is apprehensive, depressed, fears being alone and facing death, so they have a strong need to be with other people. The patient is also tired and irritable.

Physical complaints
- The patient suffers from violent pains in the facial nerves.
- They can experience painful frontal headaches, with an empty sensation in the stomach, violent stomach cramps with the stomach full of gas.
- Terrible backaches that are accompanied by pain and lameness in the cervical, lumbar and sacral vertebrae – the pains feel as if they are situated right inside the bones.
- Severe pain is also felt in all the joints, especially the knee and ankle, as well as arthritis, necrosis and ulceration, and itching all over body.
- Other symptoms include nephritis (inflammation of the kidneys) with rheumatism, gout, a persistent cold and a dry spasmodic cough.
- Women may experience itching in the vulva as well as delayed or irregular menstrual periods.

General symptoms
Use Radium bromatum to relieve the pain associated with radiation therapy for many types of cancer.

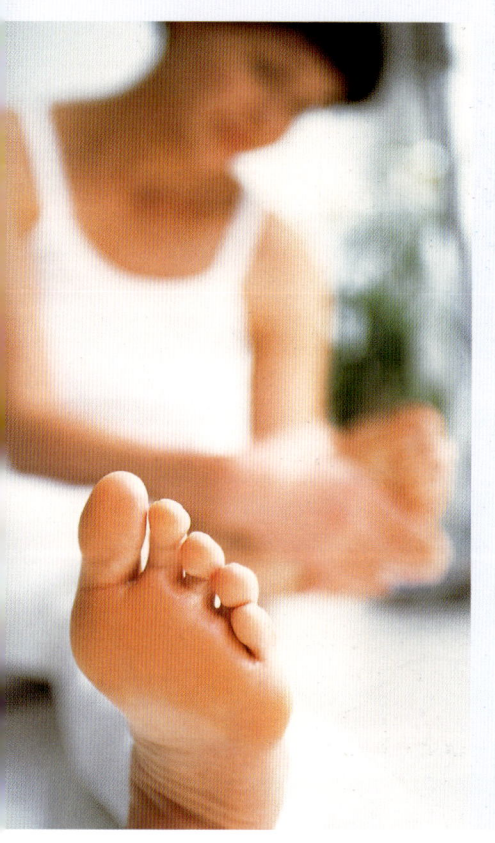

Key symptoms

The patient is depressed and fears being alone • Pain in any part of the body • Rheumatism • Stomach cramps with flatulence • Gout • Pain from radiation treatment for cancer.

The remedy Radium bromatum is useful for general and severe aches and pains in the joints as well as for rheumatism.

RHUS TOXICODENDRON

(+FA, C-C-F, CR, F, GR, Ma)
poison ivy plant*

This is a remedy for skin irritations, rheumatic pains, shingles, problems with the mucous membranes, such as cold sores, mouth ulcers and joint problems where the mucus does not protect the fluid-filled sac of the joint; also for irritability.

Mind and emotions

The patient feels extremely irritable and restless. They have a tendency to withhold feelings, to hold back affection, and be stiff and unresponsive. They also have fixed ideas and can be superstitious. They can also feel threatened without knowing why. Cares and worries are all worse at night.

Physical complaints

- The patient suffers from ailments caused by strain, lifting too many heavy items, and getting wet while perspiring.
- They can have septic conditions such as pneumonia, and infections.
- They also suffer from cramps, sciatica, stiff joints and rheumatism in cold weather, septicaemia, pustular inflammation of the eye and ulceration of the cornea.
- Respiration symptoms include a teasing cough that occurs from midnight until morning accompanied by a chill.
- They can be very thirsty with a dry throat and a craving for milk.

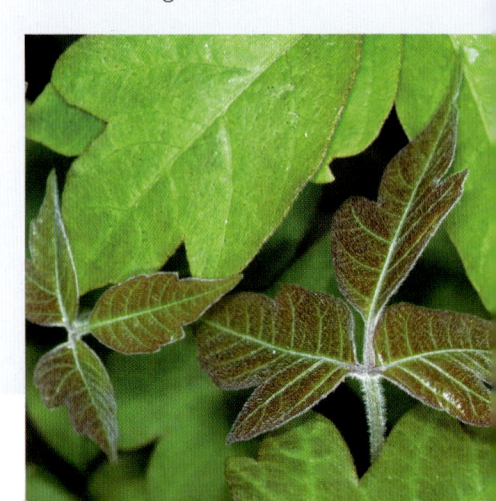

- Teeth that feel loose accompanied by sore gums, as well as a sore throat along with swollen glands.
- Men may experience swelling of the glans and prepuce, along with a swollen scrotum and intense itching.
- Women may have swelling of the vulva with intense itching.

This plant forms the basis of a remedy for skin irritations, cold sores and joint problems.

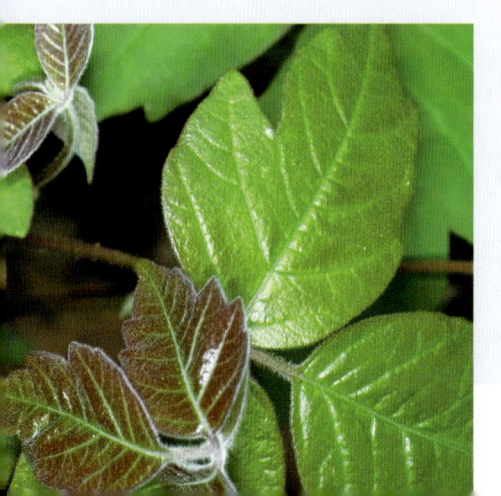

- Other symptoms include sneezing after getting wet, dislocation of the jaw with a swollen face, dysentery and heart problems caused by over-exertion.
- All pains are better for moving about.

General symptoms

Dreams that make the patient tired and feel worn out. Worse in cold, wet weather, after rain, at night and during rest. Better for warm, dry weather, motion, a change of position, rubbing and warm applications.

Key symptoms

The patient is irritable and inclined to withhold feelings • Infections and skin irritations • Cold sores • Joint problems • Problems caused by straining.

RUTA GRAVEOLENS

(+FA, CB, C-C-F, GR)
rue-bitterwort plant*

This is a remedy for complaints involving strain, flexor tendons, sprains, lameness, weakness of the joints and injured bones.

Mind and emotions
The patient feels extremely weary, as well as weak and despairing.

Physical complaints
- This remedy acts on the lining of the bone and cartilage, eye and uterus.
- Symptoms confined to the head include pains that feel as if a nail is piercing the skull and those that occur after drinking, as well as nosebleeds and eye strain followed by a headache. The eyes are red and hot, and will be painful from close work such as sewing or reading.
- The tendons in the body, and around the uterus particularly, become shortened during the seventh month of pregnancy and this remedy helps to expand them without pain.
- The chest feels weak and there are coughs with copious, thick yellow phlegm.
- Pains are felt in the nape of the neck, the back and the loins.
- Ruta graveolens is for lumbago, when the spine and limbs feel bruised and painful.
- Also used for contracture (shortening and hardening of the muscles) of the fingers

Key symptoms

The patient is weary and weak • Strains, sprains and weakness of the joints • Headache and eyestrain • Thick, yellow phlegm • Back pain • Symptoms are worse from lying down, and from cold, wet weather.

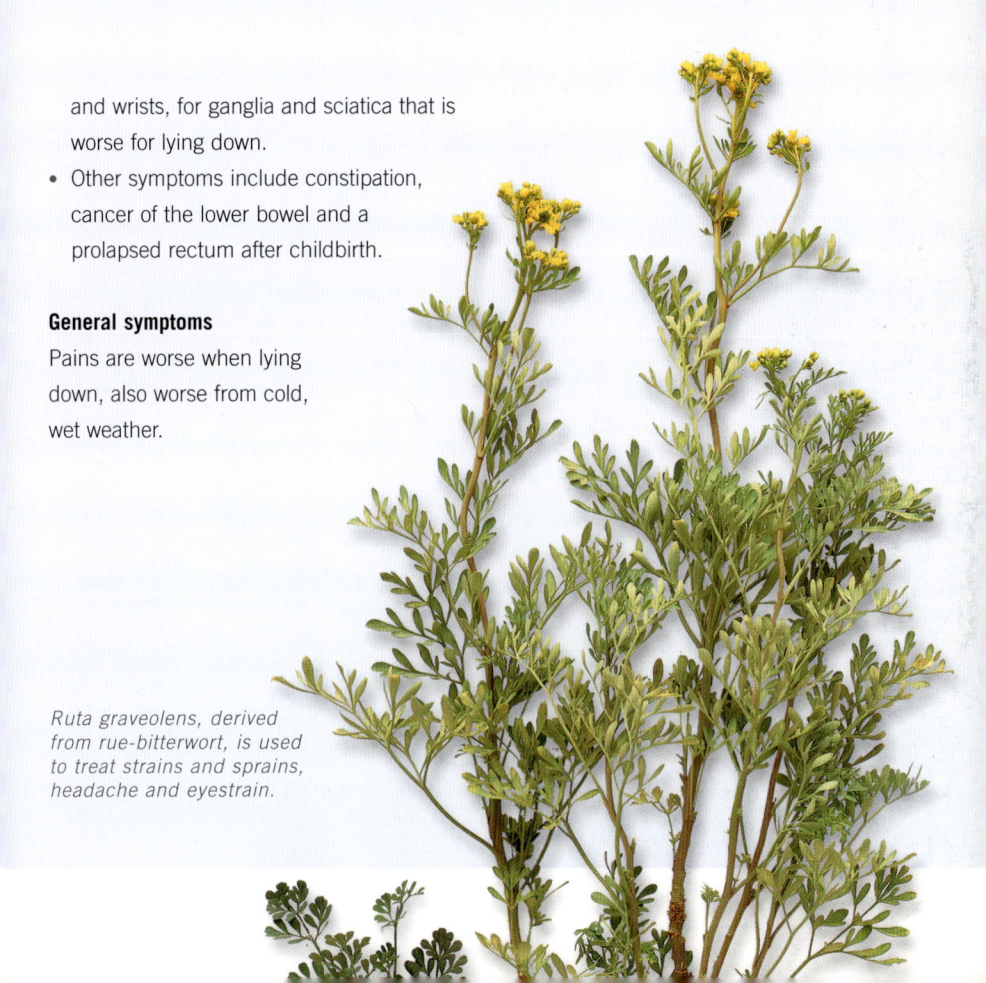

and wrists, for ganglia and sciatica that is worse for lying down.
- Other symptoms include constipation, cancer of the lower bowel and a prolapsed rectum after childbirth.

General symptoms
Pains are worse when lying down, also worse from cold, wet weather.

Ruta graveolens, derived from rue-bitterwort, is used to treat strains and sprains, headache and eyestrain.

SABINA

(+FA, CB, F, Ma) sabina tree

This is a remedy that acts on the uterus and fibrous membranes. It is also good for gout. It is used as an anti-haemorrhagic remedy during childbirth to be used in conjunction with medical treatment.

Mind and emotions
The patient is extremely sensitive when listening to music and may feel sad and weepy. They are also sensitive to every noise and long for fresh air. They are worse for warmth, touch and moving about.

Physical complaints
- The patient feels that their veins are full, distended and pulsating, which is associated with repeated haemorrhage.
- It treats growths along the mucous membranes, particularly the genitalia, and is most useful for uterine haemorrhage where there is bright red blood mixed with dark clots. Use for haemorrhage from fibroids, after a miscarriage or delivery, during a heavy menstrual period or menopausal bleeding.
- They have flushes of heat but have cold hands and feet, and crave sour, juicy, refreshing foods and drinks.
- Women may have a tendency to miscarry in the third month of pregnancy due to

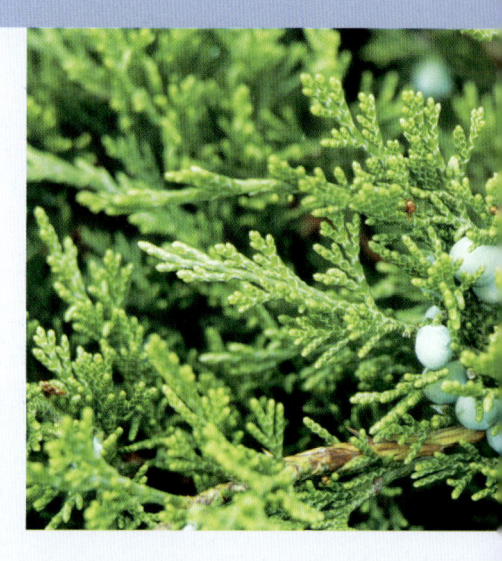

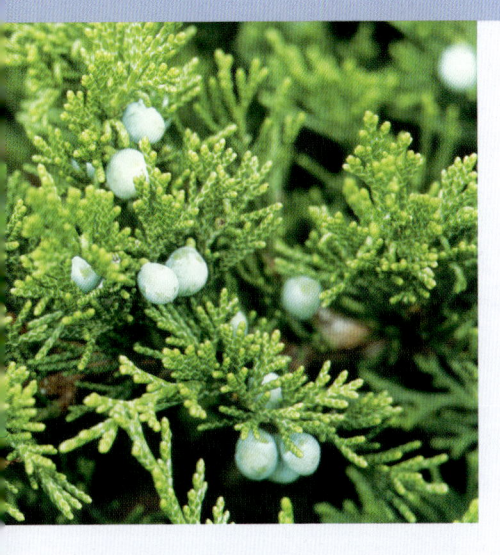

The tree Sabina is the source of a remedy for heavy bleeding during childbirth.

Key symptoms

The patient is sensitive and inclined to be sad • Heavy bleeding in women during childbirth or periods • Craves sour, juicy and refreshing foods and drinks • Miscarriage • Symptoms are better in the cool air.

atony of the uterus (where the uterus has become tired from too many births or abortions). Sabina is good for all ailments that occur after a miscarriage.

- Other symptoms include aching in the sacrum (the triangular bone in the lower back), which feels as if it is broken, bleeding between periods, and in childbirth for a retained placenta.

- Men may have inflammatory gonorrhoea with a pus-like discharge, a burning and sore pain in the glans that is accompanied by increased sexual desire.

General symptoms

Worse for the least motion, heat and warm air. Better in cool air.

SECALE CORNUTUM

(CB, D, GR) ergot fungus

Use Secale cornutum for childbirth and for old people who are weak.

Mind and emotions
The patient is weak, anxious and extremely restless. They may be inclined to want be naked in public places.

Physical complaints
- The patient experiences burning heat like fire, which makes them want to take their clothes off.
- Other symptoms include the tendency to bleed heavily, gangrene of the foot with burning sensations, bleeding that oozes and where the blood is dark and does not coagulate, and thin blood that oozes out of the uterus in between periods and at childbirth.

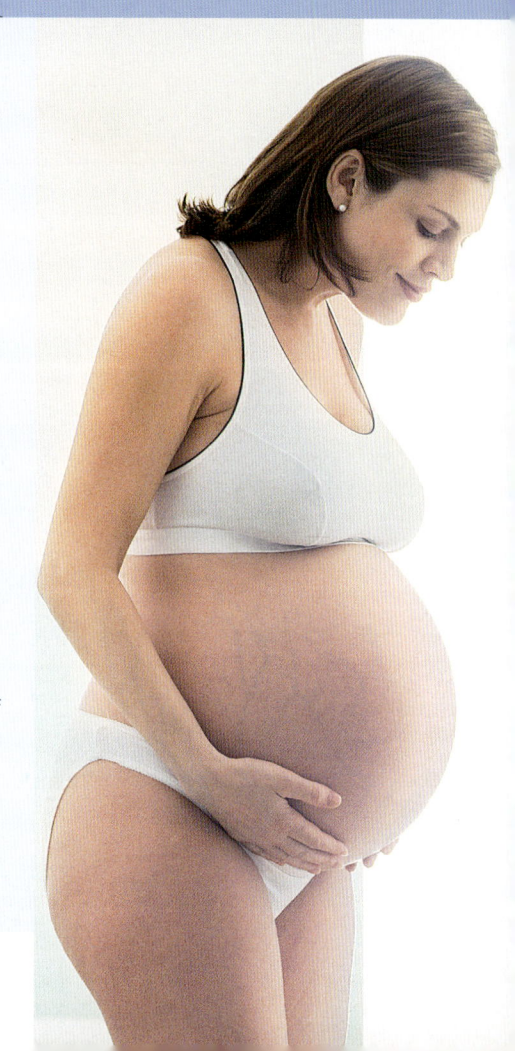

- To be used for threatened miscarriage in the third month of pregnancy.
- It also helps to expel the placenta after childbirth.

General symptoms

Icy coldness with clammy sweat and a blue tinge to the skin; the patient cannot bear to be covered. Convulsions and cramps with haemorrhage begin in the face from fright.

> **Key symptoms**
>
> *The patient is weak, anxious and restless • A burning heat felt in the body • Heavy bleeding • The patient is icy cold and clammy.*

As labour approaches, women might consider taking Secale cornutum to help expel the placenta after childbirth.

SELENIUM

(D, GR, M, Ma) selenium

This is a remedy for weakness and to alleviate the effects of ageing. It helps with strength and vitality.

Key symptoms

The patient is weak and forgetful • Old age and problems relating to ageing • Hair loss • Weakness from mental exertion, the heat or a fever.

Mind and emotions

The patient is very weak and has difficulty concentrating, so is inclined to be forgetful. They theorize constantly and have religious fantasies. Other symptoms include weariness and weakness occurring after a long fever. The patient can feel incredibly unhappy, even despairing.

Physical complaints

- The remedy will revive the body's vital forces after an illness, act as an anti-ageing tonic, and help the body recover from exhaustion due to loss of sleep.
- It is used for weakness after illness, and for hair loss from any part of the body, including eyebrows and pubic hair.
- Use Selenium as a remedy where parts of the body have become emaciated or very thin, especially extremeties such as the face and hands.
- The patient has a weak back that is worse after sex or illness.
- Men may experience a strong sexual desire accompanied by impotency, emission of prostatic fluid while walking or after a stool, or an enlarged prostate with dribbling of urine after a stool and urination.

selenium 251

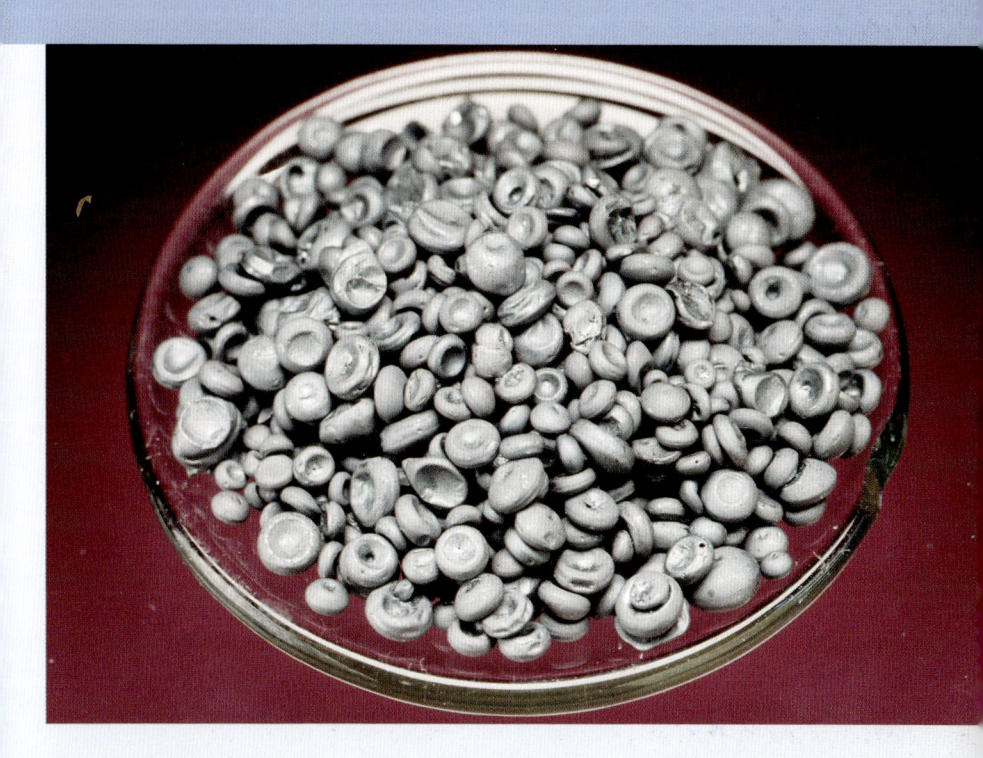

General symptoms

Weakness from mental exertion, sun and warm weather, heat, especially summer heat, and fever. Touching the hair is unbearable.

Selenium is the source mineral for a remedy to alleviate weakness, hair loss and the effects of ageing.

SEPIA

(CB, F, GR, M, Ma)
inky juice of the cuttlefish

This is a remedy primarily for women and is useful at the menopause, during pregnancy and childbirth, and at times of weakness or exhaustion.

The remedy Sepia is from the ink of the cuttlefish and is used for menopausal problems, pregnancy and childbirth.

Mind and emotions
The patient feels that they are slowing down mentally and emotionally, experiencing confusion, indifference to loved ones, and negativity about her life in every respect; she is unable or unwilling to give love and affection. She dreads being alone and is

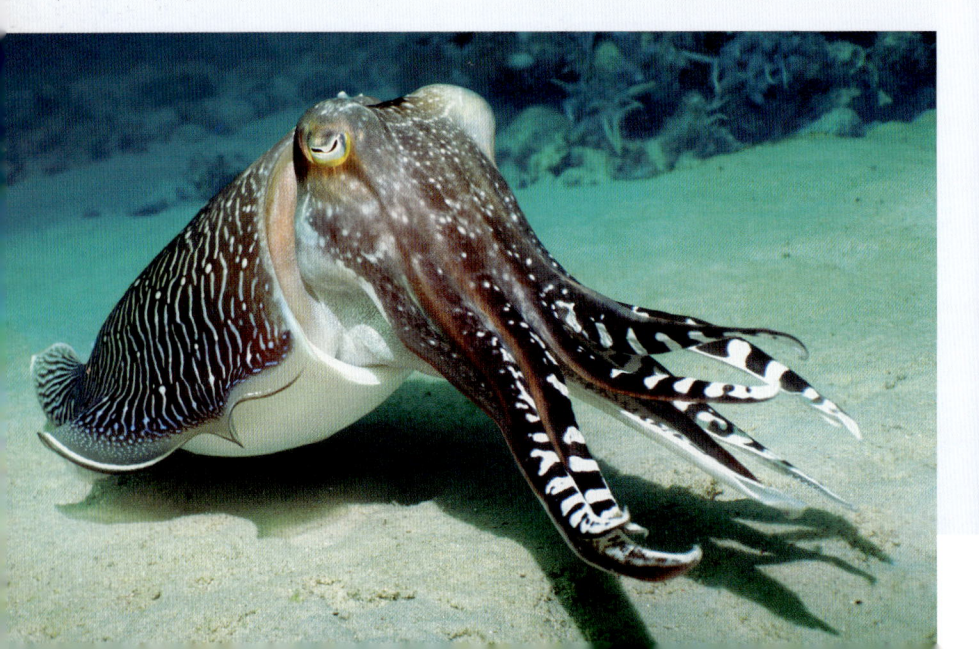

easily offended. This is a remedy for sad and unhappy women, who are miserly, defensive and uncommunicative, and who often weep, especially when compelled to give their history or tell their story.

Physical complaints

- The patient is without sexual desire and is averse or uninterested in all sexual activity; she also has fears that she will be raped, and this is often linked to a history of sexual abuse.
- Use Sepia for women who have never been well since they began taking the birth control pill.
- A sensation of emptiness will be felt in the stomach that is not relieved even after eating; the smells of food make the patient nauseous during the first three months of pregnancy.
- Other symptoms include heaviness in the eyes and uterus, with a bearing-down feeling, an itchy, dry, vaginal discharge after sex, and a prolapsed uterus.

General symptoms

Chilly at night. Being by the sea aggravates the symptoms.

> **Key symptoms**
>
> *The patient is sad and exhausted, mentally and emotionally, and dreads being alone • Exhaustion • Lack of interest in sex • Unwell since taking the birth control pill • Bearing-down feeling in the uterus • Menopausal problems • Symptoms are worse when by the sea.*

SILICA

(+FA, CR, D, GR, M) silica

Use Silica for lack of confidence, digestive problems, toothache, asthma and allergies. Also useful for helping to expel a splinter.

Mind and emotions

The patient has a deep lack of confidence and will often feel apprehensive. They are timid and delicate in character and tend to be mild and yielding as well as elegant and cultured. However, they may have many fixed ideas and thoughts, and have difficulty accepting new ones. They are precise people who like to be careful and accurate about details but have little imagination.

Physical complaints

- The patient feels worse for being cold, but perspires easily. They are also worse from suppressed sweat caused by overuse of deodorant or talc.

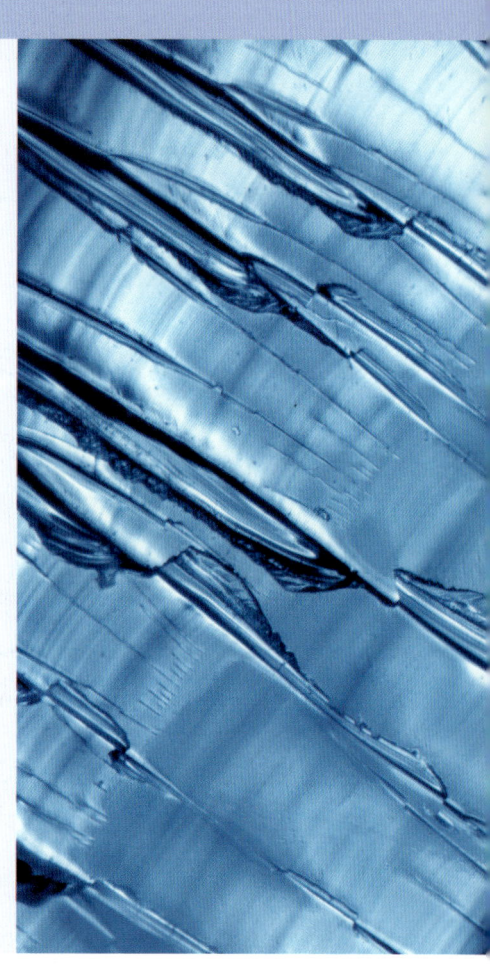

- The Silica character suffers from frequent and recurrent infections or colds, tonsillitis, bronchitis, sinusitis, boils, acne and styes, and has difficulty throwing off any of these infections.
- Generally, the patient is slow in every aspect of their life, including developing illness, and they are prone to suffering from glandular problems.
- Silica is a remedy for weak nails and hair loss, which are worse under stress. Babies can be slow to develop teeth.
- Digestive symptoms include constipation, nausea and problems with absorbing and digesting food. This is a remedy that is useful to accompany conventional medical treatment for coeliac disease.

Silica *is the source mineral for this remedy to alleviate toothache, asthma and illnesses arising from a lack of confidence.*

Key symptoms

The patient greatly lacks confidence
- *Frequent and recurrent infections or colds* • *Glandular problems* • *Weak nails* • *Asthma* • *Toothache*
- *Symptoms are worse for being cold.*

- Silica also provides the body with stamina and courage during difficult and challenging times.

General symptoms

All symptoms are made worse after vaccination against disease.

SPONGIA TOSTA

(C-C-F, CR) toasted sponge

The remedy Spongia tosta is used for colds, coughs and flu. It is also useful for children with swollen glands, and can be used for exhaustion after physical exertion for both children and adults. Spongia tosta is also a heart remedy to be used in conjunction with conventional medicine.

Mind and emotions

The patient is anxious and fearful. They are worse for moving and eating certain foods, and any exertion brings out the cough. The patient is extremely frightened that they will suffer from heart disease or even die because they have suffocated from their palpitations. They wake fearful and confused, feeling disorientated about where they are.

Physical complaints

- This is a remedy for children who are weak and pale, and who do not thrive.
- They are chilly and worse in damp weather. They also suffer dryness of the respiratory tract, but have a rattling sound in their chest.
- The patient can be asleep when an asthma attack begins so that they wake coughing and unable to catch their breath.
- They might also experience cardiac problems.
- Symptoms are worse between midnight and 2.00 a.m.
- Other symptoms include swollen, enlarged and hardened glands, as well as acute

> **Key symptoms**
>
> The patient is anxious and fearful • A weak and pale child who does not thrive • Chest problems • Exhaustion • Colds and flu • Swollen glands.

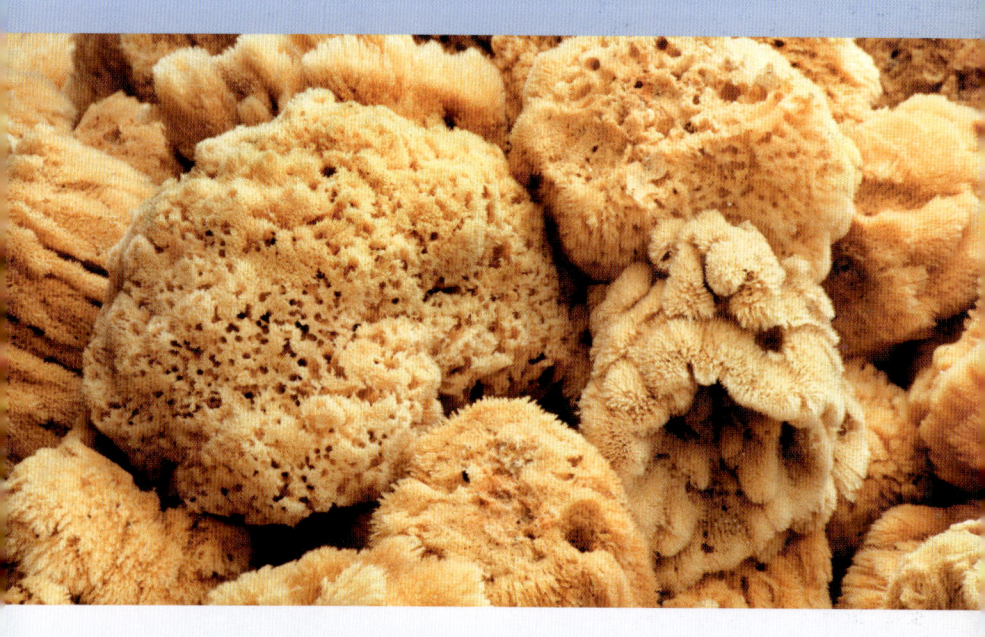

colds that settle into the larynx, resulting in further problems such as hoarseness, a dry throat and croupy coughs.
- Men may experience chronic orchitis (inflammation of the testicles) or a stitching pain in the testes that extends to the spermatic chord.

Natural sponge is the basis of this remedy for colds and flu, chest problems and for children with swollen glands.

General symptoms
Patient sleeps with head thrown backwards. Wakes suddenly after midnight with a pain in the heart and a feeling of suffocation.

STANUM METALLICUM

(C-C-F, F) tin

Use Stanum metallicum for weakened lungs where a large amount of mucus has built up in the chest, as a support therapy for conventional medical treatment.

Mind and emotions
The patient is sad and anxious, feels very discouraged and dreads seeing people. They weep and feel like crying all the time, but crying makes all the symptoms worse.

Physical complaints
- The patient has a great deal of mucus, which causes them to cough frequently and often cough up phlegm. The phlegm is copious and green, and it tastes sweet. This causes the patient to become hoarse.
- The cough is exacerbated by laughing, talking or singing and it tends to be violent and dry, especially in the evenings and at midnight.

Made from tin, the remedy Stanum metallicum is suitable for sad and anxious people who suffer from chest complaints.

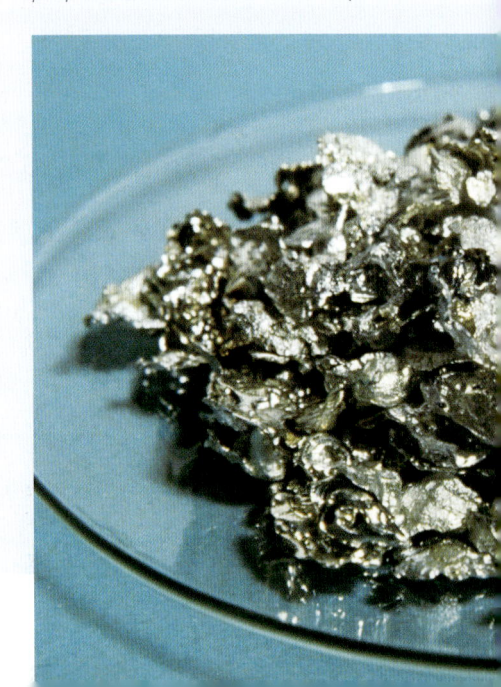

- Because of the continual coughing the chest is sore and tight and the patient feels weak and can hardly talk.
- Stanum metallicum is a remedy for a cough that accompanies flu and which comes on from midday until midnight. Breathing can be oppressive and the patient can be feverish. The arms and legs feel weak and paralysed. Fever occurs in the evening, and the patient will have exhausting night sweats.

Key symptoms

The patient is sad, anxious and weepy
- *Copious green mucus* • *Hoarseness*
- *Coughing.*

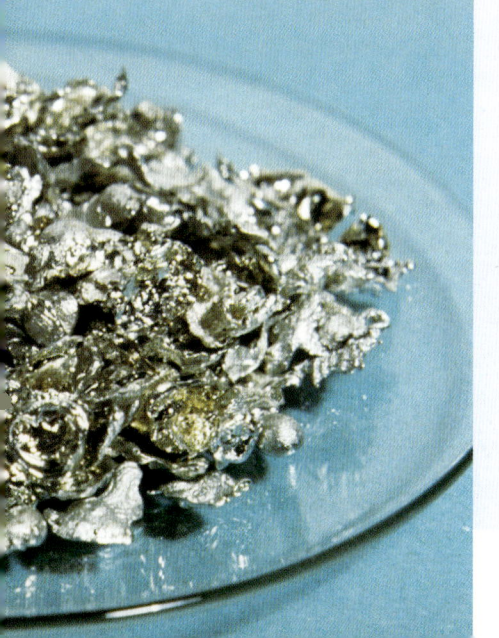

General symptoms

Perspiration after midnight until 4.00 a.m. Chest feels empty after coughing up phlegm. Asthma caused by becoming cold.

STAPHYSAGRIA

(+FA, F, GR, M)
blue delphinium flower

This is a remedy for injury to soft tissue, especially after surgery. Staphysagria is also a remedy for ailments that have been caused by emotions that have been suppressed, including those connected with sexual abuse.

Mind and emotions

The Staphysagria patient is very sensitive and has violent and passionate outbursts, which are made worse by hearing other people's opinions. It is a useful remedy for illnesses that have been caused by a person bottling up their anger inside.

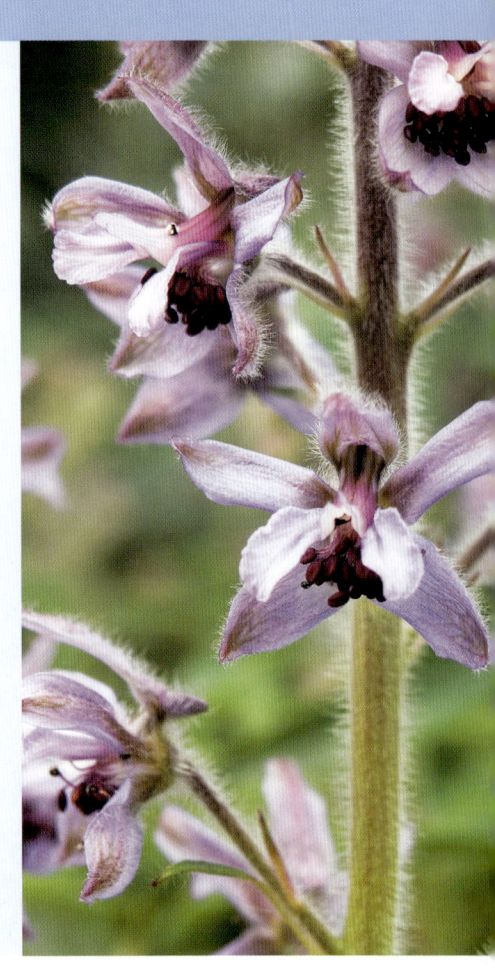

They accept the authority of others without question and are sensitive to sounds, sights, taste and touch. They are also romantic and easily disappointed, and are inclined to be very sexually aware with a history of sexual abuse, addictions to alcohol or drugs, overeating, or even overworking. They may also be constantly occupied with their children's lives.

Physical complaints

- The patient can sleep all day, but not at night and the physical symptoms are worse after sleep.
- They crave sweets, are sensitive to touch, and can tremble from anger and nervous excitement.
- Staphysagria is a remedy for cystitis after sex or after surgery.
- Other symptoms include a painful bladder and a tendency to have kidney and bladder infections and problems.

The potentized seeds of Staphysagria *(blue delphinium) produce a remedy for ailments caused by suppressed emotions.*

Key symptoms

The patient is sensitive and bottles up their anger • Sleeplessness at night • Craving for sweets • Urinary infections.

General symptoms

As this is a good remedy for any situation where there is invasive action against the body, use after dental surgery or after an operation on the soft tissues of the body such as a hysterectomy, bladder or breast surgery. Give Staphysagria for styes. It can also be given to a rape victim.

STRAMONIUM

(CB, F, GR, M, Ma) thorn apple tree

Use Stramonium for someone who is terrified or fearful. On a physical level it may be helpful in the treatment of Parkinson's disease alongside conventional medicine.

Key symptoms

The patient is full of fears and will be terrified of various imagined situations • Fright • Constipation • Lack of urination • Dim eyesight.

Mind and emotions

The patient has many fears and has experienced some form of violence in their life. They suffer from terror of the dark, certain people, from being in a war zone, under attack or seeing death. It is a useful remedy for a child who has had a violent dream. Typically, the patient awakens in fear, screaming and clinging to people close to them. Give Stramonium for all ailments that have been caused by acute fright (such as seeing a death, experiencing violence or after a life-threatening situation).

The patient has a strong desire for light and is attracted to things that glitter or reflect light. They also claim they see ghosts, hear voices and talk to spirits, or they might be overly religious. The patient is also inclined to have strange delusions about who they are.

Physical complaints

- A person who does not regularly use the toilet for either stool or urine and who rarely perspires may then suffer from other ailments that can be treated effectively with Stramonium.
- Women may suffer from abnormal bleeding from the womb, accompanied by talkativeness. Also use for convulsions that

occur after labour and for babies who have suffered traumatic or difficult births.
- Men needing this remedy may be overly interested in sex, and inclined towards indecent speech and actions, with their hands constantly on their genitals and a tendency to expose themselves.
- Also use if the patient believes they are hearing something that is not there.
- This is also a remedy for loss of vision when the patient complains that it is dark and wants the light. Their eyes will be staring and wide open with dilated pupils.
- Also if patient has an expression of terror.

General symptoms

Convulsions caused by bright lights; fainting in dark places. Fear of tunnels and other narrow places.

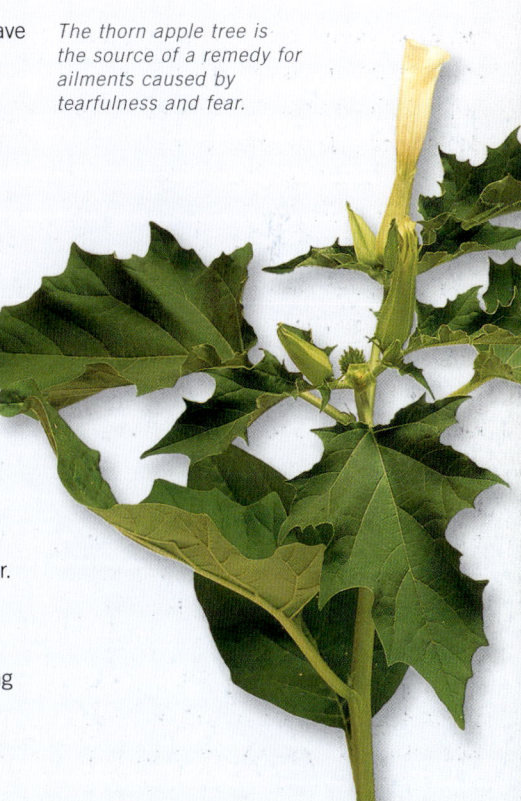

The thorn apple tree is the source of a remedy for ailments caused by tearfulness and fear.

SULPHUR

(C-C-F, D, F, GR, M, Ma) sulphur

The remedy Sulphur is useful in treating the mind and lungs, and also for skin problems, joints and the glands.

Mind and emotions

The patient is a hopeful dreamer, someone who thinks deeply about life, who is an idealist and is always theorizing. However, they are also forgetful, and wrongly believe that they are wealthy, seeing things around them as beautiful even when they are in bad repair. The patient has no focus and no depth; an idealist who is superficial and who theorizes and pontificates. This is someone who is busy all the time, irritable, very selfish and self-absorbed, and can also be lazy, easy living, untidy and rarely clean. They will also have a fear of high places and may suffer from dizziness or vertigo.

This is a remedy for ailments caused by embarrassment or anxiety about health.

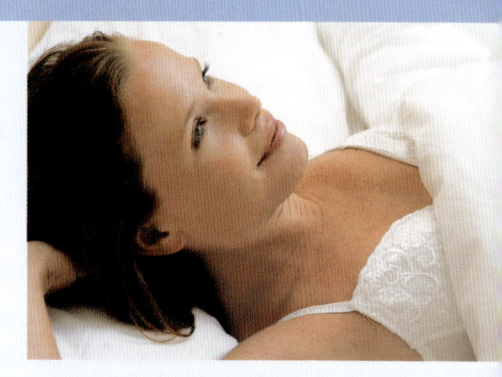

Physical complaints

- The patient suffers from sick, beating headaches that recur periodically and are worse from stooping over.
- The scalp is dry and hair tends to fall out.
- The skin burns and itches.
- The patient might have boils that are slow to develop and to heal.
- Other symptoms are burning eyes, a whizzing sound in the ears, sensitive hearing followed by deafness.
- The throat will be red and burning, and the appetite is either excessive or

Sulphur might be an appropriate remedy when the patient is a dreamy idealist.

completely gone, leaving a foul taste in the mouth and a craving for sweets.
- The patient feels very weak and faint at about 11.00 a.m. and needs to have something to eat.
- The anus itches and burns, and there will be haemorrhoids and hard stools with diarrhoea in the mornings.
- There may be burning feelings in the chest, which makes breathing difficult so that the patient requires fresh air. The patient has a loose cough, which is worse when talking or in the morning, and is accompanied by greenish phlegm.
- Rheumatic gout is also linked to this remedy, with burning in the soles of the feet and the hands at night. The patient also has dry, unhealthy skin and is thirsty.

Key symptoms

The patient is an idealist and a dreamer • Sick, beating headaches • Dry scalp • Burning and itching skin • Burning eyes or throat • Symptoms are better when the patient is active.

- Men will have stitching pains in the penis with itching genitals.
- Women may have itching genitals with a burning sensation in the vagina; they may also have cracked and burning nipples.
- Use at the end of a bout of bronchitis to help the patient to regain strength.

General symptoms

Worse for rest and the warmth of bed. Worse for alcohol and washing. Better for dry, warm weather, and for lying on the right side.

SYMPHYTUM

(+FA) comfrey plant

This is a useful remedy for injury to bones and the eyes.

Mind and emotions
No symptoms.

Physical complaints
- Use this first-aid remedy to help heal fractures, and when bones fail to knit properly (the old-fashioned name for Symphytum is 'boneset').
- To be used for pricking, stitching pains that remain after a wound has healed.
- For injury to the eyeball and pain that has been caused by this.
- Also use after amputation if the stumps of the limbs irritate.
- Useful for backaches that have been caused by too much sex.
- Symphytum is a remedy to help mend tissue together wherever it has been cut or torn apart.

General symptoms
Injuries to the eye, and broken bones.

> **Key symptoms**
>
> *Fractures • Pricking, stitching pains on a wound site • Eye injuries.*

Made from comfrey, this remedy is used for injuries to the bones and eyes.

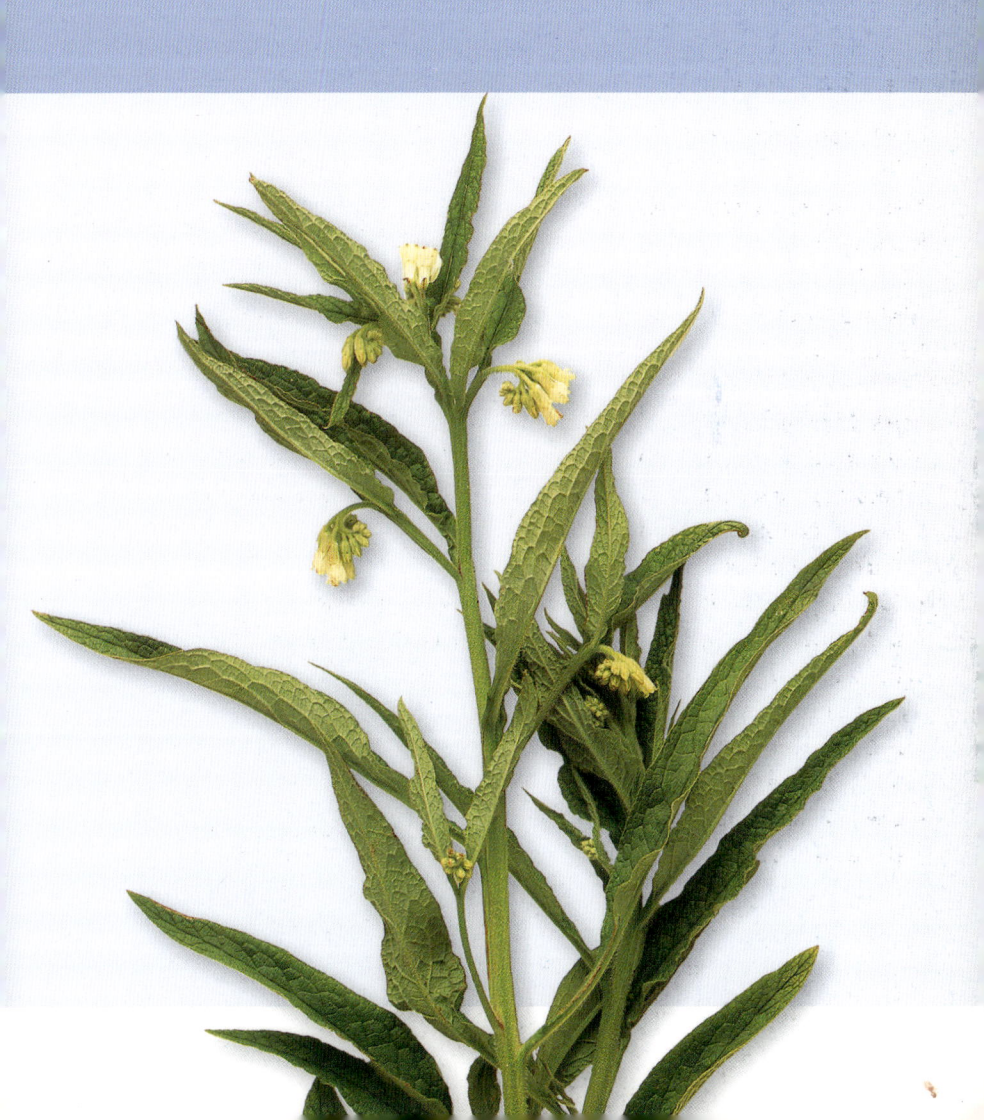

symphytum

SYZYGIUM

(D) jambul seeds

This is a remedy that is specifically for diabetes to remove sugar from the urine and should be used as a support therapy with conventional medicine.

Mind and emotions
No symptoms.

Physical complaints
- For diabetes and diabetes ulcerations. Syzygium can help to remove sugar from the urine. It is not intended to replace conventional insulin treatments but to work alongside them.
- Syzygium helps to tonify the pancreas.
- Also use for prickly heat and small red pimples that itch violently.

> **Key symptoms**
>
> *Small red pimples that itch violently • Prickly heat on the skin • Frequent thirst • Diabetes.*

General symptoms
Great thirst, weakness, loss of weight, with a frequent need to urinate. Old ulcers and skin sores.

A remedy to treat prickly heat and to accompany conventional diabetes treatments is derived from jambul seeds.

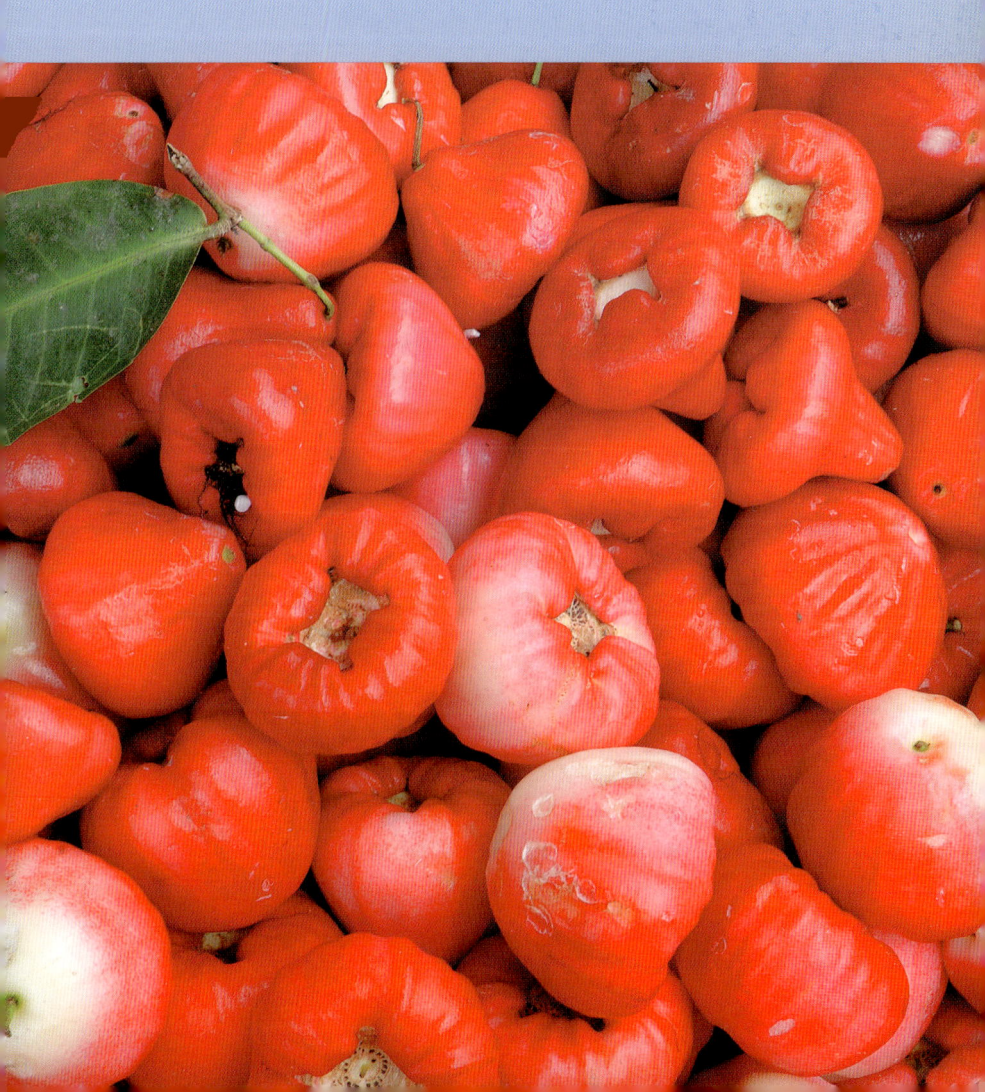

syzygium

TABACUM

(D, GR, M) tobacco leaves

This is a remedy for digestive upsets, collapse, seasickness and eye problems.

Mind and emotions
The patient feels forgetful, very low and generally discontented.

Physical complaints
- A sick headache, with dizziness and nausea, is a common symptom.
- Their face appears sunken and covered with a cold sweat.
- Symptoms of the stomach include constant nausea that is worse from smelling tobacco smoke, and the patient will vomit when they move.
- Tabacum is a useful remedy during pregnancy and for seasickness.

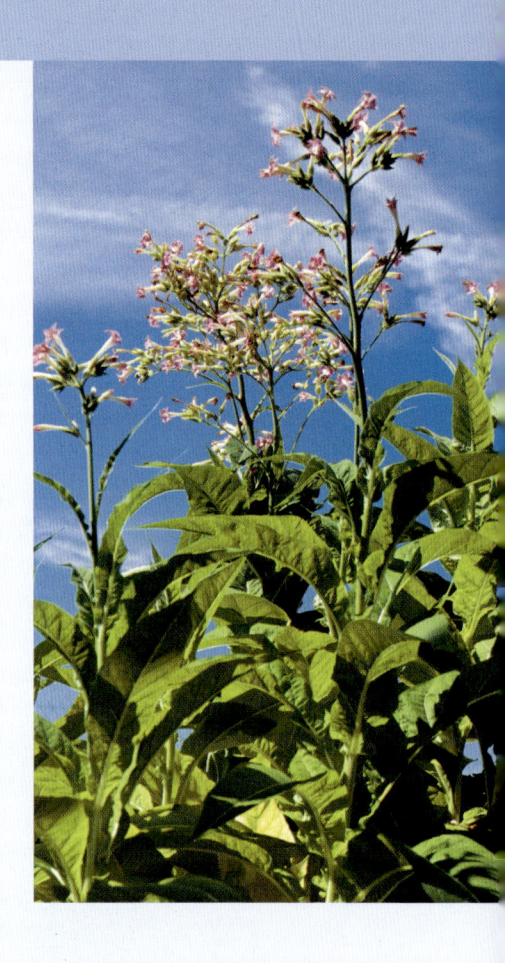

Dizziness, nausea and seasickness can be treated with the remedy Tabacum, which has tobacco leaves as its source.

- The patient will suffer from dim eyesight or blindness that comes on suddenly with wearing down of the optic nerve.
- Other symptoms include constipation or diarrhoea that is sudden and watery, accompanied by nausea and vomiting, extreme weakness with a cold sweat, palpitations, and an intermittent and feeble pulse.
- People who suffer from angina pectoris that is caused by shock or violent exercise may benefit from using this remedy with their medical treatment.

General symptoms

Worse for opening their eyes when feeling ill. Worse for extreme heat or cold. Better uncovered and in fresh air.

> **Key symptoms**
>
> The patient is in low spirits and discontented • Sick headache with dizziness and nausea • Nausea that is worse from smelling tobacco smoke • Seasickness • Symptoms are worse for extreme heat or cold.

TARANTULA CUBENSIS

(M, D, F, GR) cuban spider

The remedy Tarantula cubensis is predominately a remedy for overactive children but it is also very useful to calm someone who is dying and who is agitated and afraid.

Mind and emotions

The patient is extremely restless and needs to be moving constantly, although motion makes all the symptoms worse. They might feel they want to jump and climb, and that they have boundless energy. Always in a hurry, the typical Tarantula cubensis patient is very impatient and their hands and legs will always be moving. They love music, especially a good rhythm, dancing, horse-riding and massage, although being overexcited causes them to lack control mentally and physically.

Inclined to be cunning and devious, there is often a sense of threatening, violent and unexpected behaviour, which might be destructive, that is characteristic of the Tarantula cubensis person. They are guided by their whims and act impulsively. They enjoy laughter, but also play pranks and jokes, and will do absurd things.

Physical complaints

- The patient is chilly but loves the fresh air; they love spicy foods, and are worse for being touched although they feel better when massaged.
- Their body twitches and jerks and they are very thirsty for cold water.
- The genitals are inclined to be sensitive.
- The patient is often constipated, accompanied by anxiety and restlessness.

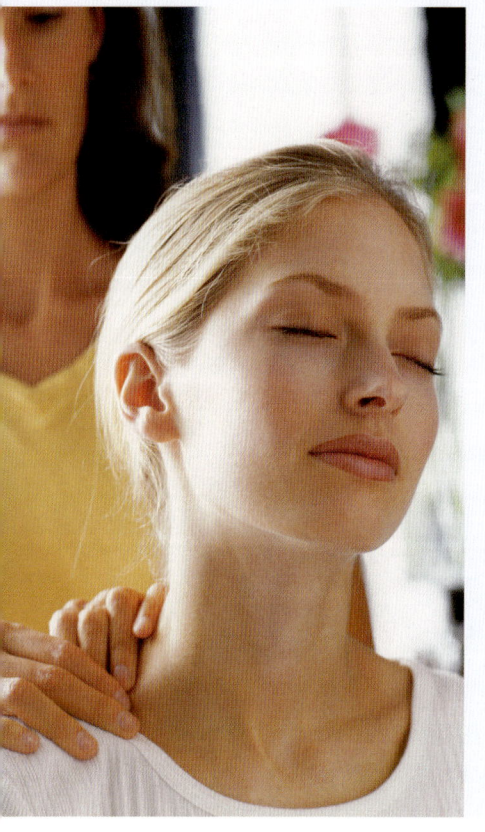

> ### Key symptoms
>
> The patient is restless and impatient • Feels chilly but prefers fresh air • Twitching and jerky movements • Thirsty • Constipation.

General symptoms

Extreme sensitivity to the tips of the fingers, with a painful spine. Touch creates pains elsewhere in the body. Hyperactive children, and people who are agitated and afraid at the end of their life. Give Tarantula cubensis to someone at the end of their life to help them pass on in a more gentle way.

When a person's symptoms are generally worse for touch but improve when gently massaged, Tarantula cubensis is a useful calming remedy.

TARACUM

(D) dandelion plant

This is a specific remedy for liver problems. Taraxacum will tonify the liver and can be used in conjunction with conventional medicine to help cancer of the bladder.

Mind and emotions

The patient is gloomy when unoccupied, worrying about their health and feeling isolated from the outside world. They can also be overly concerned about others so that they care little about themselves.

Physical complaints
- The patient suffers with jaundice of the skin caused by hepatitis or an enlarged liver.
- They have sharp stitching pains on the left side of the body and their bowels feel as if they will burst.
- They are constipated and have neuralgia of the limbs. They will also sweat heavily during the night.

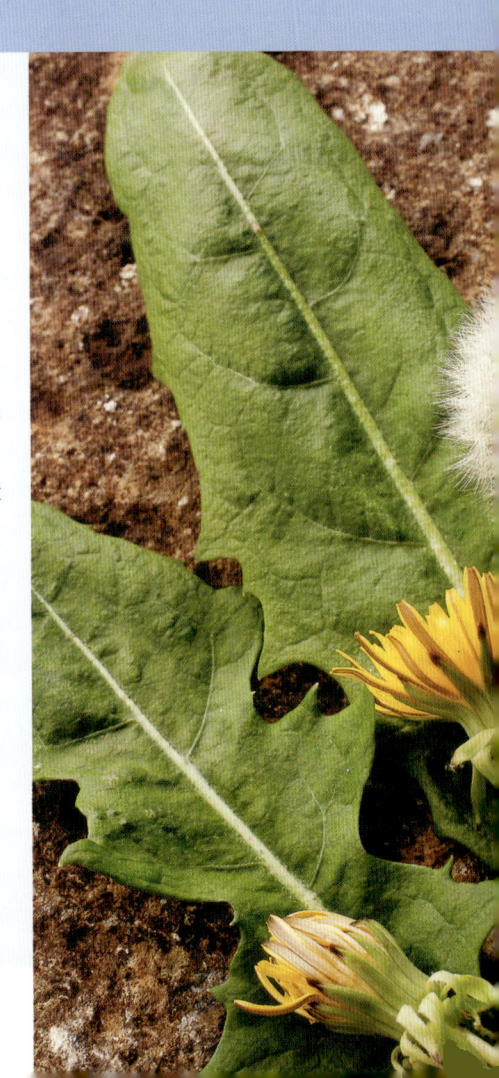

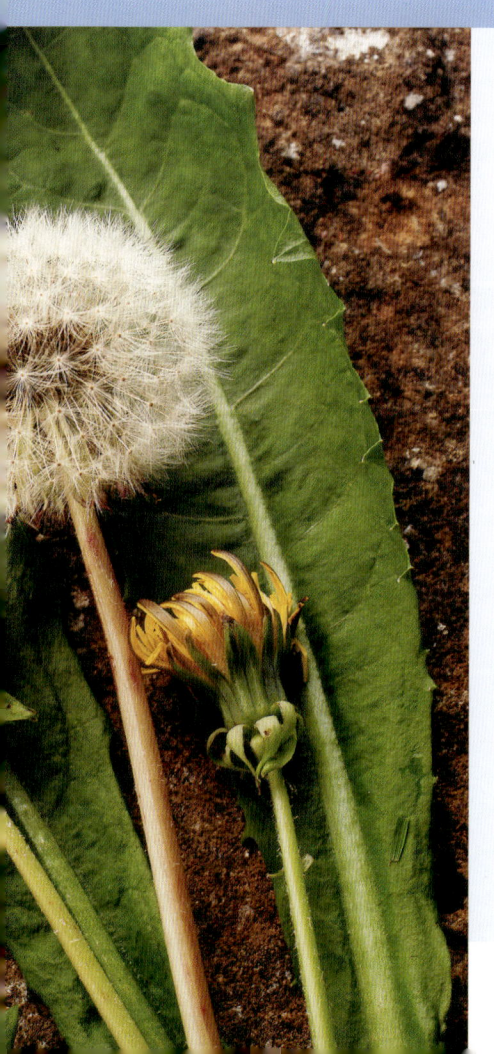

A remedy derived from dandelion is suited to people who worry about their health.

- Their tongue is covered with a white film, and they will have lost their appetite; there is also a bitter taste in the mouth with burping and flatulence.

General symptoms

Worse for resting, lying down or sitting in a chair. A useful remedy to accompany cancer treatment, as it treats the liver.

> **Key symptoms**
>
> *The patient is gloomy and needs to be busy • Sharp pains on the left side of the body • Uncomfortable bowels • Heavy perspiration at night • White coating on the tongue • Constipation.*

THUJA OCCIDENTALIS

(M, C-C-F, Ma, F, D, GR)
arbor vitae, white cedar

The remedy Thuja occidentalis is suitable for many conditions. It works on the skin, blood, gastro-intestinal tract, genitalia, kidneys and brain. It is also a remedy for warts, fibroids and tumours in conjunction with conventional medicine.

Mind and emotions

The patient has fanciful ideas and believes they are superhuman; they are inclined to be fanatical and may have religious delusions, believing in divine intervention so that they do not see the need to take any responsibility for themselves. They have fixed ideas and become anxious about minor or imaginary things. They also feel that their body is frail. They are self-contained, polite and appear to be conventional. However, they suffer from low self-esteem and feel that they are unlovable and that people would not love

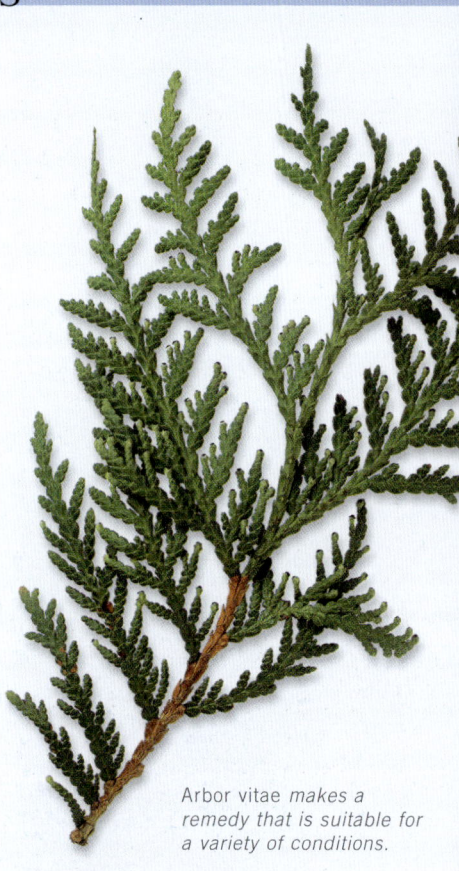

Arbor vitae makes a remedy that is suitable for a variety of conditions.

them if they knew who they really were. So that they will be accepted they imitate others. Their outer appearance is very important to them. They may have dreams of falling and of the dead.

Physical complaints

- The patient has copious yellow-green discharges, which can be a sign of suppressed gonorrhoea.
- Other symptoms include pain in small areas, various kinds of warts and polyps on the skin, and also chronic urinary or ovarian problems.
- This is a good support remedy for fibroids, tumours and endometriosis.
- Men may have erections that are troublesome during stool, with an itching and sweating penis.
- Women may have condylomata (raised growths) on the uterus or vagina, inflammation of the ovaries, itching during urination, and a vagina that has a burning sensation while sitting.

Key symptoms

They patient is anxious about minor things • Warts and growths on the skin • Yellow-green discharges • Back injuries.

General symptoms

Back injuries that are worse for jarring, ridges in the nails and whitlows on the hands that appear after vaccination. There may also be lots of perspiration on the body although none on the head.

URTICA URENS

(+FA, D, F) stinging nettle

The remedy Urtica urens is used for skin irritation with burning and stinging and is a support remedy for gout.

Mind and emotions
No symptoms.

Physical complaints
- The patient suffers from stinging and burning pains.
- This is a remedy for acute gout, hives, rheumatism or arthritis, to use with conventional medicine.
- The patient is worse for eating shellfish and may have an allergic skin reaction where there is burning and itching.
- Digestive symptoms include diarrhoea that has been caused by eruptions that have become suppressed; pungently smelling urine that causes itching.
- Breastfeeding women may have swollen breasts with an absence of milk for no apparent cause.

General symptoms
Worse for eating highly acidic foods such as shellfish. Snowy air aggravates.

> ### Key symptoms
> Stinging and burning pains • Hives, rheumatism, gout or arthritis • Symptoms are worse for eating shellfish.

Stinging nettles when in flower are used to make this remedy for stinging and burning pains, rheumatism and arthritis.

urtica urens

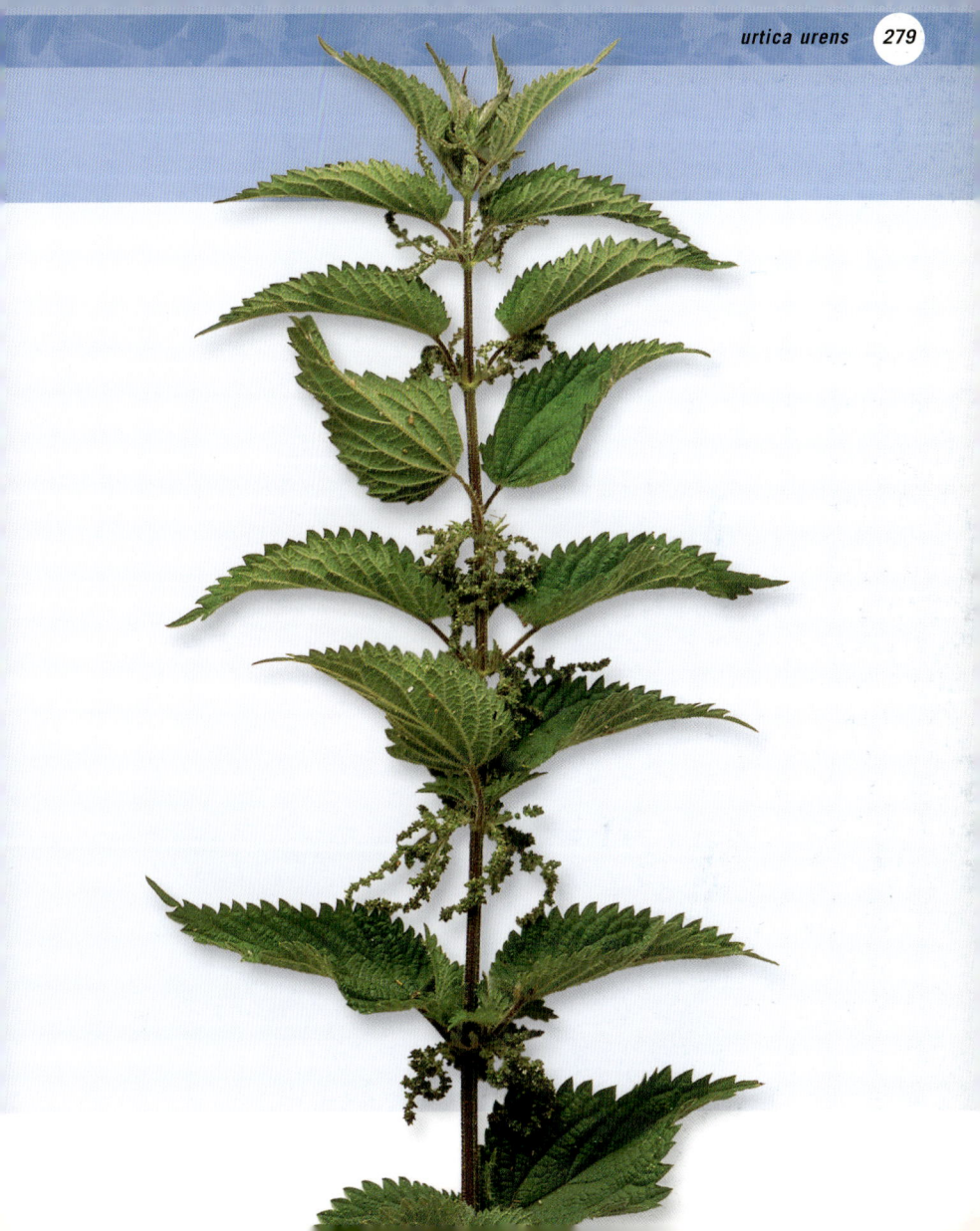

VERATRUM ALBUM

(D, F, GR, M) white helleborus

This is a remedy for a wide spectrum of symptoms ranging from mental problems to cholera-like symptoms with diarrhoea. It also helps the body to recover from surgery.

Mind and emotions

Veratrum album is a remedy for hyperactive minds. The patient suffers from mental overstimulation, overactivity and restlessness. Hard working, restless and high-spirited, they are ambitious and use every means to reach their goal, and they also strongly believe that they are special. Flattering and affectionate, they will embrace everyone in the room, but can also be scornful and hard on people who work for them, while being agreeable to superiors and people they fear. They can also be inclined to feign sickness in order to get sympathy from others. They have fears about their position in society or within the family.

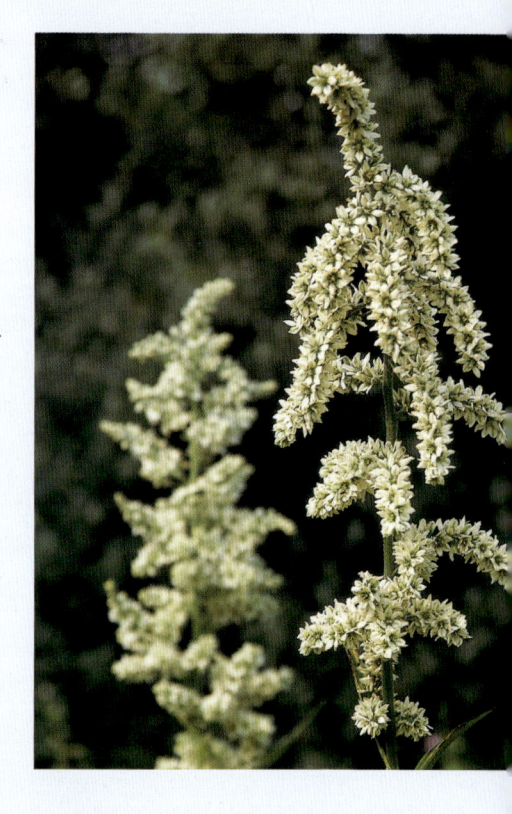

veratrum album

Key symptoms

The patient is overactive and restless.
• Cold in places or all over, and with cold perspiration • Craves acidic fruits, salt and cold drinks • Spasms and cramps.

Use this remedy for someone who is incapable of speaking the truth, as well as for mental instability, depression, indifference and feeling abandoned. Ailments that are caused by injured pride are also helped with this remedy.

White helleborus is the source of a remedy suited to overactive people. It covers a wide range of symptoms.

Physical complaints

- The patient may be very cold in specific places or generally all over and will also have cold perspiration.
- The patient craves acidic fruits, salt and cold drinks.
- They also suffer from a sudden sinking feeling, with spasms and cramps.
- This is a remedy for cholera with excessive diarrhoea and watery stools.
- Pain that produces delirium, vomiting and diarrhoea simultaneously will also benefit from Veratrum album.

General symptoms

Convulsions with coldness of the body and a ravenous appetite.

VIBURNUM OPULUS

(F) high-bush cranberry

This is a general remedy for cramps and possible miscarriage.

Mind and emotions

The patient is very restless and nervous during her menstrual periods and finds she can't keep still.

Physical complaints

- The patient suffers from spasms and painful cramps.
- This is a remedy for a threatened early miscarriage, which should always be referred to a doctor.
- The patient has constant nausea, which is relieved only by food. There are sudden cramps and colicky pains.
- The menstrual periods can be too late and too scanty, lasting just a few hours and accompanied by an offensive odour and cramping pains extending down the thigh. The area around the ovaries feels heavy and congested, with aching in the lower back and the lower front of the abdomen.
- The patient needs to urinate frequently and has a stiff and sore feeling at the nape of their neck.
- The back feels as if it will break from pain.

General symptoms

Worse lying on the affected side, in a warm room, in the evening and night. Better in fresh air and for resting.

Key symptoms

Restless and nervous during periods • Spasms and cramps • Nausea, relieved by food • Late and scanty periods • Symptoms are better for air and rest.

viburnum opulus 283

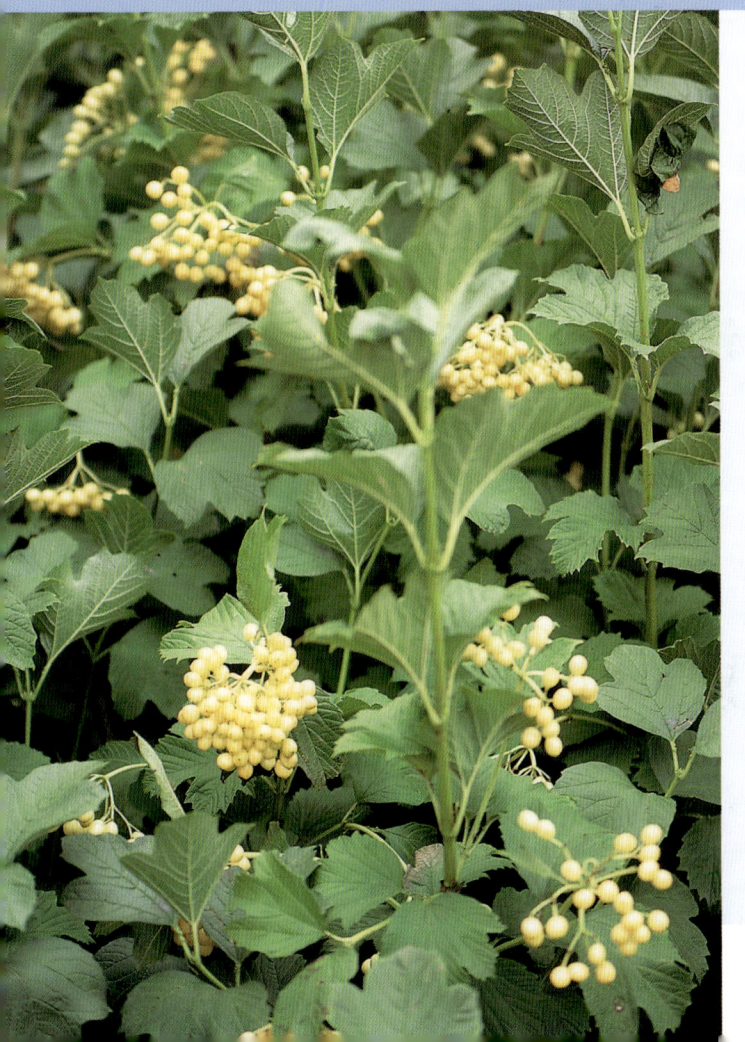

Viburnum opulus, from the berry-bearing shrub, is good for cramps and miscarriage.

VIOLA TRICOLOR

(+FA, CR, F) wild pansy

This is a remedy for ear problems in children. It is also used for measles, worms, snake bites and bee stings. Viola tricolor is also a remedy for carpal tunnel syndrome where the median nerve, which runs from the forearm into the hand, becomes pressed or squeezed at the wrist.

Mind and emotions

The patient is tense, nervous and suffering from sudden exhaustion. They have serious thoughts and their head rules their heart. They have a weak memory and their thoughts often wander.

Physical complaints

- An excellent headache remedy.
- Viola tricolor is also good for earache in children.
- The patient knits their brows together because of a tightness felt in their head.
- It is also a remedy for the pain, tingling and numbness in the thumb and fingers caused by swelling in the carpal tunnel pressing on the median nerve. This can make it difficult to grip things.

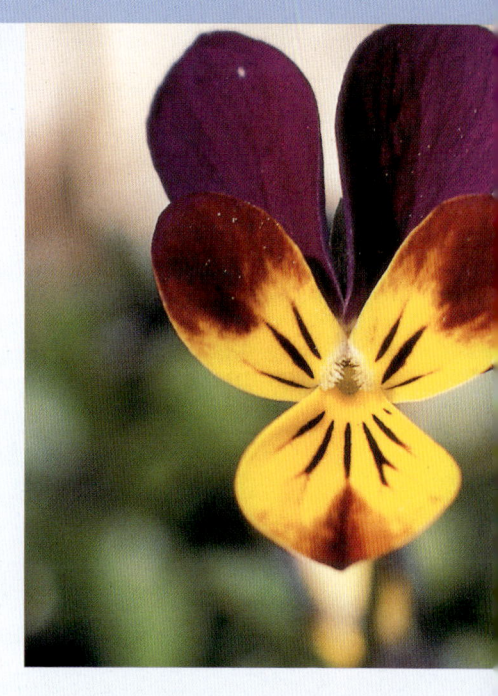

viola tricolor

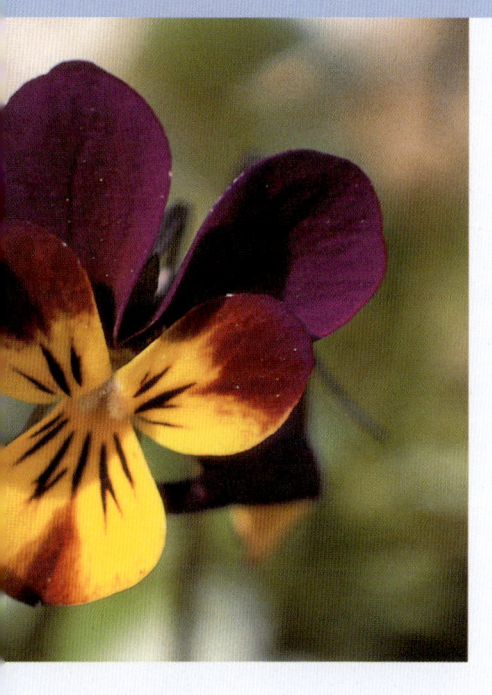

Key symptoms

The patient is tense and nervous. They have a poor memory • Headache • Earache in children • Tight feeling in the head • Measles.

This remedy for ear problems in children as well as snake bites and bee stings uses the wild pansy.

General symptoms

Measles, where the skin is hot and dry and the palms moist, and a sensation of burning occurs in small spots; to accompany conventional medical treatment.

VISCUM ALBUM

(D, GR, M) mistletoe

The remedy Viscum album is used for mental and emotional problems and the sudden onset of pain.

Mind and emotions

The patient dwells on the past. They are negative and full of dark, persistent thoughts. They suffer with depression, are tired, sad and worse for consolation. Although worn out and apathetic towards others, the patient is restless. They are oversensitive, have an aversion to people and want to be left alone. They have a tendency to go to the extremes and can be very fearful of open spaces, public places, buildings and the telephone. They are also overly sensitive to change and to new surroundings.

Physical complaints

- The patient's pains are caused by sudden spasms, such as angina pectoris, asthma, palpitations, an abnormally rapid heartbeat and explosive stools.
- They are extremely weak and have tired and restless legs.
- They are chilly, even near a source of heat, and are lacking in vital warmth.
- They fall asleep late and wake early, and their sleep is not deep enough.
- They suffer from dull, pressing, hammering and bursting headaches.

> **Key symptoms**
>
> *The patient is depressed and oversensitive, with negative thoughts • Pains caused by sudden spasms • Tired and restless legs • Feels chilly • Insufficient sleep • Hammering headaches.*

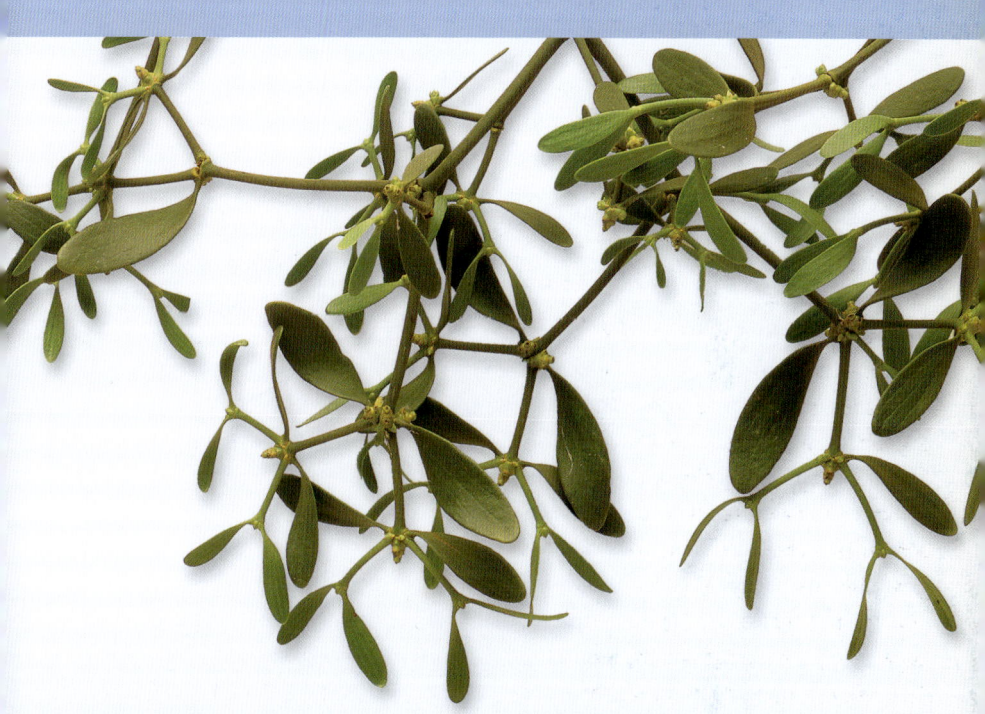

General symptoms

Patient experiences a sensation of a glowing coal under the right shoulder blade. Pain in the lower back and stiffness in moving. Good for arthritis of the knee.

A treatment for pain that appears suddenly, as well as emotional problems, is derived from mistletoe.

ZINCUM METALLICUM

(D, F, GR, M, Ma) zinc

This is a remedy for someone who is thoroughly exhausted emotionally, physically and mentally.

Mind and emotions

The patient is mentally exhausted and unable to express themselves freely. However, they constantly complain and moan; they can't let go of the things that bother them. This is a remedy for ailments that are caused by loss of sleep, fright, stress, exhausting diseases and alcoholism.

Physical complaints

- The patient suffers from increased weakness and restlessness.
- There are suppressed discharges such as: coughing up phlegm, foot sweat, periods, milk and perspiration.
- The patient suffers from a lack of vitality and weak nerves as well as poor digestion.

> **Key symptoms**
>
> *The patient is exhausted emotionally and physically • Poor digestion • Symptoms are worse for alcohol.*

- Women feel better when they have regular menstrual periods.
- Men and women feel better when they can clear their throats of phlegm when they cough, making the lungs more functional.
- The patient is worse for alcohol and cannot tolerate the smallest amount of wine.
- They can suffer from vertigo, headaches, a red face, weakness, weariness, asthma, confusion, constipation or diarrhoea and also coughs.
- The digestive symptoms include nausea, vomiting bitter mucus, burning in the

zincum metallicum

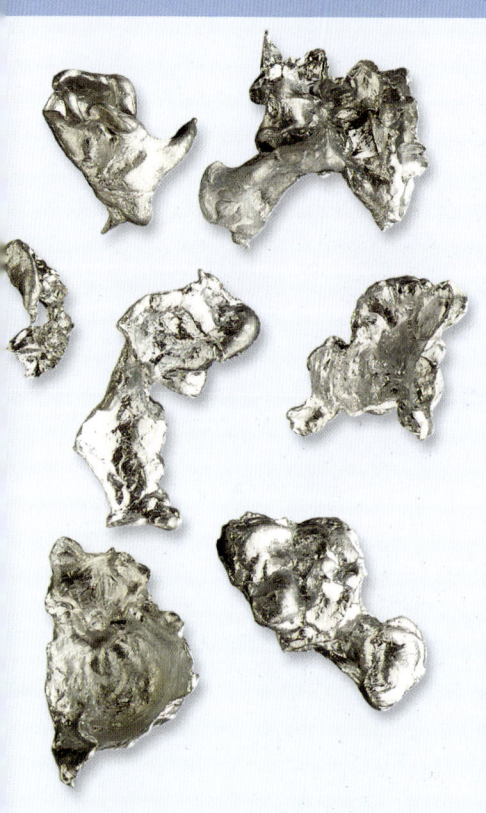

The mineral zinc forms a remedy for treating mental and physical exhaustion.

stomach, greediness when eating and where the patient cannot eat fast enough, pains after a light meal, an enlarged liver or constipation.
- This is a remedy to help a person with anorexia, alongside appropriate professional treatment.
- Women may experience ovarian pain, especially on the left side, painful breasts, and painful and sore nipples. Complaints improve during a menstrual period.
- Men may have testicles that are swollen and drawn up.

General symptoms
Varicose veins. Eczema in someone who is anaemic and highly emotional. General weakness and weariness. The patient is unable to throw off illness due to a build-up of toxins in the body that stops the immune system from working properly.

ZINGIBER OFFICINALE

(C-C-F, D, GR, M) ginger

This is a remedy for poor digestion, sexual problems in men and respiratory problems.

Mind and emotions
The patient has fanciful dreams. They fear something will happen. They are very friendly and easy-going.

Physical complaints
- Those needing this remedy are chilly, with poor digestion, always thirsty and have a dry mouth.
- They suffer from diarrhoea and are worse after having eaten vegetables and fruit, especially melons.
- This is a remedy to treat symptoms of nausea and indigestion.
- The patient is extremely hoarse and is unable to talk.
- Also use Zingiber officinale to treat asthma during the night.

> **Key symptoms**
>
> *The patient has fanciful dreams, is agreeable in nature but sometimes fearful • Feels chilly • Diarrhoea • Thirsty • Symptoms are worse from eating fruit and vegetables.*

- Men may find that the remedy helps painful erections.

General symptoms
The patient has weak joints. Their back is painful and they have cramps in the soles of their feet.

Made from ginger root, the remedy Zingiber officinale soothes poor digestion, diarrhoea and nausea.

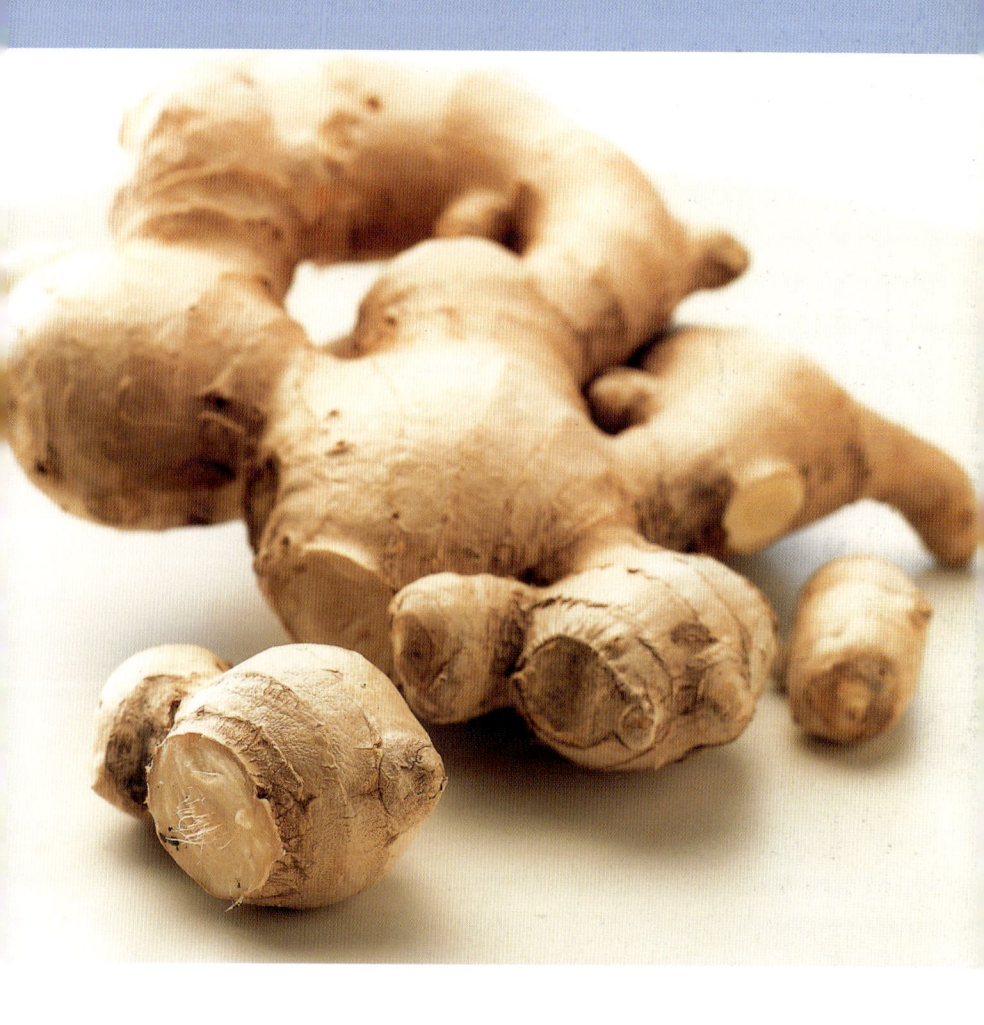

zingiber officinale

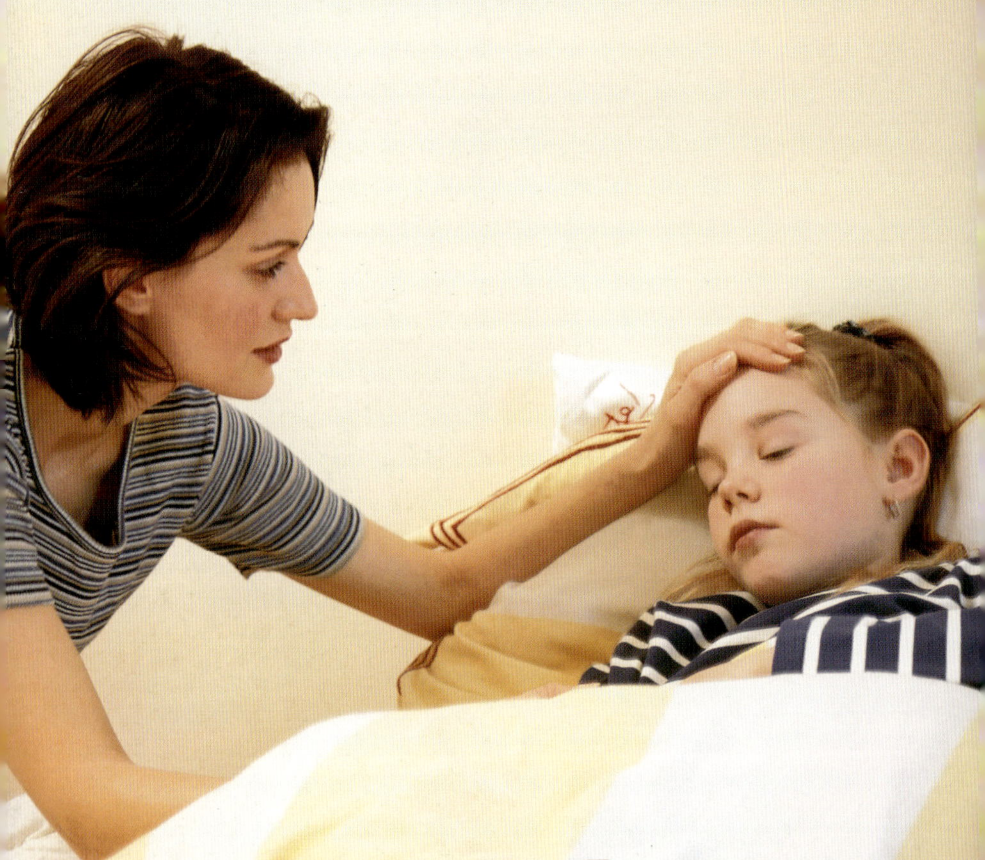

PART THREE

treating acute and chronic conditions

how to self-prescribe

In this part of the book you will find a list of common conditions that respond well to homeopathic treatment. A number of remedies may be listed for each condition, so refer to the remedy entry in the Materia Medica section (pages 54–291) to determine which one best addresses your symptoms.

Refer back to the section on dosage in How to Choose a Remedy (pages 38–39) so that you can decide which potency to begin with. Take your chosen remedy as follows:

- If you decide a 6X remedy is appropriate, repeat the remedy every two hours until your condition improves. You should see an improvement after a few doses or over a few days. When the condition stops being troublesome stop taking the remedy.
- A 12C potency should be taken two times in a day until the condition has stopped.
- If you choose a 30C potency, take once in a day and wait to see if the condition has abated. If necessary take another dose the next day, but do not repeat the dosage if the condition is beginning to improve.

If you continue to take a remedy after symptoms have stopped you may possibly create that condition again by using too much of the remedy.

MONITORING IMPROVEMENT

All treatment should begin with a single dose of a remedy. Wait and watch to see how the symptoms change. If there is no apparent change, consider repeating the dose again before trying another remedy. If a remedy fails to act after a few doses as noted above you may want to consider whether another remedy is better suited to your condition.

Danger signs

If there are symptoms that are out of the ordinary and persist following treatment, such as a very high fever, projectile vomiting, diarrhoea or other acute symptoms, please consult your doctor immediately.

In acute cases you may give a single remedy two or three times every few minutes. As the symptoms change spread the remedies out until the condition has righted itself. Once the symptoms have disappeared stop taking the remedy.

When you treat children you should expect to see an improvement in their symptoms very quickly. Homeopathic remedies can transform a crying and unhappy child, with fever or pain, very rapidly. Once their symptoms have stopped you must stop giving the child the remedy. If the symptoms do not subside after giving a remedy you should call your doctor.

Remember: any time you have an acute emergency call your doctor.

Note: *Remedies marked with two asterisks (**) are recommended for specific uses and do not appear in the Materia Medica.*

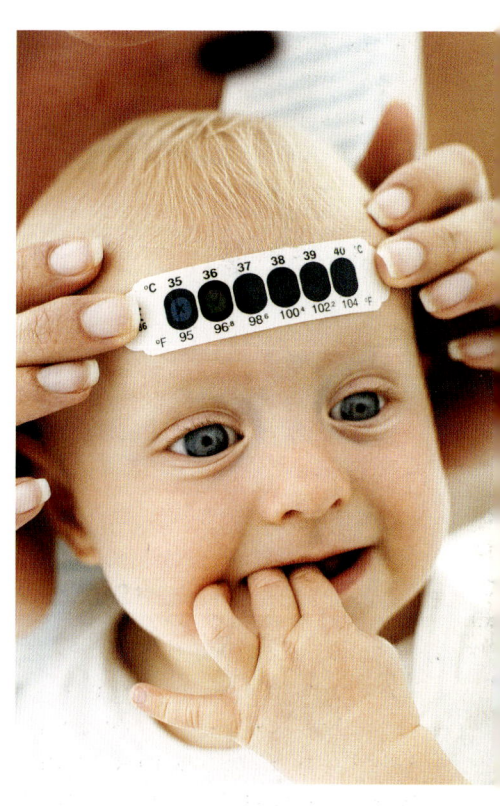

Monitor a child's condition constantly, as you should see an improvement soon after administering the remedy.

circulatory and respiratory systems

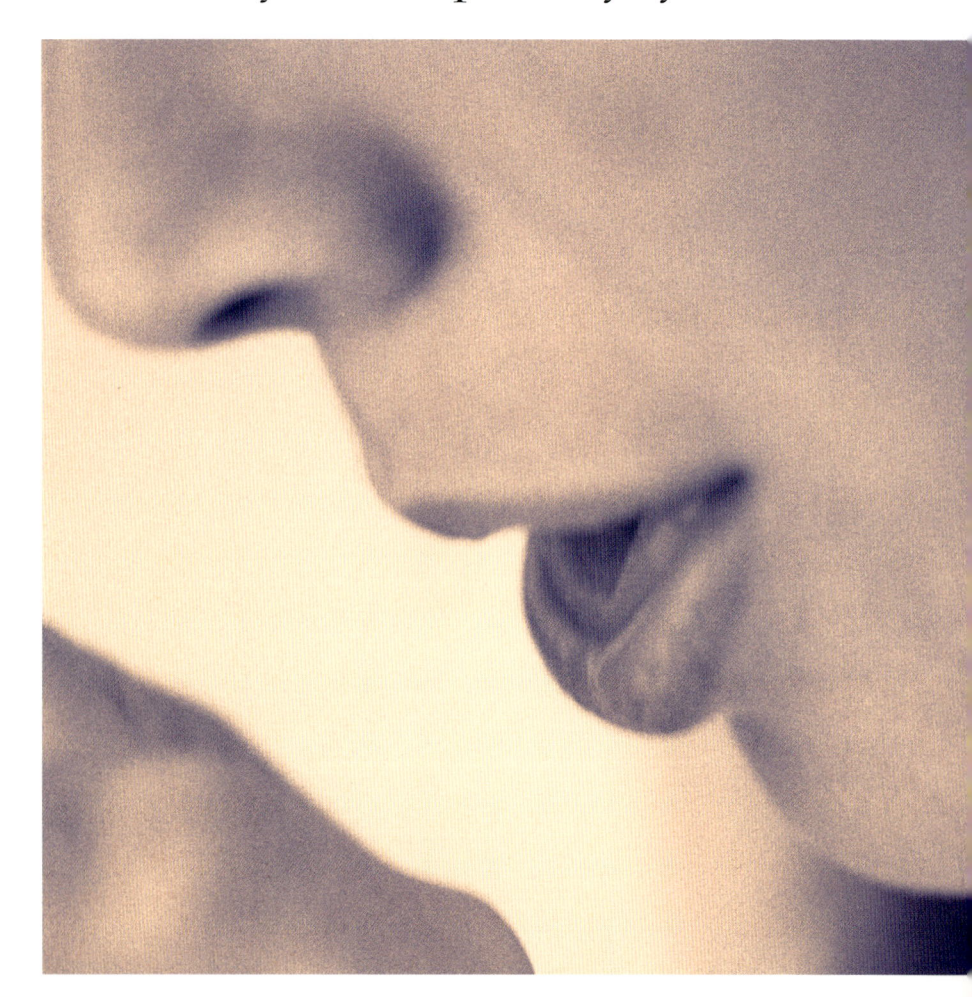

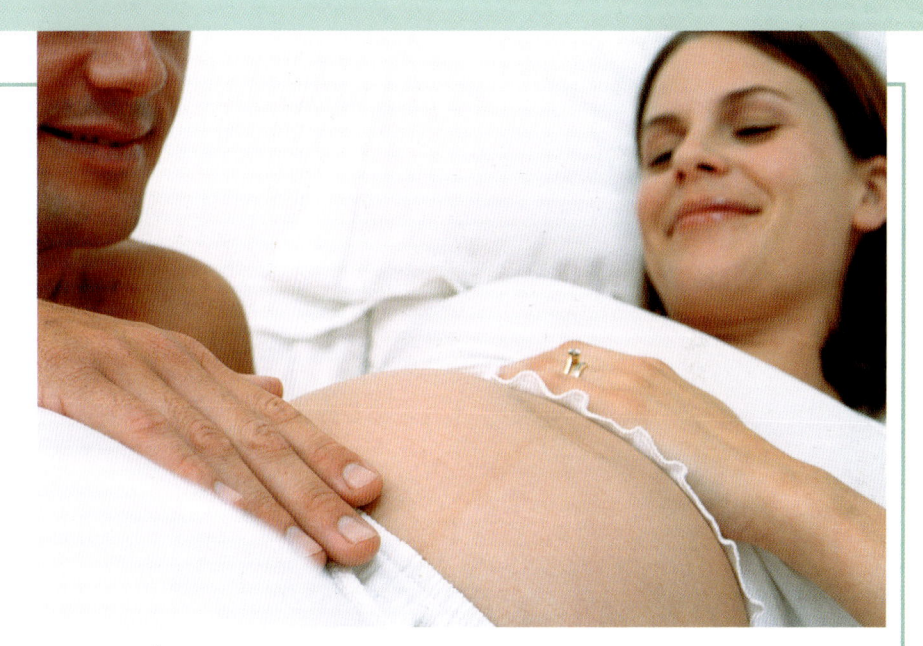

anaemia

When haemoglobin is very low anaemia occurs. This can be a sign of a more serious condition so consult your doctor with symptoms of tiredness and pallor.

- **Calcarea carbonica** for people who are overweight and gain weight easily, are prone to diarrhoea, weakness and dizziness.

Anaemia can occur in pregnancy, as the baby uses all the iron it needs.

- **Ferrum metallicum** For cases where a breastfed child is iron-deficient, also for a child with poor nutrition, or who fails to thrive. It increases the body's ability to absorb iron. For pregnant women who are anaemic. For those who are losing blood in their stool.

asthma

The characteristics of asthma are recurrent breathlessness and wheezing. This is a serious condition and should be seen by a physician. These remedies may be helpful uring an attack:

- **Aconite** For asthma with sudden onset, especially from fright, chill winds and exposure to cold.
- **Antimonium tartaricum** For asthma with heavy wheezing.
- **Arsenicum album** For attacks that come between midnight and 2.00 a.m. accompanied with panic and restlessness.
- **Ipecac** Nausea and mucus accompany the attack.
- **Veretrum album** Asthma with cold sweats, nausea and vomiting.

bronchitis

Bronchitis is a serious condition, indicated by a persistent cough that may produce large amounts of phlegm. Consult a doctor.

- **Aconite** To be used at the beginning of symptoms. It can stop a fever and prevent the disease from spreading to the chest.
- **Antimonium tartaricum** To be used when the cough rattles deep in the chest.
- **Arsenicum album** For those with a nasty cough that will not go away, restless and worse after midnight.
- **Bryonia alba** For dry, hacking coughs, headaches and pain in the chest.
- **Hepar sulphuricum** For wet coughs with yellow mucus.
- **Ipecac** For coughs with vomiting and nausea.
- **Kali bichromicum** For sticky, thick mucus that is hard to bring up.
- **Pulsatilla** For weepy children, who are coughing up yellow mucus.
- **Sulphur** Used at the end of the illness this will help the patient to revitalize energy and regain strength. Give one single dose.

coughs

Coughts can be caused by irritation of the airways, excess mucus or viral infection.

- **Bryonia alba** When the cough is dry, painful and comes in fits.
- **Calcarea fluorica** For a croup-like cough, with spasms.
- **Cuprum metallicum** For spasmodic fits of coughing and tightness in the chest.
- **Drosera rotundifolia** For sudden and violent coughing.
- **Hepar sulphuricum** When a croup-like cough comes after midnight.
- **Ignatia** When a croup-like cough is accompanied by fright.
- **Phosphorus** With hoarseness, loss of voice and glassed-over eyes.
- **Spongia tosta** Persistent coughing that is worse at night, particularly with children.

chilliness

A shivering attack with pale skin and goose pimples can often precede a fever.

- **Aconite** When the patient has been exposed to draughts and chill winds. Give at the first sign of a chill to prevent colds or flu.
- **Arsenicum album** When accompanied by a desire to sit next to the fire or radiator.
- **Calcarea carbonica** With cold hands.
- **Hepar sulphuricum** When chilliness is intense, with shivering.
- **Sepia** When chilly at night.

catarrh (excess mucus)

Catarrh is a condition where the mucous membrane in the nose or throat becomes inflamed, often due to infection or allergy.

- **Calcarea fluorica** When the patient has a head cold with thick, yellow discharge.
- **Kali bichromicum** When there is a stringy, glue-like discharge.
- **Pulsatilla** When there is thick, yellow discharge, weakness and fretting.

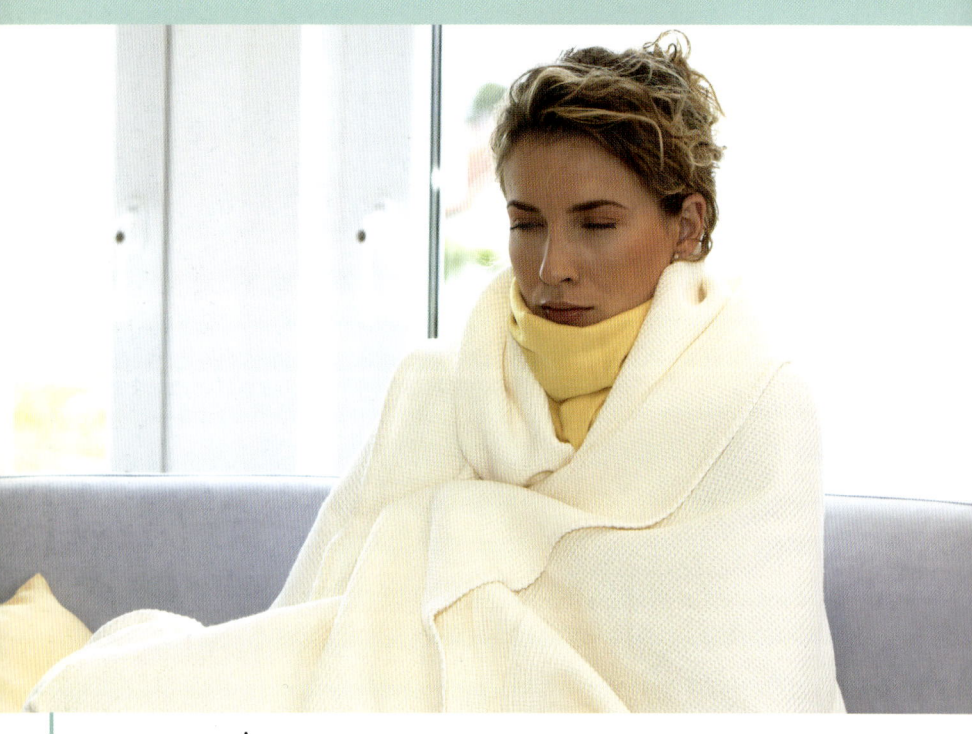

pneumonia

This serious condition results from infection and is due to inflammation of the lungs. It is important to consult your doctor with symptoms of pneumonia.

- **Aconite** For the first stages of pneumonia, with shaking chills, then fever. The skin is hot and dry, and there is no sweating. Breathing is difficult and the patient becomes restless and fearful. Coughing is painful and the phlegm may be pink.

Numerous remedies help treat pneumonia alongside conventional medicine.

- **Bryonia alba** For pneumonia in acute stages. It is useful for pain and pressure in the chest, pleurisy and all sensations that are worse for movement. There is also anxiety and thirst.
- **Chelidonium majus** For infants with pneumonia that begins as bronchitis with a deep but strained cough. The child is red-faced and short of breath with apathy during the day and anxiety at night.
- **Ferrum phosphate** Use this cell salt for pneumonia in the summer in infants who also suffer from dehydration and blood in the phlegm.
- **Hepar sulphuricum** For the middle stages of pneumonia brought on by cold draughts. There is purulent mucus leaving the child weak and unable to talk.
- **Pulsatilla** Pneumonia with a loose cough, weakness and apathy.
- **Sulphur** For the hot patient with rapid breathing and faintness. The patient feels pressure on the chest that makes breathing, coughing and spitting difficult.

colds and influenza

Inluenza is characterized by headache, fever, muscle ache and fatigue. Colds have mucus, coughing and sneezing, and may be accompanied by flu symptoms, such as aching muscles and a headache. A strong immune system is your best defence.

- **Aconite** To be used at the first sign of flu or a cold. Accompanied with restlessness, fear and thirst. Must be given in the first 12 hours of onset. After this treatment, look for other remedies.
- **Allium cepa** For running noses and eyes, when the discharge is burning.
- **Arsenicum album** Flu symptoms with tossing and turning, anxiety, restlessness and a thirst for sips of water.
- **Belladonna** When there is a sudden onset of symptoms, the child is hot, dry and thirstless. They may be red-faced, have dilated pupils and be very uncomfortable.
- **Bryonia alba** Flu symptoms with tension and irritability. All symptoms are worse for movement. The patient is thirsty, has a headache and aching bones.

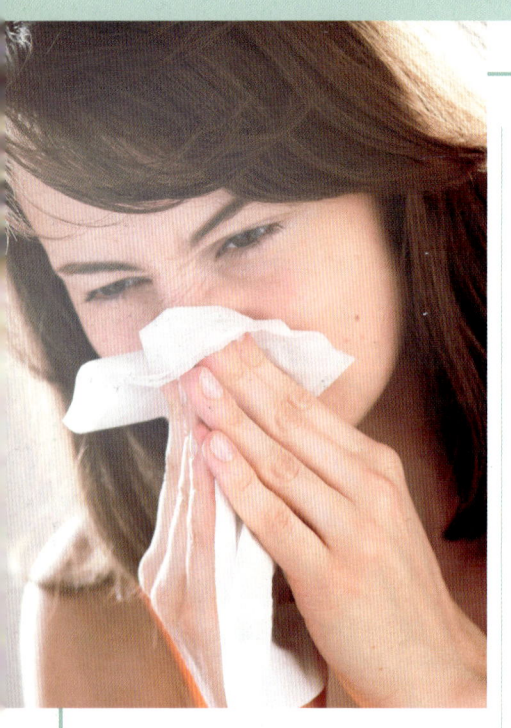

Two of the most common illnesses are colds and flu, which can be alleviated by homeopathic remedies.

- **Gelsemium** For colds and flu due to anticipation, overwork and exhaustion.
- **Ferrum phosphate** Use this cell salt at the beginning of a cold.
- **Hepar sulphuricum** For a left-sided sore throat with a cold.
- **Kali bichromicum** For colds and sinusitis with tough, stringy mucus.
- **Natrum muriaticum** Where there is thin, watery, profuse nasal discharge.
- **Nux vomica** For nasal congestion that is worse at night but becomes runny during the day. The discharge may be burning and the patient is irritable and impatient.
- **Pulsatilla** For a cold accompanied by thick yellow mucus.
- **Rhus toxicodendron** For symptoms with stiffness and restlessness that may occur after heavy exertion or exercise. Symptoms are worse in cold weather.
- **China officinalis** Give for recurrent bouts of flu.
- **Dulcamara**** For colds and flu that come on in the summer or autumn.
- **Eupatorium perfoliatum** For colds and flu that make the bones and muscles ache and the chest feel sore. The patient is thirsty and suffers from coughs.

hoarseness/laryngitis

Overuse of the voice from talking or singing, or an upper respiratory tract infection, can create hoarseness. Inflammation of the larynx can result in hoarseness or loss of voice. Persistent hoarseness should be checked by a doctor.

- **Carbo vegetabilis** For when the weather is cold and damp.
- **Phosphorus** When hoarseness is accompanied by laryngitis.

sinus disorders

When infection causes inflammation of the membrane lining the facial sinuses this condition is called sinusitis.

- **Kali bichromicum** When there is excess mucus with stringy discharge.
- **Natrum muriaticum** When there is great pain in the face and head, sometimes accompanied by nausea.
- **Silica** When the pain starts at the back of the head and settles over the face.

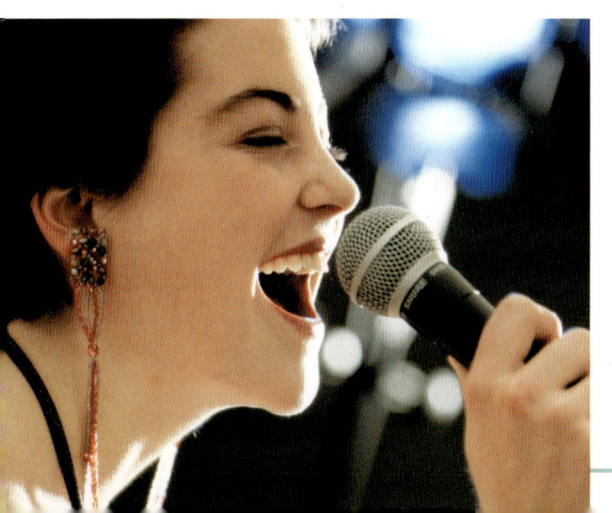

Hoarseness can be caused by overuse of the voice when singing or talking.

digestive system

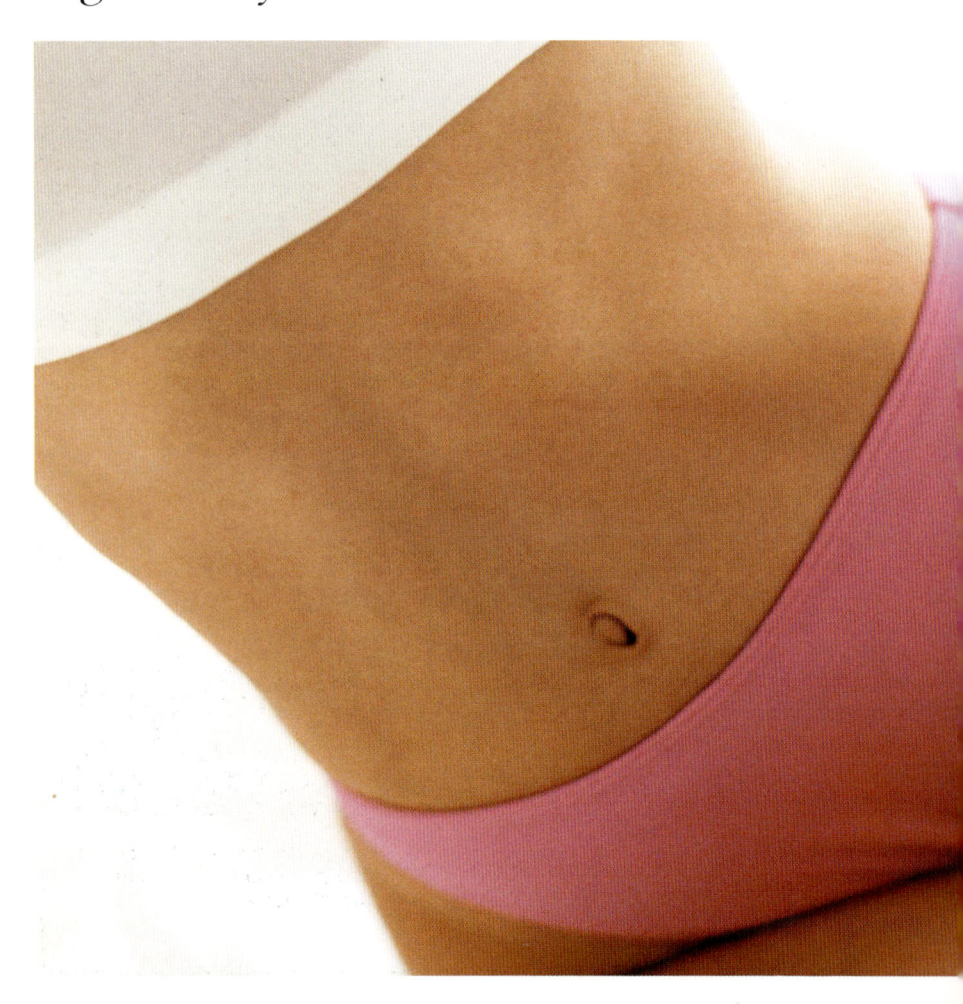

loss of appetite

When people are ill they lose their appetite and their metabolism slows down for healing to begin. A sign of health is when they start to become hungry. A persistent loss of appetite, however, should be checked by your doctor.

- **Arsenicum album** A constant craving with a loss of appetite.
- **Ignatia** Aversion to all food; hunger stops the person from sleeping.

bad breath (halitosis)

Persistent bad breath may be a symptom of mouth infection, sinusitis or a lung disorder.

- **Kali phosphoricum** When there is a bitter taste in the mouth on waking.
- **Mercurius solubilis**** When there is a metallic taste in the mouth.

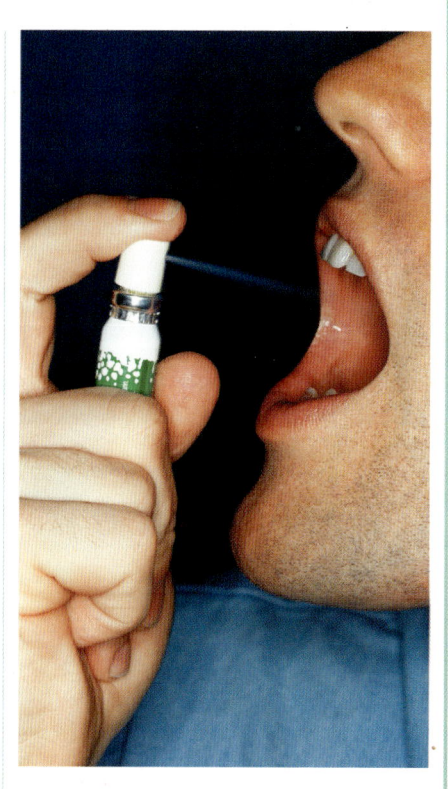

If you find you frequently have bad breath this can be a sign of poor oral hygiene or underlying health problems.

abdominal pain

Overeating or diarrhoea may cause abdominal pain. Women may also experience pain during the menstrual cycle or due to cystitis.

- **Bryonia alba** When food feels like a stone in the stomach and the patient feels better after resting. The feeling may be accompanied by a headache and a feeling of biliousness.
- **Lycopodium** When the stomach feels bloated and the patient also experiences gas after taking a small amount of food such as a light meal or a snack.
- **Nux vomica** When there is gas and colic after eating rich food and drinking alcohol.

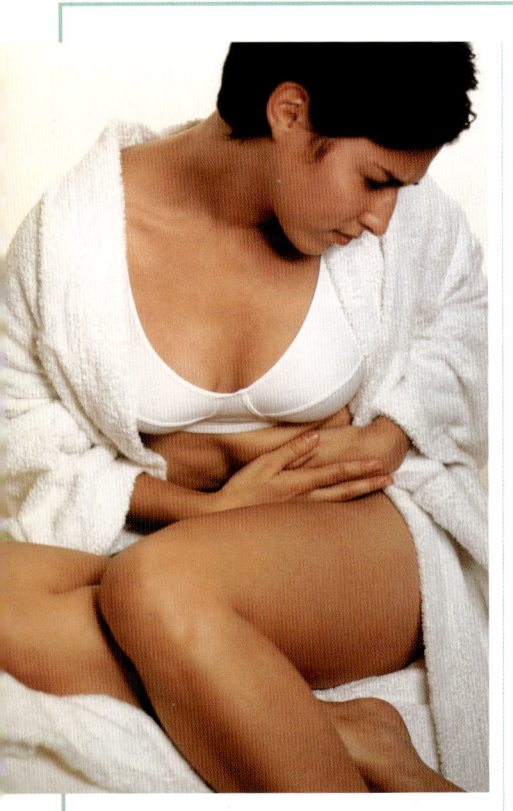

Abdominal pain can be caused by overeating, diarrhoea or menstruation.

acid reflux

When acidic fluid from the stomach is regurgitated into the oesophagus, causing a burning feeling, this is known as acid reflux. It is associated with heartburn.

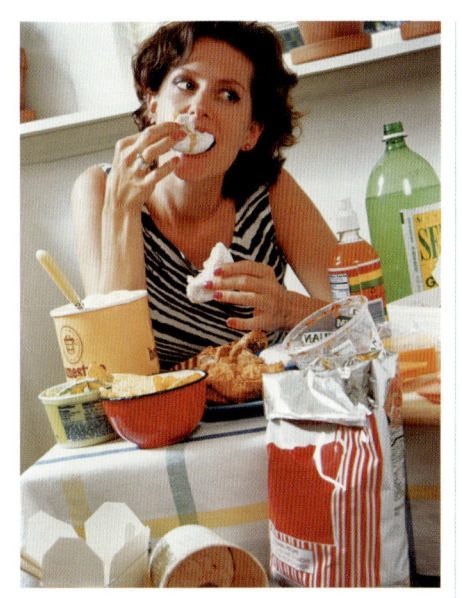

An excessive appetite can lead to other health problems if unchecked.

- **Arsenicum album** For chronic acid reflux or persistent indigestion.
- **Magnesia phosphorica** For distress from medications or from acidity during pregnancy. For babies with colic.

appendicitis

Some cases of abdominal pain are caused by appendicitis, which is caused by acute inflammation of the appendix. This is an acute situation that requires consulting your doctor. To ease the pain use:

- **Iris tenax**** For intense pain in the lower right side of the abdomen and tenderness to pressure on one side. Use 3X to 30C every two hours.

appetite, excessive

When people are out of balance they can have very strong appetites and find they eat to excess.

- **Calcarea carbonica** When there is a feeling of emptiness even after eating.
- **Ferrum phosphate** Use this cell salt when the appetite is excessive and then is followed by a complete loss of appetite.
- **Lycopodium** Excessive appetite, even at night and easily satisfied.

constipation

Try these remedies to relieve temporary constipation, but always seek medical advice if the condition persists.

- **Alumina** For hard, persistent constipation, often brought about by eating canned food.
- **Bryonia alba** For hard, dry stools, often because of dehydration. The patient is often thirsty.
- **Lycopodium** Constipation with much gas but no movement.
- **Nitric acid**** For painful movements with a sharp feeling and bleeding.
- **Nux vomica** The first remedy for constipation, when people become angry, irritable and their bowels are sluggish or there is incomplete movement.
- **Sulphur** When there is hard stool, straining to evacuate, alternating with diarrhoea.

Although it is healthy to drink plenty of water, consult your doctor if you find you are excessively thirsty.

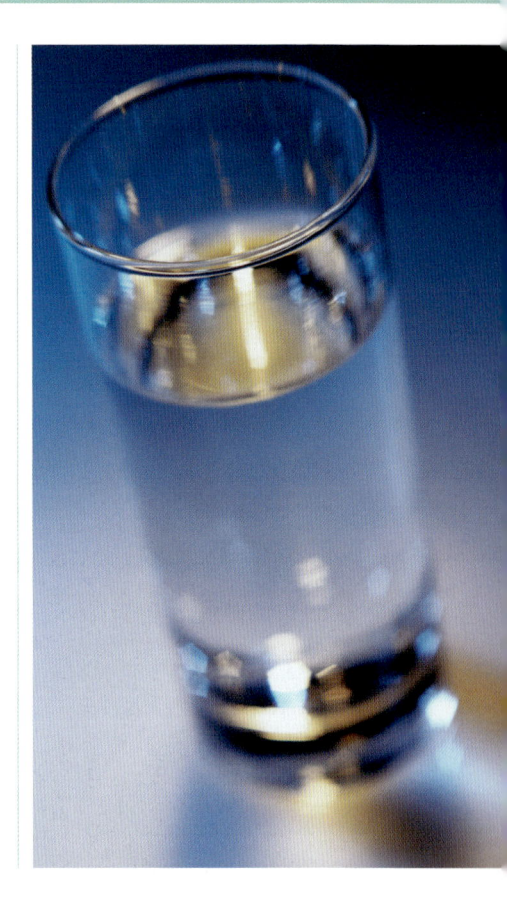

thirst (excessive)

Excessive thirst is often associated with colds and infection. It may also be a sign of diabetes or other serious diseases, so it is important to consult your doctor if you are always thirsty.

- **Aconite** When there is a high temperature.
- **Bryonia alba** When there is a craving for cold drinks.
- **Natrum muriaticum** When there has been an excessive use of salt.
- **Rhus toxicodendron** When the mouth and throat are dry, craving milk.

lack of thirst

A strange, rare and peculiar symptom is a lack of thirst, especially when a person is very hot, even feverish, as they are in Belladonna cases. Lack of thirst is a symptom we use to detemine the correct remedy to prescribe: it is used to decide whether Bryonia alba or Belladonna is appropriate for a fever, for example.

- **Apis mellifica** When the throat is swollen.
- **Gelsemium** When there is a high temperature.
- **Pulsatilla** When the mouth is dry.

dyspepsia

This is the medical term for indigestion and may be caused by eating too much, too quickly, or by stress. Please consult your doctor if the condition persists.

- **Argentum nitricum** When the symptoms come from the nervous anticipation of future events.
- **Carbo vegetabilis** When there is gas, and the patient craves fresh air and is chilly.
- **Lycopodium** When symptoms appear after small amounts of food, with pain, between 4.00 and 8.00 p.m.
- **Phosphorus** When there is an acute sensation of burning.

food poisoning

The usual characteristics for food poisoning are stomach pain, vomiting and diarrhoea. Incidents should be reported to your doctor.

- **Arsenicum album** When it is clear that sickness comes from spoiled food, and the patient has diarrhoea and is vomiting.
- **Carbo vegetabilis** When the poison comes from tainted fish.

hiccups

The common complaint of hiccups can be very uncomfortable and sometimes prolonged. The following remedies can help to alleviate the discomfort.

- **Arsenicum album** When they arise from drinking cold water.
- **Ignatia** Brought on by shock and fear, after crying or fits of hysteria.

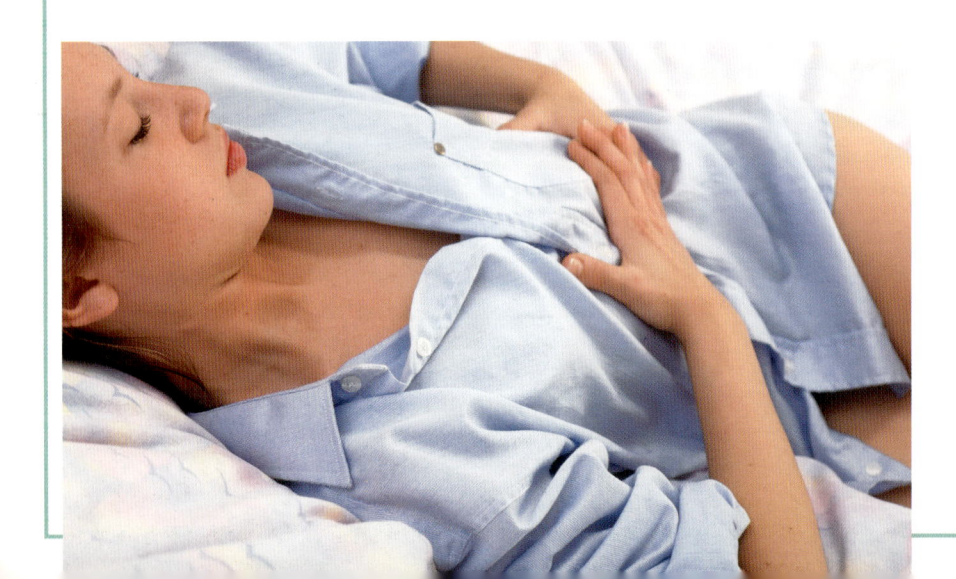

- **Magnesia phosphorica** Gagging and hiccups all day and night.
- **Natrum muriaticum** For cases of acute and severe hiccups.
- **Pulsatilla** Brought on after cold drinks.
- **Vertrum viride**** Spasms with hiccups.

nausea and vomiting

If the patient is nauseous and vomiting this may be the sign of serious illness.

- **Aethusa**** Specifically for milk allergies, especially in babies. The patient is weak with a painful stomach.
- **Antimonium tartaricum** When there is nausea, vomiting and faintness, with sweating and a disgust for food; vomiting of liquid as soon as it is taken, and the patient has no thirst.
- **Arsenicum album** Useful for nausea and vomiting accompanied by diarrhoea. Also for food poisoning.
- **Bryonia alba** When there is vomiting of solid food and the patient needs to keep still as movement makes the vomiting start again.
- **Carbo vegetabilis** Where there is pain in the middle of their stomach, which is bloated with gas.
- **Ignatia** For nausea due to emotional stress.
- **Ipecac** Helps to stop projectile vomiting and nausea.
- **Nux vomica** When there has been excessive overeating and excessive drinking, vomit is sour smelling, the stomach worse for any pressure, and the patient is irritable and chilled.
- **Pulsatilla** When vomiting is due to a suppressed menstrual period or a chill in the stomach. The stomach craves rich, fatty foods such as mayonnaise, butter and pastry; patient craves cold water and cool air.

Vomiting, diarrhoea and stomach pain can indicate food poisoning. Homeopathy can help while awaiting medical assistance.

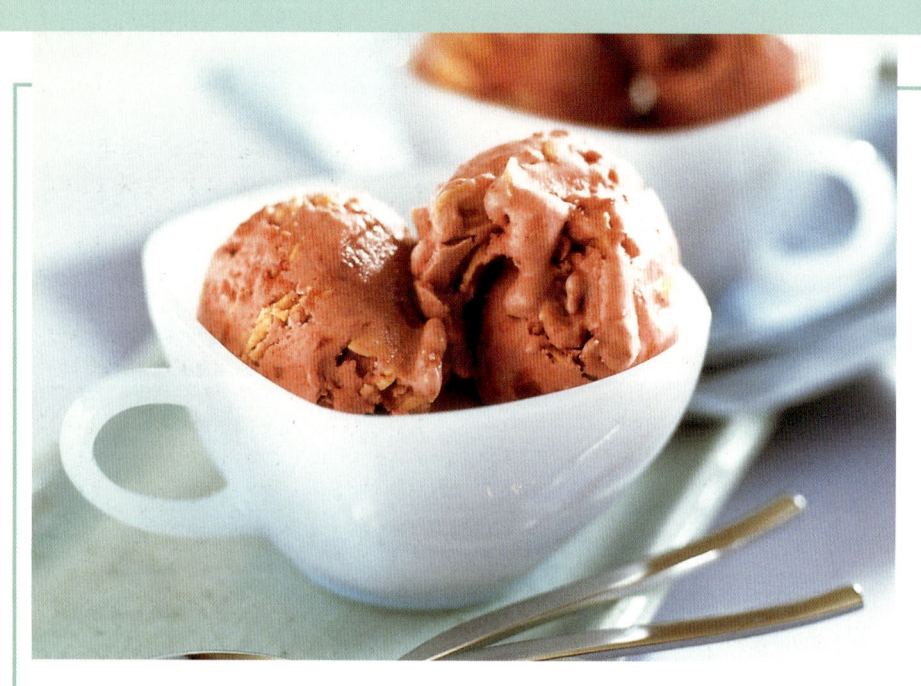

Prescribe Pulsatilla for people who get tummy aches after eating ice cream.

stomach aches

See also Abdominal Pain (page 306) and Dyspepsia (page 309) for further information.

- **Aconite** For people who drink cold water and then vomit. The stomach is hard.
- **Antimonium crudum** For vomiting after drinking milk.
- **Lycopodium** Rumbling, gas and distension, burping and pain.
- **Pulsatilla** Slow digestion from eating too rich food. People who love ice cream and get tummy aches afterwards.

diarrhoea

Short bouts of diarrhoea can be caused by rich foods that upset the system or by tummy upsets that are passed from one person to another. However, persistent diarrhoea needs to be referred to your doctor. (See also Food Poisoning on page 310)

- **Arsenicum album** For severe diarrhoea that burns and scalds the skin. This can be from exposure to toxic food, too much sun, or cold food and drink on a hot day. Symptoms are worse after midnight. Always give after diarrhoea and vomiting to rebalance the acidity in the system, even after several days of no symptoms.
- **Chamomilla** For diarrhoea with teething. The patient is irritable, restless and changeable. A keynote symptom for Chamomilla is that the patient will have one apple-red cheek and one white cheek.
- **China officinalis** For diarrhoea that is worse from fruit, causing pale, white stools. Worse at night.
- **Gelsemium** Diarrhoea from anticipation, excitement and fear. Copious stools, green in colour.
- **Phosphorus** Painful diarrhoea filled with mucus where the patient is exhausted.
- **Podophyllum** For projectile diarrhoea and cholera. Worse in the morning, watery and foul. It occurs after eating and during teething in infants.
- **Pulsatilla** For diarrhoea worse from eating fats and starch. Changeability is the keynote symptom. The patient will complain, weep and cling.
- **Sulphur** For offensive diarrhoea with undigested food particles and burning and itching of the skin.

musculoskeletal system

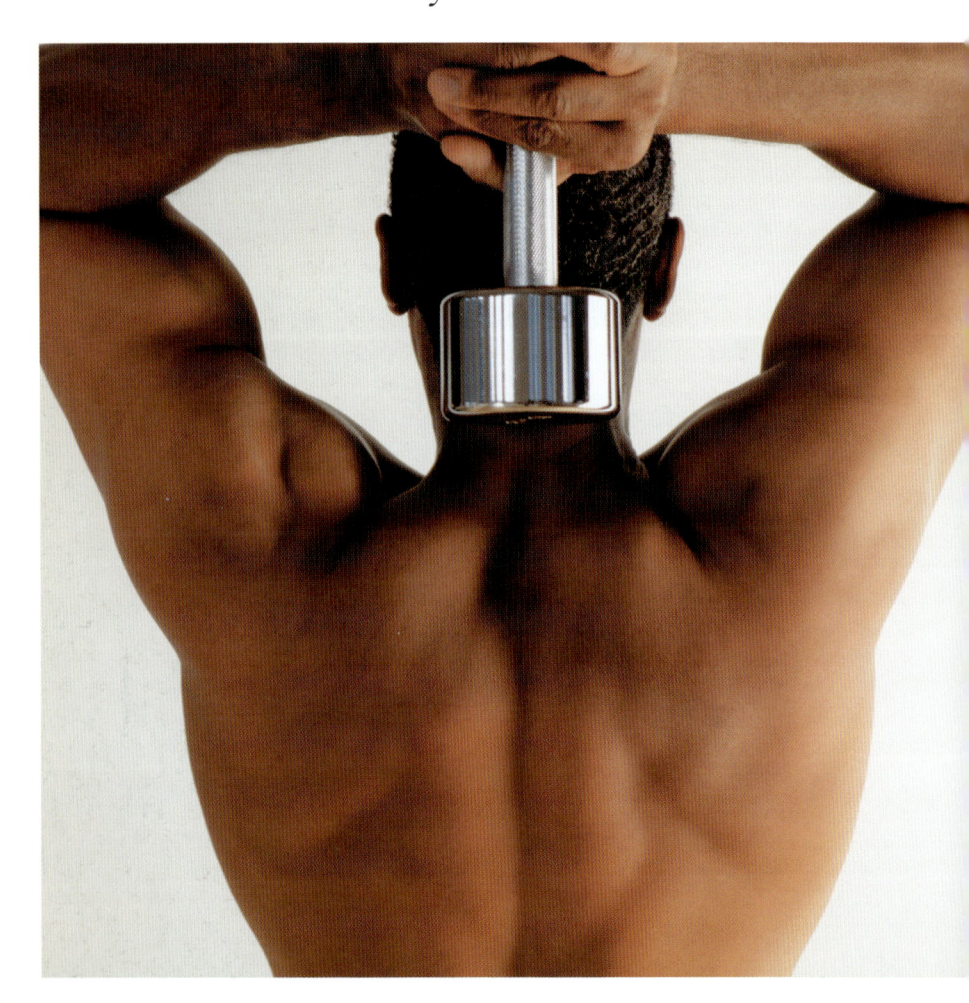

crushed fingers and toes

Please consult your doctor or emergency facilities immediately. The following will help in the meantime:

- **Arnica montana** To alleviate the symptoms of shock associated with this injury.
- **Hypericum perforatum 6X** Taken internally every five minutes for 15 minutes, or until the pain subsides.

cramps (muscle)

Contractions of the muscles causing cramp are common conditions, but if they persist you should consult your doctor.

- **Arnica montana** When cramps are in the calf and are caused by exhaustion.
- **Arsenicum album** For cramps in the calf muscles.
- **Cuprum metallicum** For cramps in the legs and feet with contracted muscles; for cramps in fingers and toes.
- **Ledum palustre** For any type of cramp.
- **Nux vomica** When cramp starts at night, affects the soles of the feet and the person feels the need to stretch.
- **Rhus toxicodendron** When cramps occur only during the day and while sitting.

backache and spine problems

Although there are many minor problems that cause backache it can also be a symptom of a more serious condition. Check with your doctor.

- **Arnica montana** When there is extensive bruising.
- **Hypericum perforatum** When the nerve endings of the coccyx are injured.
- **Ignatia** For pain with a strong emotional component where the structure of one's life breaks down and there is grief.
- **Kali carbonicum** For lower back pain.
- **Ruta graveolens** For pain resulting from overstraining the muscles and when the bone feels bruised.

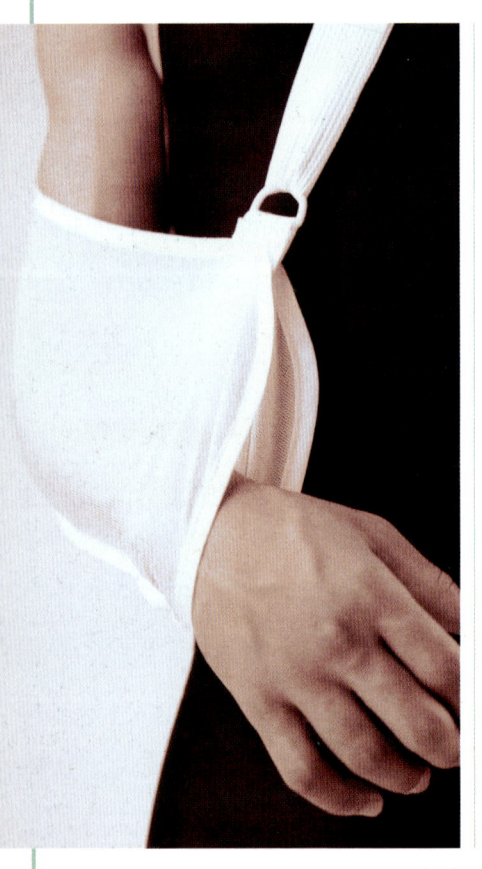

sprains

There are a number of remedies that can alleviate pain after a strain and help the damaged area to heal.

- **Arnica montana** For all injuries accompanied by acute pain and tenderness to the area.
- **Rhus toxicodendron** For ruptured ligaments and tendons. Give Rhus, Ruta graveolens and Arnica montana together for acute situations and relief of pain.
- **Ruta graveolens** Good for all sprains to tendons and ligaments, and for inflammation of the joints.

dental problems

These remedies may help toothache as well as strengthening teeth. A dentist should be consulted for ongoing problems.

A severe sprain will benefit from rest. Take a remedy such as Rhus toxicodendron or Ruta graveolens to help it to heal.

- **Aconite** Useful when there is fear of visiting the dentist.
- **Apis mellifica** When there is swelling, inflammation and pain.
- **Arnica montana** To alleviate dental shock and to control pain and bleeding.

Oral hygiene ensures healthy teeth. When problems occur homeopathy can help.

Useful tinctures

There are two herbal tinctures that help teeth and gums. They are: Calendula tincture (to heal a pulled tooth) and Fragaria tincture (to strengthen weak and bleeding gums).

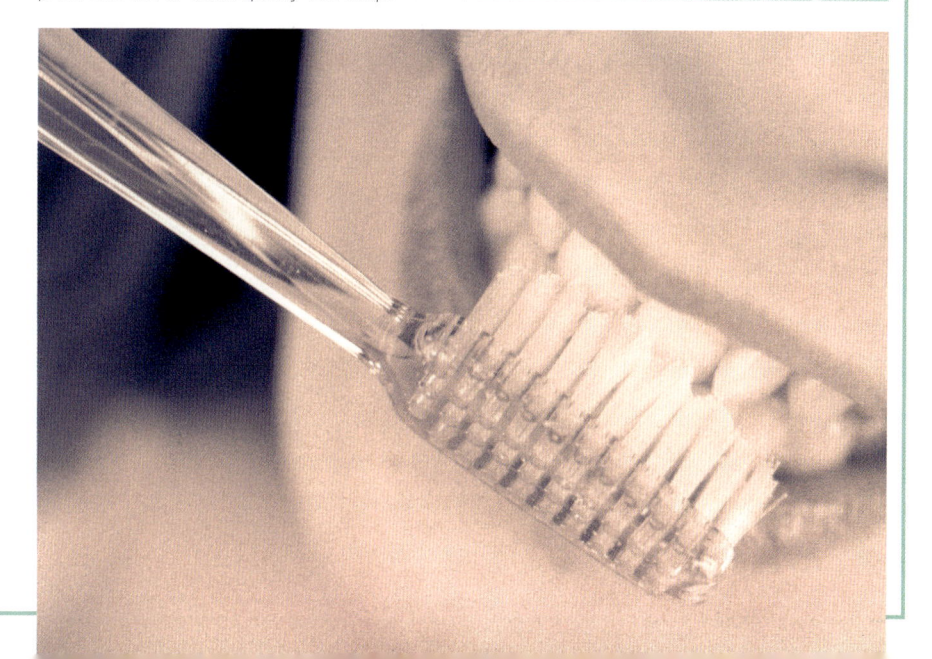

- **Calcarea carbonica** To strengthen teeth and prevent decay in children with early decay symptoms. Give one dose monthly to help with teeth. Use a 6X only for this treatment. Also use when the pain of toothache is made worse with cold drinks and air.
- **Calcarea fluorica** For teeth in poor condition.
- **Chamomilla** When there is great sensitivity to pain, especially in young people.
- **Hypericum perforatum** For sharp darting pains following drilling. Whenever there is nerve pain.
- **Kreosotum** When there is a toothache without any signs of inflammation or gumboils.
- **Mercurius solubilis**** When there is no clear indication other than pain.
- **Phosphorus** For excessive bleeding following drilling or tooth pulling.

sciatica

Sciatica pain radiates along the sciatic nerve, affecting the buttock and thigh.

- **Rhus toxicodendron** For discomfort that is worse in cold, damp weather and at night.

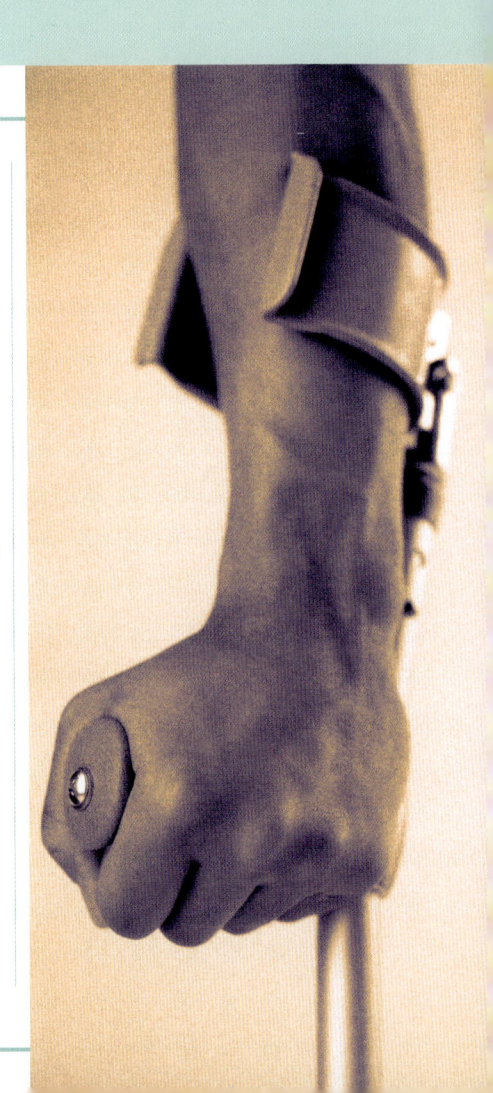

painful joints

The following remedies may help alleviate the symptoms of rheumatism and arthritis, which cause pain, stiffness and swelling in the joints, most commonly in the hands and feet, but any joint may be affected (see also Arthritis opposite).

- **Belladonna** When joints are swollen, stiff and painful.
- **Rhus toxicodendron** When there is rheumatism and pain.

bones (fractures, bruising)

Please consult your doctor or accident and emergency department for broken bones. Use remedies as a support measure.

- **Arnica montana** For a bruised feeling in the bones and for the shock of a break.

Using crutches helps a broken leg to heal. A remedy will help the body repair itself.

- **Calcarea phosphorica** For slow-mending fractures or pain when bones grow quickly.
- **Ruta graveolens** To mend bone injuries well.
- **Symphytum** For broken bones, to aid healing.

arthritis

Homeopathic remedies work well for the relief of discomfort and pain associated with arthritis. For more intensive treatment see your homeopath for constitutional care having first spoken to your doctor.

- **Apis mellifica** When the joints swell and are red and painful
- **Arnica montana** When the joints feel bruised.
- **Bryonia alba** When there appears to be no relief from pain.
- **Pulsatilla** When the pain shifts from joint to joint or extremity to extremity.
- **Rhus toxicodendron** When you awake with stiff joints that feel better on movement. Symptoms are worse in damp weather.
- **Ruta graveolens** When the limbs feel tender and sore.

sensory and nervous systems

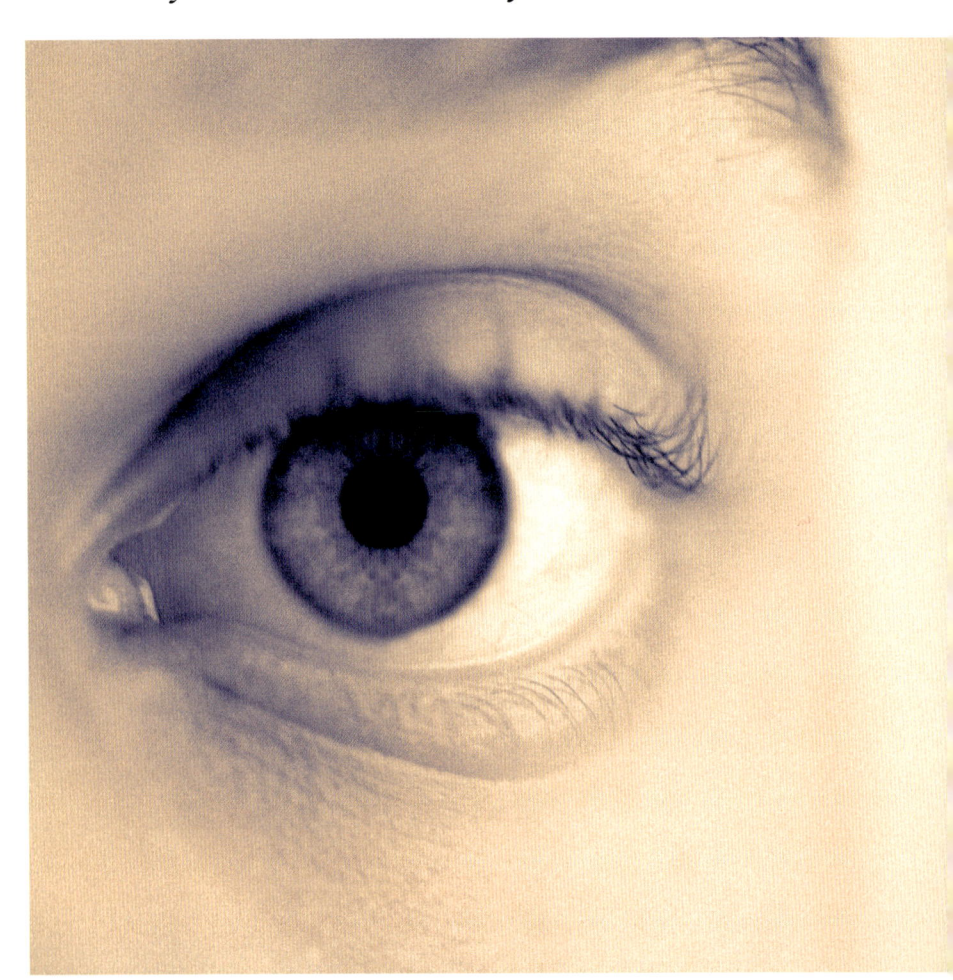

concussion

Always seek medical attention after any head injury that results in loss of consciousness, even if only temporary.

- **Arnica montana** For treating shock, injury and bruising.
- **Helleborus niger**** For headache from injury and lethargy.
- **Hypericum perforatum** Persistent, sharp pains in the head
- **Natrum muriaticum** For depression following a head injury.
- **Natrum sulphuricum** A specific remedy given for all head injuries, past or present.

convulsions

A doctor should be consulted immediately. These remedies are for temporary relief when you are not near a doctor.

- **Aconite** For convulsions that are caused by fright or fever.
- **Belladonna** For convulsions from high fever where the patient is flushed, pupils are dilated and the child may be delirious
- **Chamomilla** For convulsions during teething.
- **Cuprum metallicum** For convulsions brought on by whooping cough, when the fingers and toes are in spasm.
- **Ignatia** For convulsions from grief and emotional turmoil.

eye strain

If you suffer from eye strain this may be due to fatigue or sight problems. Consult your optician.

- **Apis mellifica** When the eyelids are puffy and swollen.
- **Euphrasia** When the patient is unable to bear the light.
- **Hamamelis virginiana** For foreign objects in the eye.

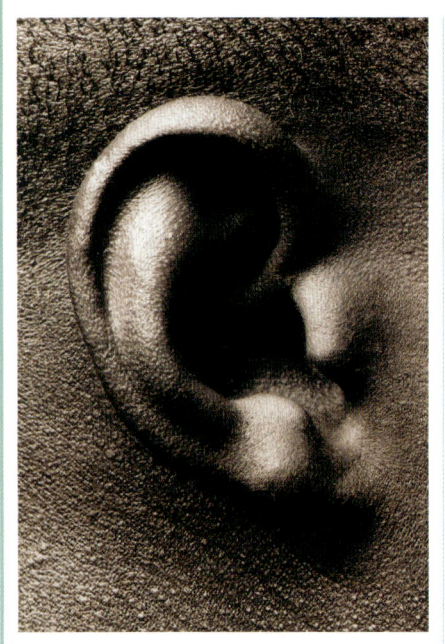

earaches

An earache may indicate an infection, which needs medical attention if it does not quickly disappear.

Some people can be particularly susceptible to ear discomfort or infections. A number of remedies might be appropriate.

- **Belladonna** For red, hot, throbbing ears.
- **Bellis perennis** For earaches that come on suddenly, where other symptoms are a red face, a red and swollen ear canal, and a throbbing ear.
- **Calcarea carbonica** For chronic, mild, ear infections.
- **Chamomilla** For fussy, irritable children who scream, yell, and toss and turn with pain.
- **Silica** For the later stages of recurrent ear infections.
- **Ferrum phosphate** Use this cell salt for painful, early stages of ear infection, often with fever.
- **Hepar sulphuricum** For splinter-like pain in the ear and an aversion to touching the ear.
- **Mercurius solubilis**** For severe earaches with a ruptured drum and purule discharge. Medical assistance is essential.
- **Pulsatilla** This treats the emotional state of the child. The child is mild, soft, whimpery and weeping. Worse in the evening, craving attention and to be held.

exhaustion

Although exhaustion can occur from time to time for a number of reasons, frequent exhaustion can also be symptomatic of a more serious condition. Please check with your doctor if you are experiencing the long-term effects of exhaustion.

- **Arnica montana** When exhaustion comes after physical exertion.
- **Arsenicum album** When exhaustion comes on after a sickness.
- **Kali phosphoricum** When exhaustion comes after mental effort, or any time you need to keep the blood sugar elevated for long periods of activity, such as long-distance driving, childbirth or studying for exams.

fainting

If fainting persists you should consult your doctor as it may indicate more serious problems. Select a remedy, then administer it to the patient every ten minutes until they have recovered.

- **Aconite** or **Chamomilla** When fainting comes about from pain. Use Chamomilla in childbirth.
- **China officinalis** When fainting is caused by the loss of blood.
- **Coffea cruda** When there is fainting from over-excitement.
- **Ignatia** When there is fainting due to an emotional upset.

When a person faints a remedy can be placed just under the lip.

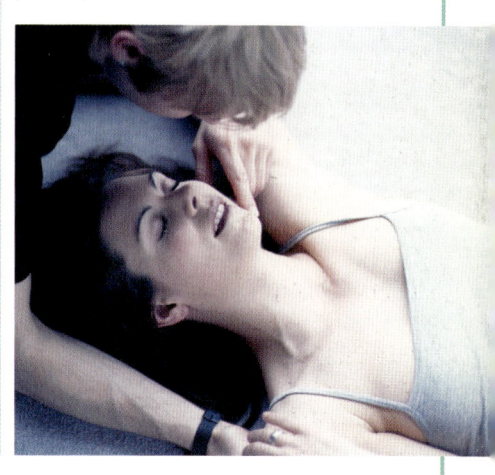

- **Nux vomica** When fainting is caused by the sight of blood.
- **Pulsatilla** When there is fainting from walking into a hot, stuffy room.

heat exhaustion (heatstroke)

Serious cases of heat exhaustion will need medical treatment.

- **Aconite** For fever, accompanied by confusion and dullness.
- **Belladonna** For heatstroke causing a throbbing headache. Child will be hot and red, with dry skin.
- **Cuprum metallicum** Treats children who sweat copiously, lose too much salt and get cramps in their stomach and legs.
- **Gelsemium** For heatstroke with giddiness.
- **Glonine**** For heatstroke with severe headaches and copious sweating.

motion sickness

Sickness when travelling by car is a common problem, especially with children.

- **Calcarea carbonica** For overweight and chilly children who suffer from motion sickness with nausea, vomiting and headache.

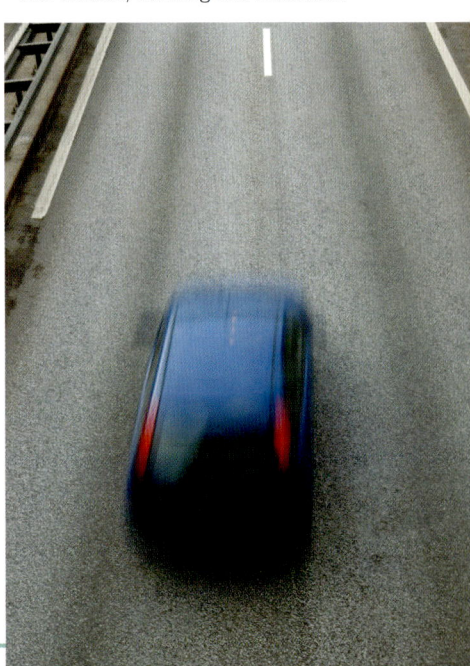

Use a homeopathic treatment to reduce your child's feelings of motion sickness.

- **Cocculus indicus** For all types of motion sickness with headache, dizziness and nausea.
- **Ipecac** Continuous nausea that is not relieved by vomiting and is caused by any movement.
- **Tabacum** Nausea and vomiting.

seasickness

Remedies can help sufferers overcome the symptoms of seasickness.

- **Cocculus indicus** When there is nausea, dizziness, a feeling of faintness and a loss of direction. When travelling by sea take the remedy a few minutes before departure, then one dose every hour.
- **Petroleum** When there is nausea accompanied by saliva in the mouth, and vomiting and dizziness that is better when having food in the mouth.
- **Tabacum** When there is nausea and vomiting, and when the patient feels icy cold, has a sinking feeling in the stomach and is made worse for the smell of tobacco smoke.

air-travel sickness

Sickness during air travel can be particularly distressing for sufferers, but can be helped with the following remedies.

- **Aconite** When there is restlessness and fear.
- **Arnica montana** For recovery from jet lag.
- **Belladonna** When the symptoms of air sickness appear.
- **Bryonia alba** When the least movement upsets the patient.
- **Ipecac** When movement causes nausea and vomiting.
- **Nux vomica** When there is irritability about movement and jarring.
- **Phosphorus** For recovery from jet lag.

neuralgia

The term neuralgia refers to pain caused by the irritation of, or damage to, a nerve. Migraine is a common form of neuralgia.

- **Actaea racemosa**** When pains disappear during the night and reappear during the day.

- **Belladonna** When the face is flushed and hot, and the pain is throbbing.
- **Bryonia alba** To use when the migraine has already started.

nose (nosebleeds, running nose)

During a cold the nose usually runs profusely. Remedies can help the illness to move through the body with little distress. Also, children and old people, especially, can suffer from sudden nosebleeds.

- **Arnica montana** For a nosebleed that is caused by a blow.
- **Ferrum phosphate** Use this cell salt for nosebleeds in children.
- **Gelsemium** For a running nose during colds and flu.
- **Hamamelis virginiana** For frequent nosebleeds.
- **Natrum muriaticum** For a nose running constantly without stopping.
- **Phosphorus** For nosebleeds accompanied by profuse bleeding.

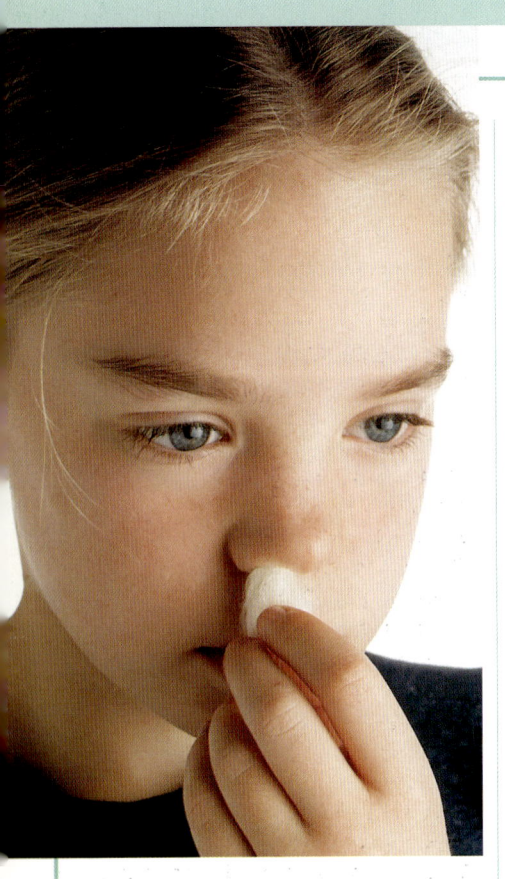

Children can often suffer with sudden nosebleeds. There are several suitable remedies that can be prescribed.

headaches

A headache can arise from dehydration, colds and flu, fatigue or stress. (See also Neuralgia on page 325.) Persistent or severe headaches should be checked by a doctor.

- **Aconite** When there are sudden, violent pains with a burning sensation, as if the brain is in boiling water. The pain is intolerable, there is throbbing in the temples, the patient is restless, fearful and thirsty.
- **Arsenicum album** When the headaches reoccur periodically and the patient is weakened by them. Sometimes the pain is relieved by vomiting. There is great thirst and the patient will take frequent sips of cool water. The patient is restless and fearful, but feels better for moving.
- **Belladonna** When there is sudden pain, and a throbbing, bursting sensation; the pain is worse for moving, bending and moving the eyes. The head is hot, and the face is flushed. The patient cannot bear light or noise. Headache often begins in the afternoon and lasts throughout the night.
- **Bryonia alba** When a headache comes on from eating rich food or from too much exertion and is accompanied by great thirst or no desire for movement of any kind; is worse on the left side, and the patient lingers in bed.
- **Gelsemium** When a headache comes on with acute sickness or great exhaustion, begins in the nape of the neck, and settles over the eyes. It is often worse on the right side. The patient feels heavy, sleepy and drowsy. Sometimes the person is shivery with chills, shows no thirst, and feels better after vomiting.
- **Glonine**** When pains are violent, pulsating, throbbing, or bursting; made worse by light and bending the head backwards. These headaches are always made worse by exposure to the sun or heat. The patient will actually grab their head in pain. They are flushed and hot to the touch. They cannot bear to be touched and feel better in the cold air and with cold applications.
- **Natrum muriaticum** When the headache feels like there is hammering inside the head; a stitching pain in the head, and a sore, bruised feeling around the eyes, and when

movement makes the headache worse. Headache starts in the back of the neck, and spreads all over the head. It can be a blinding headache, often associated with PMS (pre-menstrual syndrome) or with mental exertion.
- **Nux vomica** When the headache is accompanied with vomiting and nausea caused by eating rich food and drink or excessive anger. The headache feels as if a nail is being driven into the head. The patient is worse with conversation, excitement or movement, and is very irritable and chilly. Almost always constipated as well.
- **Pulsatilla** When the headache is in the temples and the head is hot. It is better for cold applications and fresh air. This is often associated with delayed or suppressed periods. The patient is dizzy when bending over and feels worse in a stuffy room or in an area with noise and light.

sleep problems

Contact your doctor with insomnia and sleep problems, which are often caused by stress. These remedies may be helpful.

- **Aconite** Restless from frights causing the patient to thrash about in bed; when there is twisting and turning and the person can't seem to settle.
- **Arnica montana** For when overly tired and unable to settle down.
- **Arsenicum album** For restless people who wake between midnight and 2.00 a.m.

Useful tinctures

There are two herbal tinctures that help with sleep. They are: Avena sativa (16 drops in water before bed) and Passiflora incarnata (five drops in water will help children sleep well).

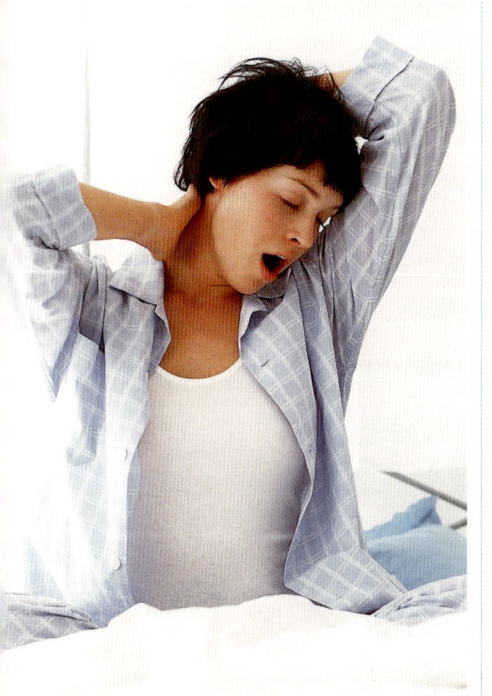

Lack of sleep caused by insomnia is distressing and can lead to stress-related illness and difficulty working in the day.

- **Belladonna** For nightmares, jerking and twitching before falling asleep.
- **Ignatia** Where there is much yawning and the person is unable to sleep.
- **Phosphorus** Frequent nightmares that create sleep problems.
- **Sulphur** For hot people who kick the covers off the bed.

shingles

This is an infection of the nerves in certain areas of the skin. It causes a painful rash. Please see a doctor with these symptoms, as they can be very serious.

- **Rhus toxicodendron** For when the scalp is affected by shingles.

skin

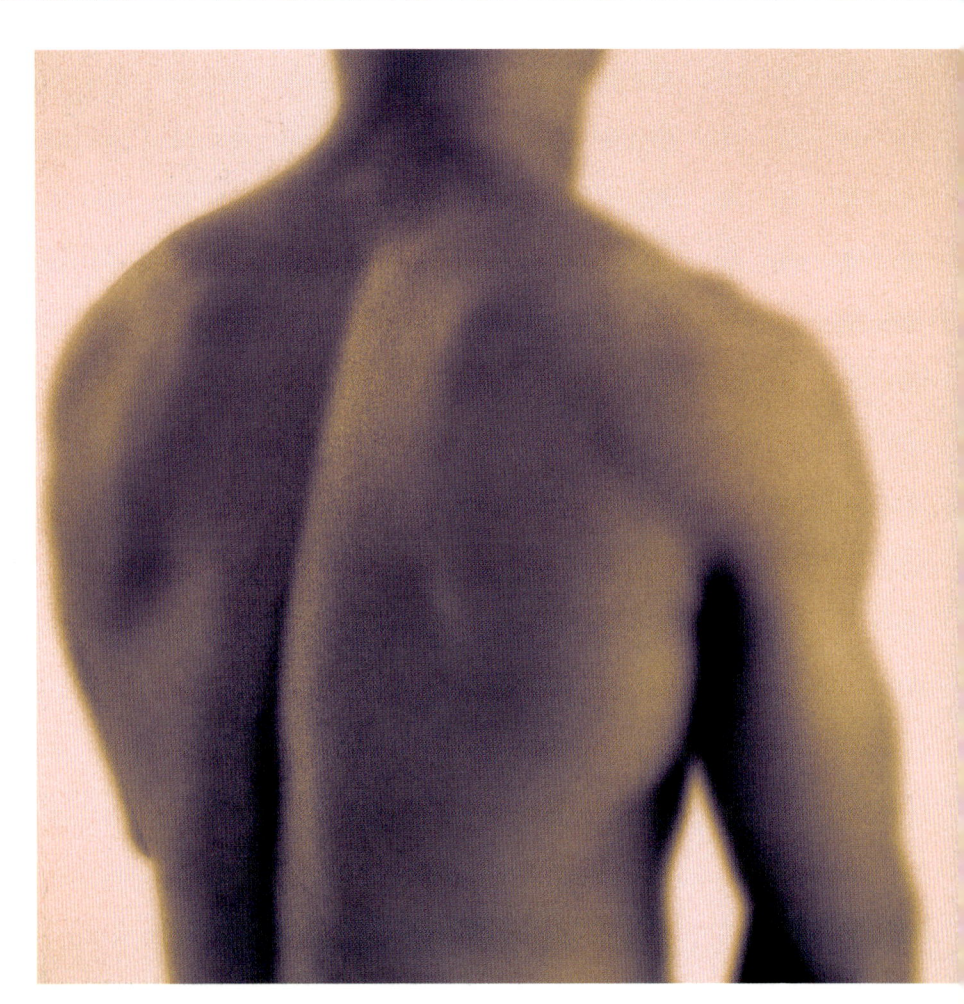

blisters

Do not burst blisters as this may cause infection in the skin beneath. The treatment below may help.

- **Causticum** Use morning and evening. Reduce the intake as symptoms decrease.

> **Useful ointment**
>
> Treat blisters topically with Calendula ointment.

abscesses

For general care bathe affected parts in Calendula tincture or rub with ointment along with the indicated homeopathic remedy below.

- **Belladonna** When irritation is accompanied by redness and throbbing pain.
- **Hepar sulphuricum** When there is pus and the skin is sensitive to touch.
- **Hypericum perforatum** When the skin is tense and painful.
- **Mercurius solubilis**** For mouth abscesses.
- **Silica** After discharge of pus, use three times a day for three days as a cleanser.

acne

There are many different types of acne. If symptoms persist see a homeopath or consult your doctor.

- **Belladonna** For people with red faces.
- **Hepar sulphuricum** Where many pustules are present.
- **Pulsatilla** For people with fair complexions.
- **Silica** When the skin becomes scarred from pustules.
- **Sulphur** In cases that resist conventional treatment of any kind.

bites

The remedies below may help both insect and animal bites. If the bites do not respond to treatment or if you have a painful infection consult your doctor.

- **Apis mellifica** For insect bites and stings where there is burning, or a stinging pain made worse by the application of heat. For bites that are red, swollen and irritated.
- **Cantharis vesicatoria** Suitable for insect bites with serious inflammation with burning that is worse for touch and better after massage.
- **Hypericum perforatum** For insect bites, to bring the swelling down.
- **Ledum palustre** When there is a tick, spider, cat or dog bite, with puncture of the flesh, this remedy is excellent for relieving symptoms. Also for when there is numbness, sensitivity to being touched, and pain that is relieved by cold applications.

Wasp and bee stings can be extremely uncomfortable. Take a remedy as soon as possible to reduce the effects.

Useful tinctures

There are two herbal tinctures to use for insect bites. They are Arnica tincture or Calendula tincture, to be applied topically for all insect bites.

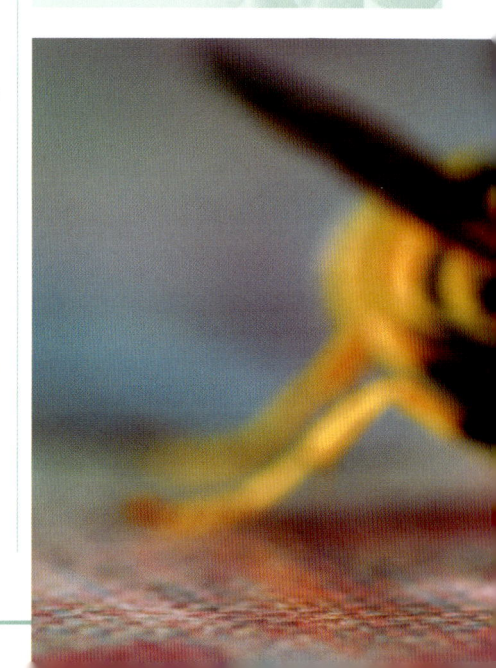

abrasions and cuts

Serious cuts should be attended to in an emergency room or be seen by a doctor, but use these remedies as support measures for all cases in an emergency.

- **Arnica montana** To stop the bleeding.

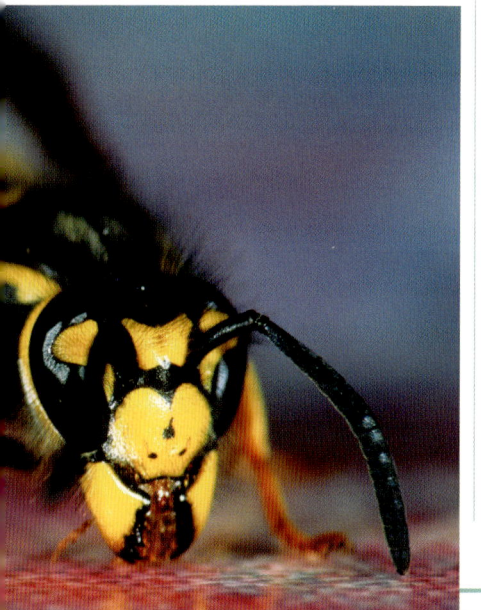

Care of minor cuts

Clean the wound, cover it and moisten with a few drops of Calendula tincture several times a day. Hypericum cream helps cuts heal without sepsis. A must in any homeopathic first-aid kit.

boils

Usually boils develop in an infected hair follicle. Do not burst a boil as you may spread the infection.

- **Apis mellifica** For boils that are red and swollen, hot and stinging.
- **Arnica montana** Where skin is bruised.
- **Arsenicum album** Pus-filled boils that burn.
- **Calcarea sulphurica** For boils in crops.
- **Hepar sulphuricum** For boils that need to be brought to a head and the pus discharged.
- **Mercurius solubilis**** For boils in the ear.
- **Sulphur** For boils that are slow to develop and slow to heal.

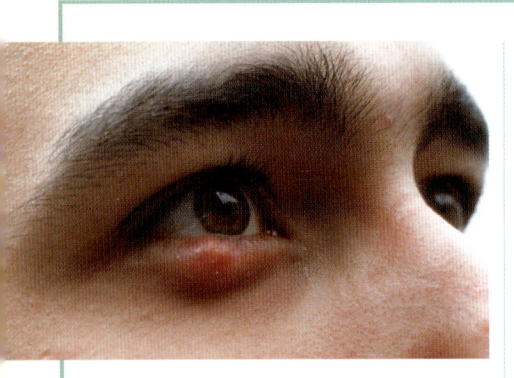

If a stye develops on the eyelid use a compress of hot water to soothe it.

stye

Styes can develop near the eyelashes and are the result of infection. Compresses can help: soak a soft cloth in cold water and press onto the stye.

- **Apis mellifica** For styes that sting and are better for a cold compress.
- **Calcarea carbonica** For styes on the right eyelid in chilly, overweight children.
- **Cheldonium majus**** With yellow discharge and eyelash loss on the right lower lid.
- **Graphites** For recurrent styes on the lower lid and a burning pain in the eye.
- **Hepar sulphuricum** When the eyelids are swollen and painful, and feel bruised.
- **Hypericum perforatum** For styes of the lower left eyelid with a sharp, sticking pain.
- **Lycopodium** For chronic cases of infected styes, worse on the left eye.
- **Phytolacca decandra** Styes that are hard, round, swollen, thick, with reddened eyelids.
- **Pulsatilla** Inflamed and painful styes.
- **Staphysagria** For styes on the left upper eyelid that are painful and swollen.

black eye

If a blow is serious it should be examined by a doctor. The treatments below may help with a resulting black eye.

- **Arnica montana** Give every hour for up to five doses.
- **Ledum palustre** For bruising that is relieved by cold applications.
- **Symphytum** Give every hour for five doses if there is pain in the eyeball.

ringworm

The term ringworm refers to certain kinds of skin infections marked by ring-shaped, reddened, scaly or blistery patches that appear on the skin

- **Apis mellifica** For symptoms of itching and burning that are better for cold applications.
- **Bacillinum**** Use in 200C potency for three weeks, giving it once a week. This is a specific for ringworm.
- **Sulphur** For children who wash rarely, with unhealthy skin, poor digestion and irritability.

Useful creams

An Iodine or Calendula tincture will work as a topical antiseptic to help control ringworm.

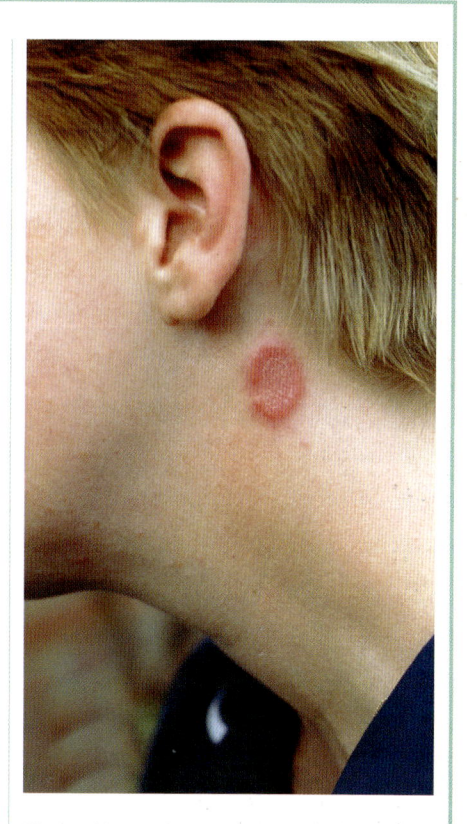

The ring-shaped skin infection known as ringworm can be very uncomfortable.

mouth ulcers (apthae)

Ulcers are often a sign that the patient is run down. They can be helped with remedies as well as eating plenty of fresh fruit and vegetables.

- **Baptisia tinctoria**** For small, painful ulcers when children refuse to eat because of pain in their mouths.
- **Borax** For mouth ulcers on the tongue and inside the cheeks. The patient is restless, nervous and sensitive.
- **Magnesia carbonica** For chronic sores in weak, allergic and hypersensitive people.

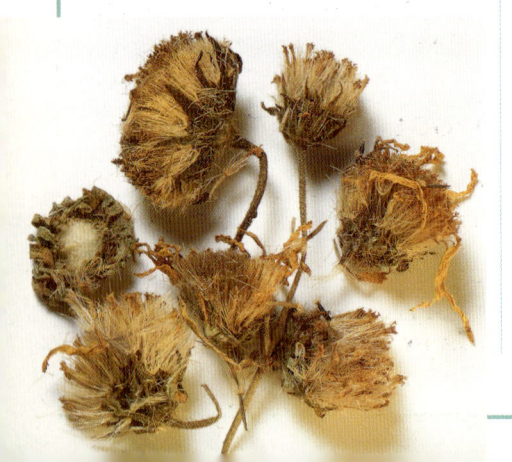

bruising

If a bruise does not fade after about a week, or if bruises appear for no reason, consult your doctor.

- **Arnica montana** For bruising that results from falls, injury or trauma. Arnica montana can be given every two to three minutes to help ease the pain and take away shock. As symptoms ease spread the treatment to every two hours. Arnica montana will bring the bruising out and the skin will be discoloured, but the deep trauma will be released and the pain diminished.
- **Hypericum perforatum** For bruising to toes, fingers and nerve endings.
- **Ruta graveolens** For bruised feelings to the bones and tendons.

Arnica flowers (shown here dried) are potentized to make a popular first-aid remedy for bruises.

conjunctivitis (pink eye)

This inflammation of the eye's membrane is generally caused by infections associated with colds or allergies.

- **Argentum nitricum** For yellow discharges from the eye.
- **Arsenicum album** For burning, watery discharges.
- **Euphrasia** For a watery discharge that burns; for irritation and soreness to the eye.

Ledum palustre can help minor wounds, such as this cut finger, to heal.

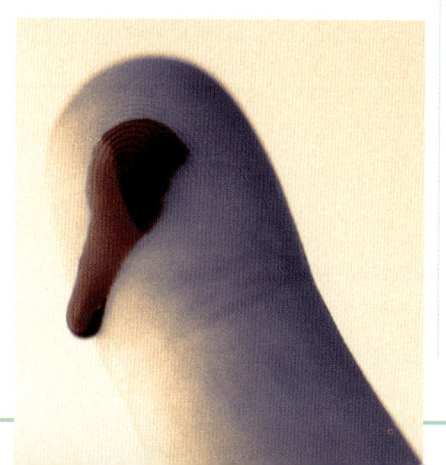

warts

Warts are harmless but can be stubborn to get rid of. In homeopathy, warts are considered to signal that a constitutional remedy is appropriate and you are best advised to contact a homeopath if these remedies below fail to work.

- **Calcarea carbonica** For multiple warts that itch and bleed.
- **Kali muriaticum** For warts on the hand that occur after vaccination.
- **Natrum muriaticum** For warts on the palms of the hands.
- **Thuja occidentalis** This is a specific remedy for warts.

wounds

Serious wounds should be seen by a doctor.

- **Ledum palustre** For puncture wounds. Take five doses on the first day then three doses the next.

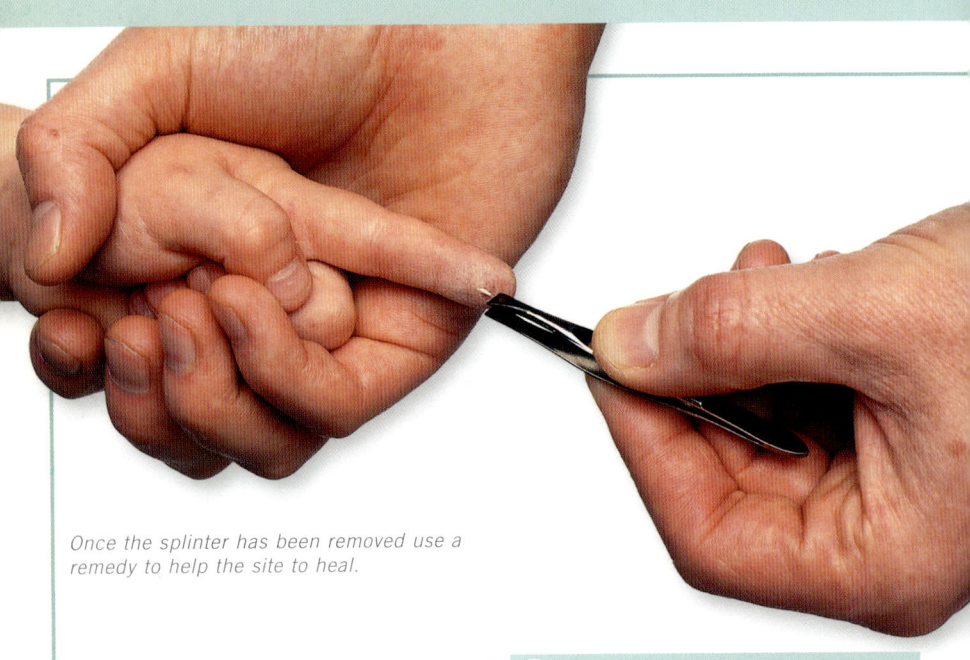

Once the splinter has been removed use a remedy to help the site to heal.

splinters

Use sterilized tweezers to avoid infection when removing splinters. The remedies below may help the healing process.

- **Ledum palustre** Use if the splinter has penetrated deeply into the skin.
- **Silica** To expel the splinter.

Useful tincture

Use Calendula tincture immediately to clean out wounds and to use after removing a splinter.

skin problems (general)

People who have dry, sensitive skin may find these remedies helpful.

- **Argentum nitricum** When the skin is blotchy.
- **Calcarea carbonica** When the skin feels better when scratched.
- **Graphites** When the skin is cracked and there is weeping eczema.
- **Mercurius solubilis**** When the skin itches and is worse when hot.
- **Sulphur** For when the skin itches and begins to burn.

Useful cream

Use Rescue Remedy cream to alleviate discomfort (see page 376).

eczema

Consult your doctor if you suffer with eczema. It is sometimes caused by an allergy, so isolating and avoiding the irritating substance may solve the problem. Stress can also be a factor. For the homeopathic treatment of eczema avoid using a cortizone cream or taking steroids, but do not stop taking any medical treatment without consulting your doctor.

- **Sulphur** For burning, red, itchy and unhealthy-looking skin.
- **Graphites** For oozing, crusty types of skin irritation.
- **Petroleum** For cracked, dry and rough skin.
- **Mezerium**** For painful, small, bumpy eczema that is not found on the face.

burns

Serious burns must always be treated by trained medical staff.

- **Arnica montana** To remove the shock effect of burns. Take with one of the other remedies that follow.
- **Cantharis vesicatoria** To be taken every two minutes for the relief of burns. Cantharsis can stop blistering if taken in time.
- **Causticum** For painful scars and to help them to heal.
- **Hepar sulphuricum** For burns that have not been kept clean and have become infected.
- **Kali bichromicum** For complementary treatment of serious second-degree burns.
- **Urtica urens** For the stinging pain of burns.

sunburn

It's wise to wear a hat and protective clothing and seek shade during the hottest parts of the day. You can find sun creams made without chemicals and using natural and organic ingredients at your health-food store. Severe cases of sunburn need medical treatment.

- **Belladonna** When the skin is red, hot and throbbing, and where the patient has no apparent thirst.
- **Cantharis vesicatoria** After a day in the sun when the patient has been highly exposed to the sun's rays.
- **Cuprum metallicum** For use if sweating and cramping occur.

Sunburn is not only painful but is also potentially dangerous, as skin cancers can form in years to come.

skin 341

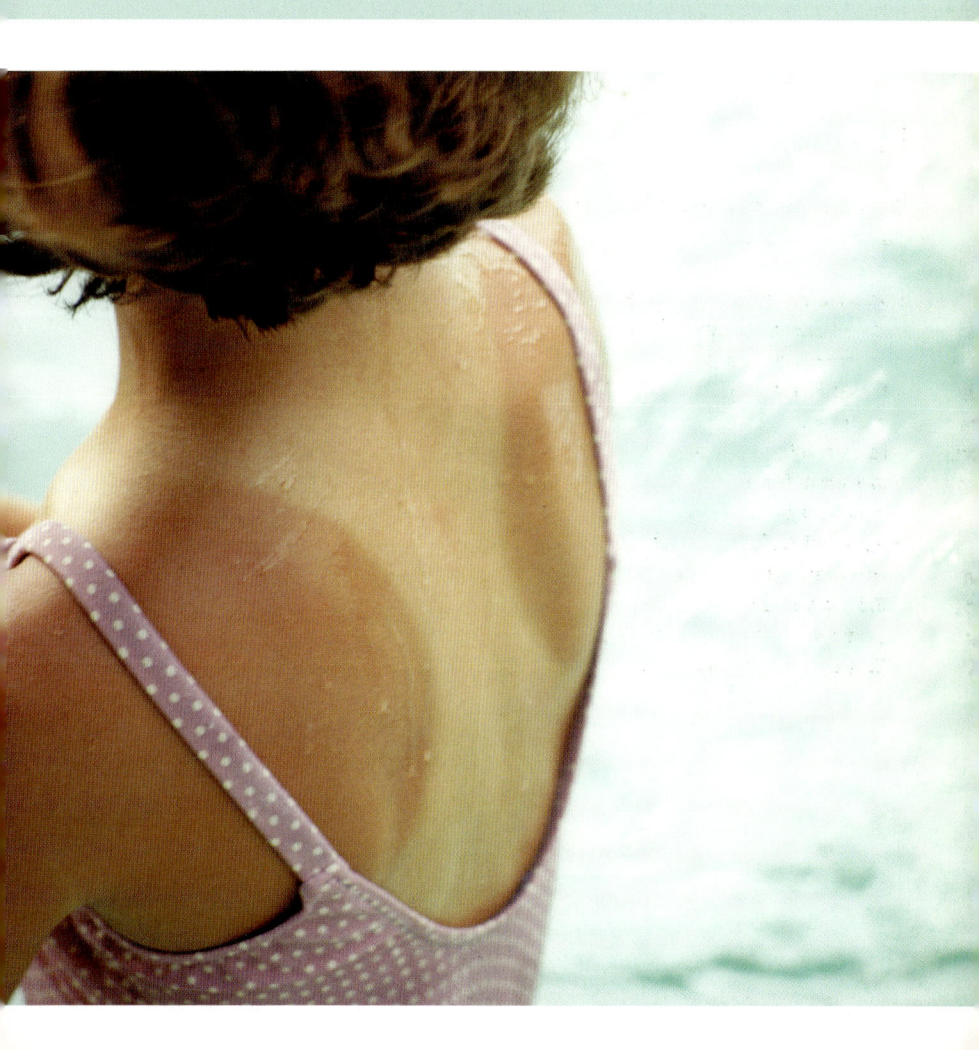

treating acute and chronic conditions

moods and emotions

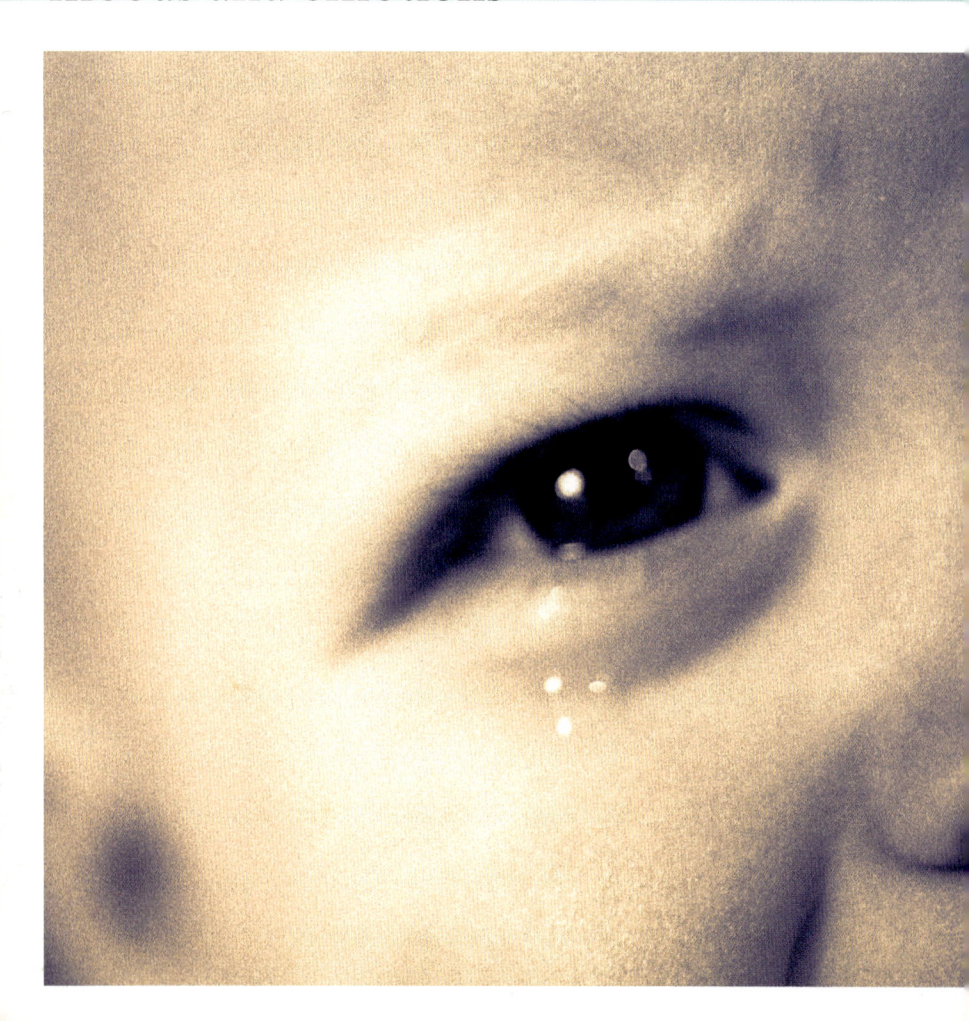

apprehension (anxiety)

There are many conditions and situations that can provoke apprehension. When these situations take away your vitality and energy these remedies can help you considerably. However, if anxiety becomes a regular occurrence you should contact your doctor for professional guidance.

- **Argentum nitricum** For anticipatory anxiety before an event such as an exam, a speech or an important event that causes anxiety.
- **Gelsemium** For apprehension accompanied with fear, diarrhoea and trembling.

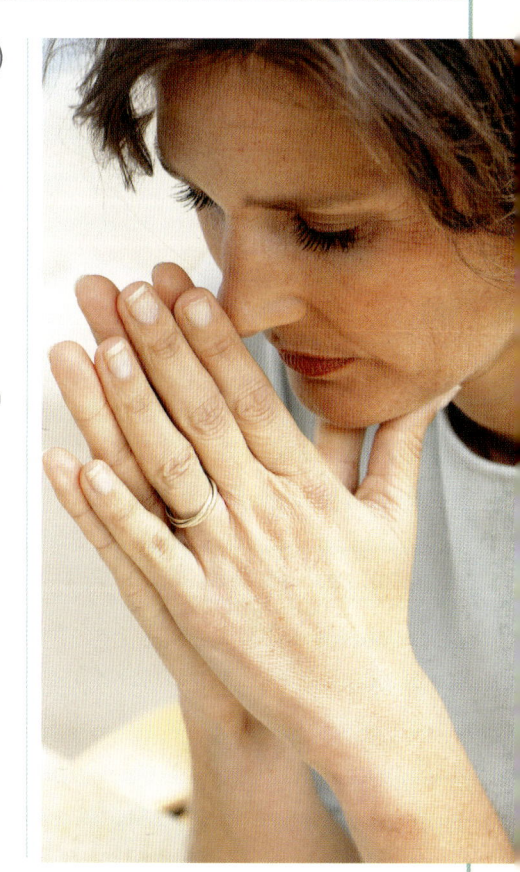

Feelings of apprehension and anxiety can be helped by taking Argentum nitricum or Gelsemium.

bereavement (grief)

This may arise at any time one experiences loss. This can also be for losses felt acutely in the past that have not disappeared with time. Use for family members at a funeral or when a loved one is ill in hospital, or when hearing upsetting or sad news. It is better to allow the feelings to come to the surface rather than to suppress them.

- **Aconite** When death comes quickly and friends or family are in shock.
- **Ignatia** For grief that lingers; when there is silent brooding, sadness, hysteria, or deep crying.
- **Natrum muriaticum** When there is deep depression from grief and the patient shuns consolation and wishes to be alone.
- **Phosphoric acid** When grief turns to indolence, indifference, despair or apathy.

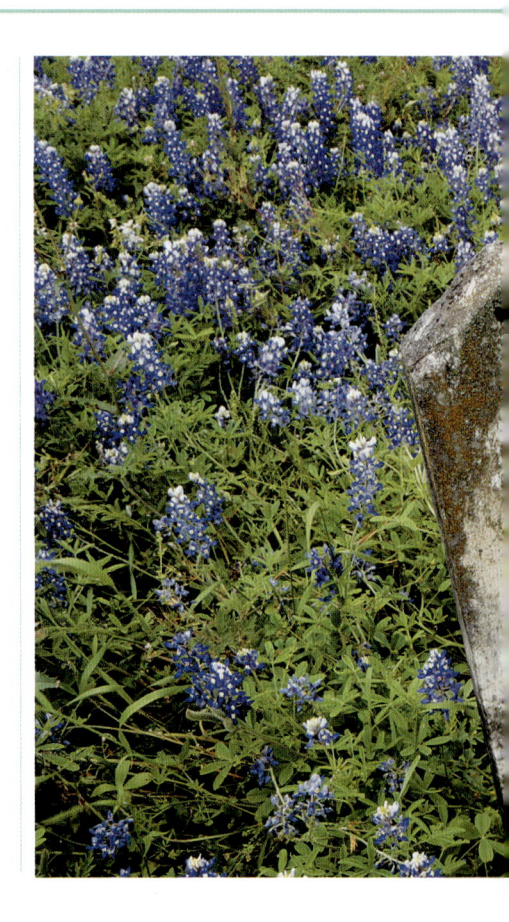

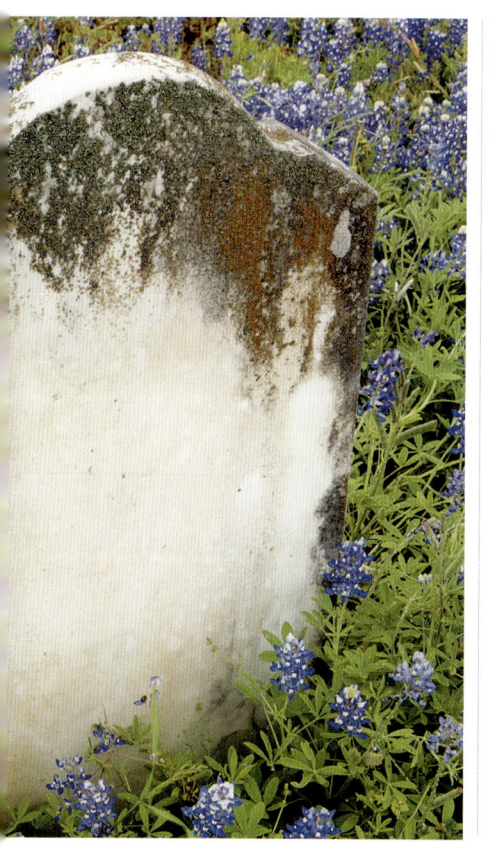

fear

This is a treatment for immediate fear. Do not use for long term, persistent fear, as this needs professional help. Consult your doctor in these cases.

- **Aconite** When fear comes on after a frightening experience.
- **Argentum nitricum** When fear comes from having to be in crowds or in front of a group.
- **Arsenicum album** When fear becomes terror (of death, crowds or a bad experience).
- **Phosphorus** Where there is fear of thunder or of darkness.

Homeopathic remedies can help you cope with the terrible pain of grief.

reproductive system and pregnancy

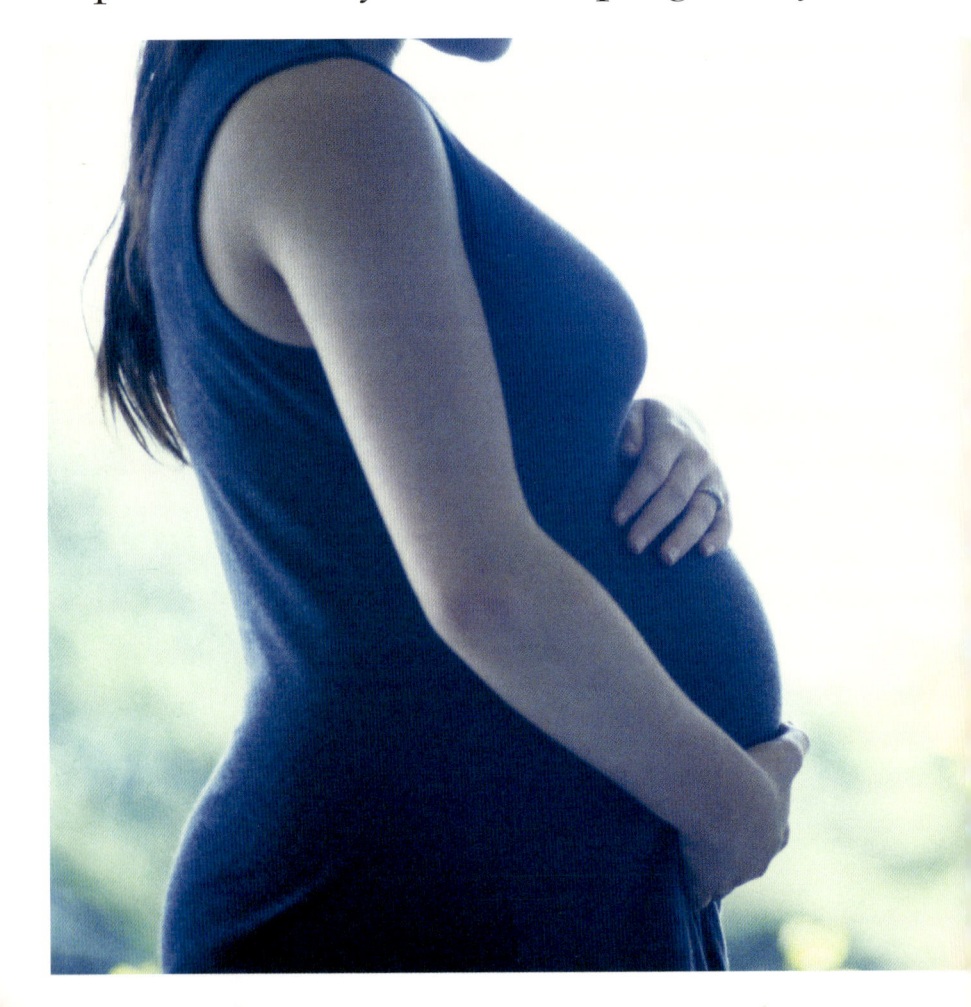

cystitis

Women, particularly, can suffer from cystitis, which is caused by inflammation of the inner lining of the bladder. The condition is characterized by the urge to pass water accompanied by pain. Always drink plenty of water if you suffer from cystitis, and consult your doctor if the condition persists or becomes particularly uncomfortable.

- **Apis mellifica** When it is painful to urinate and there is a stinging feeling, and the patient is not thirsty.
- **Belladonna** When it is painful to urinate and there is a stinging feeling and a fever.
- **Cantharis vesicatoria** When there is frequent urination and a burning feeling.
- **Chamomilla** When there is great sensitivity to pain, especially in young people.
- **Lycopodium** When there are pink deposits in the urine.
- **Pulsatilla** When symptoms shift from place to place and the patient is upset.

menstrual pains

Homeopathy can help with many common symptoms that women experience during the menstrual period. The remedies below are particularly effective.

- **Calcarea carbonica** When the breasts are tender and swollen.
- **Calcarea phosphorica** When the period is accompanied by headaches, arrives too early or is excessive in young girls.
- **Lycopodium** When depression accompanies the period.
- **Magnesia muriatica** When there are cramps before and during a period.
- **Natrum muriaticum** When sad and irritable before and during a period.
- **Pulsatilla** When tearful with painful breasts.

morning sickness

The following remedies may help if you suffer from morning sickness in pregnancy. All remedies should be given in a 30C potency, repeated no more than every two hours. Take as needed; when symptoms disappear, stop taking the remedy.

- **Ipecac** The woman's tongue is clean and pink with no yellowing or discoloration but nausea is constant.
- **Nux vomica** The woman craves stimulants, such as curries and spices. She is irritable with her partner and other children. She can be constipated or be violently sick.
- **Pulsatilla** The woman craves food that disagrees with her. She longs for rich food that is hard to digest. The food lies in the stomach and feels like a stone.
- **Sepia** The woman feels much worse at the sight and smell of food. She is oversensitive to smells, and better for motion, such as a brisk walk. She is often constipated.

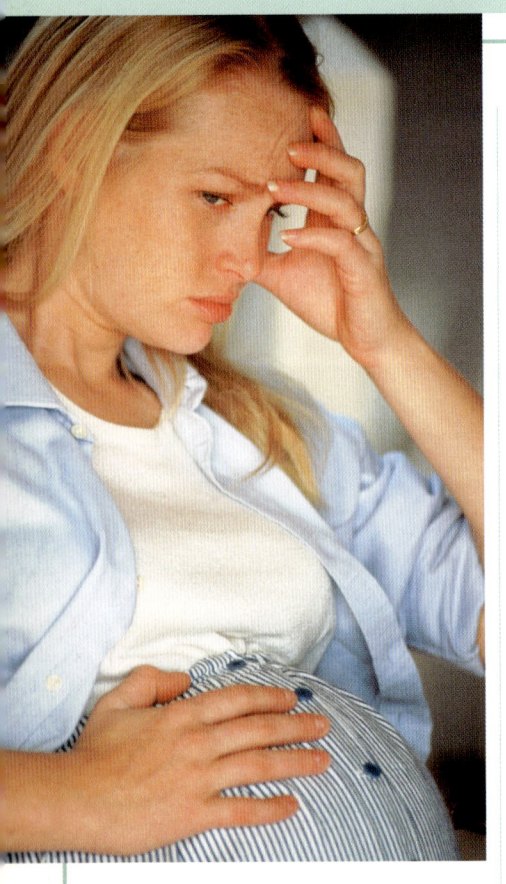

Morning sickness during pregnancy can be disabling. Several remedies can help.

A blocked milk duct during breastfeeding can become infected, leading to mastitis. A remedy will help relieve the condition.

mastitis

Mastitis is an inflammation of breast tissue, often caused by blocked milk ducts or a bacterial infection. The remedies below should be taken in 30C potency.

- **Belladonna** Mastitis resulting from too copious flow of milk. Mother feels shaky, hot but not thirsty, with swollen, tender, hard breasts. She can be emotional and delirious, with a flushed face and hot, dry skin.
- **Bryonia alba** For when the patient is hot, feverish and thirsty. The mother is worse for motion and better for pressure. She has shooting pains in her breasts, which are hot, swollen and hard.
- **Phytolacca decandra** Mastitis that is caused from excessive flow of milk. Nipples are so sensitive that the baby's sucking produces pain which can radiate to the mother's whole body. The nipples are raw and burning.

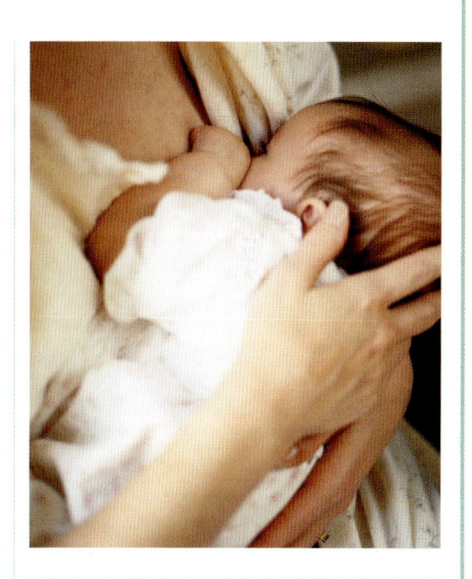

Useful tincture

Use two drops of Phytolacca tincture in a little water to bathe the breasts as well as taking the remedy Phytolacca decandra.

injury and surgery

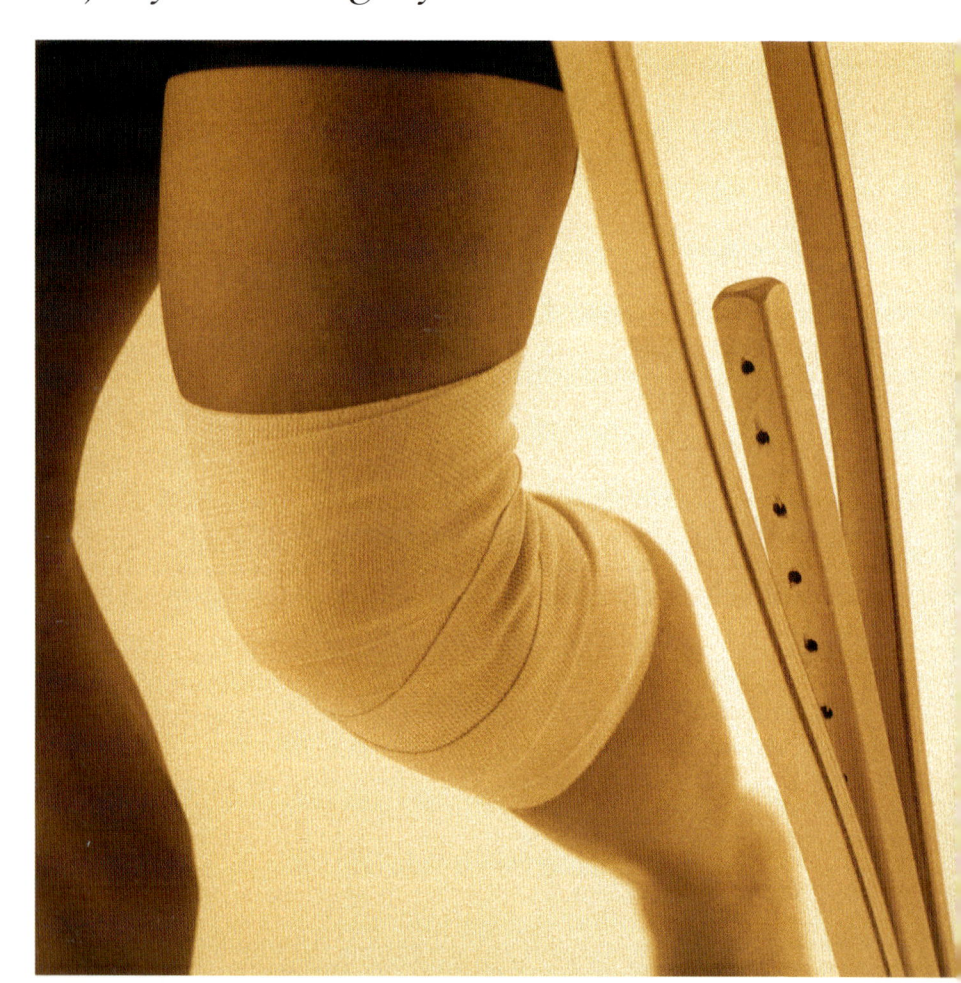

accidents

Contact your doctor or nearest accident and emergency department immediately for anything other than minor accidents. The following remedies may help with minor accidents only.

- **Arnica montana** For injury, shock and trauma where there are no symptoms of fear.
- **Aconite** For shock, injury and trauma where there is fear.

Support therapy

Use Rescue Remedy (see page 376) as well as your chosen remedy for relief of fear and trauma after surgery.

surgery

Homeopathy can help someone to recover after they have undergone surgery. These remedies can be repeated every 15 minutes to hourly. When the symptoms are relieved stop the remedy.

- **Arnica montana** To remove shock and trauma from the body.
- **Bellis perennis** A remedy which helps with the repair of soft tissue that becomes damaged during surgery.
- **Phosphorus** Give this remedy after surgery for clearing the anaesthetic from the system.
- **Veratrum album** For physical recovery from surgery.

babies, children and immune system problems

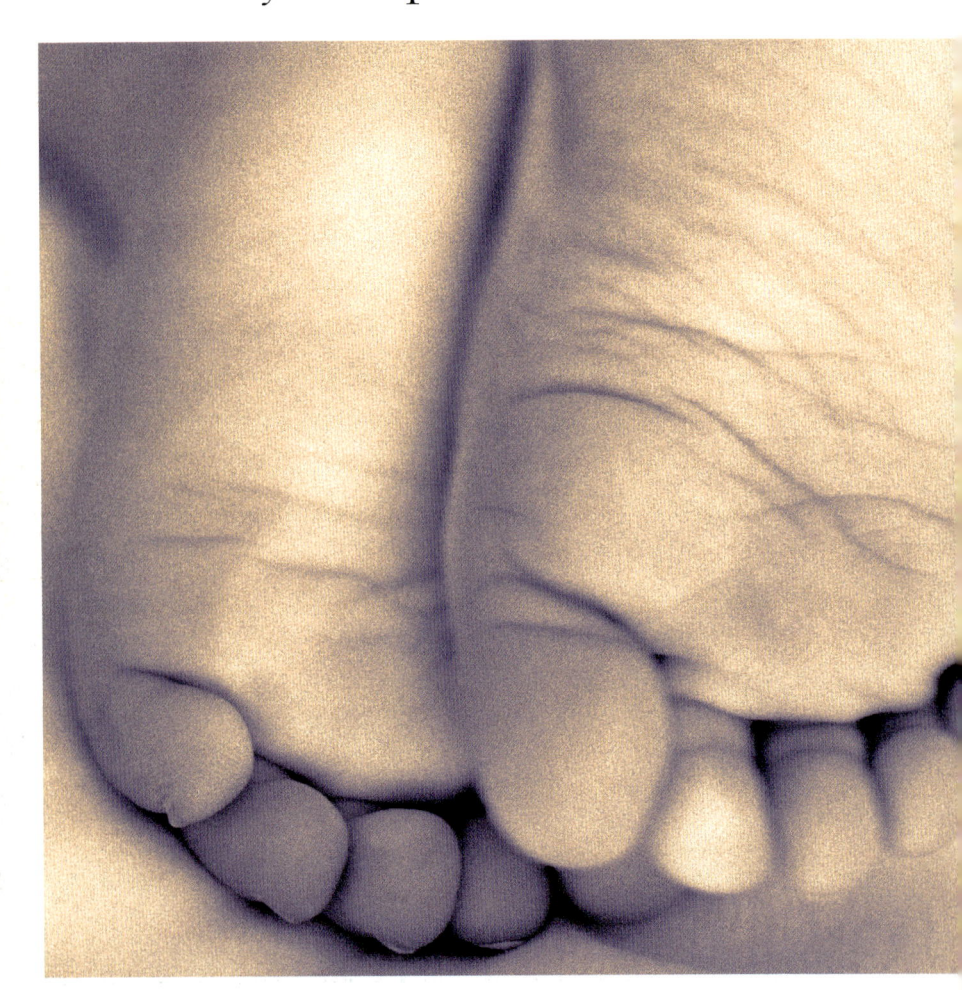

teething

A baby can become very distressed and irritable when he or she begins teething, and it can be a difficult time for the mother as well.

- **Aconite** For fearful and distressed babies.
- **Belladonna** For convulsions due to teething.
- **Borax** For teething accompanied by tiny ulcers in the mouth, or thrush.
- **Calcarea carbonica** For late teething. Where there is diarrhoea with green stools as a result of teething.
- **Chamomilla** For irritable and crying babies who want to be picked up and held.
- **Mercurius solubilis**** For excessive drooling during teething arising from sore gums.
- **Silica** For slow teething and sensitive gums with blisters.

As the first teeth push through the gums the baby can become upset. Homeopathy offers gentle pain relief.

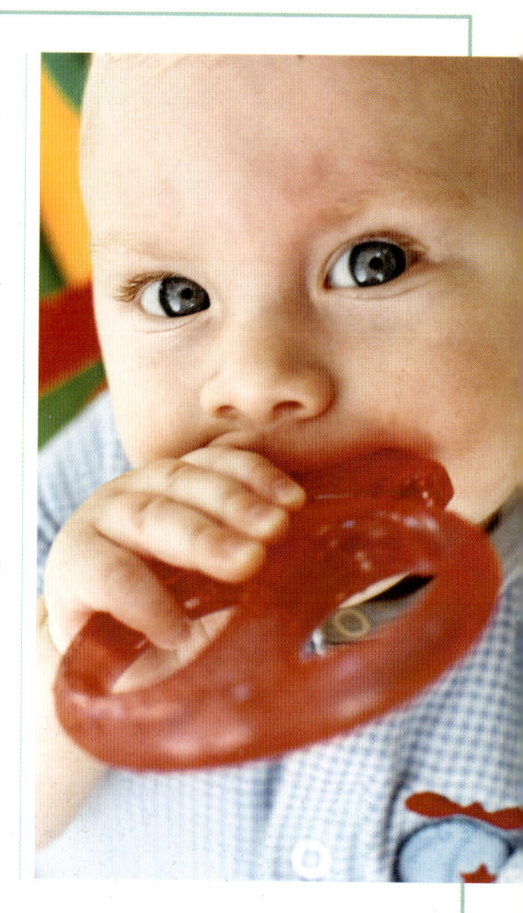

croup

Infants and young children may suffer from croup, which is characterized by a barking cough and hoarseness. Persistent croup needs a doctor's attention.

- **Aconite** For the sudden onset of symptoms that usually occur in the middle of the night. The cough is dry and barking, and the baby chokes and gags. Often dry skin and fever follow. The baby can be anxious and fearful.
- **Belladonna** For attacks when the patient is red, flushed and hot to the touch, with glassy eyes. The cough is often explosive and painful, and leaves the patient hoarse.
- **Hepar sulphuricum** For croup that comes from dry, cold winds. The baby chokes and there is a rattling sound in the chest. It feels as if a fish bone is caught in the throat.
- **Kali bichromicum** Stringy mucus that is difficult to cough up is the key symptom for this remedy.
- **Phosphorus** The patient is hoarse and unable to speak; talking and coughing are painful.
- **Spongia tosta** For dry coughs that are not accompanied by mucus.

colic

Infantile colic is the extreme end of normal crying behaviour. The cause is not known but some suspect that it is due to spasms in the intestine. The baby is irritable and cries or screams excessively.

- **Aethusa**** For colic caused by sensitivity to breast milk.
- **Chamomilla** For angry, irritated children.
- **Cina** For colic with gas; often the child also has worms.
- **Magnesia carbonica** For colic that is better for heat and pressure.
- **Pulsatilla** For gentle, unhappy babies who need to be held, rocked and moved often.

cradle cap

Cradle cap is a common condition in babies where thick yellow scales occur in patches over the scalp. It is harmless unless the scales become infected. Please see your doctor if the condition worsens or looks inflamed.

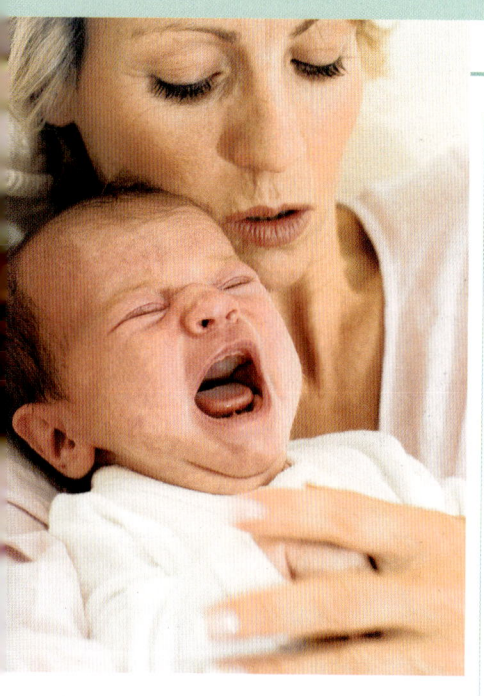

Colic in very young babies is a distressing condition for baby and parent alike. The baby screams and cannot settle.

- **Sulphur** For a scruffy, oily skin and scalp. The child is hot tempered and hot skinned.
- **Thuja occidentalis** For skin infections in a cooler, calmer child.

nappy rash

When a baby's skin becomes irritated by substances in the urine or faeces he or she will develop nappy rash, which is very uncomfortable. Aim to keep your baby's skin dry for as long as possible to prevent its occurrence.

- **Sulphur** This remedy is good for red, irritated skin conditions with cracked skin. The child is often hot and irritable.
- **Thuja occidentalis** This remedy is better suited to quiet, calm children who suffer with skin irritation.

adenoids (for children only)

Swelling at the back of the throat above the tonsils can cause adenoid problems. If your child experiences persistent symptoms please consult your doctor.

- **Baryta carbonica** For children who are underdeveloped.
- **Calcarea carbonica** For overweight and clammy children who sweat at night.
- **Calcarea phosphorica** For thin children with enlarged adenoids.
- **Sulphur** Give to hungry children who dislike bathing and who have enlarged, obstructing adenoids.

tonsillitis

A person will have tonsillitis when there is inflammation of the tonsils caused by infection. Please consult your doctor if these symptoms do not disappear within a moderate period of time.

- **Baryta carbonica** For small children with large tonsils that suppurate and are painful.
- **Calcarea carbonica** For swollen tonsils and swollen cervical glands (found at the base of the throat just above the shoulders).
- **Hepar sulphuricum** For tonsils with a yellow discharge, patient is better for hot drinks.

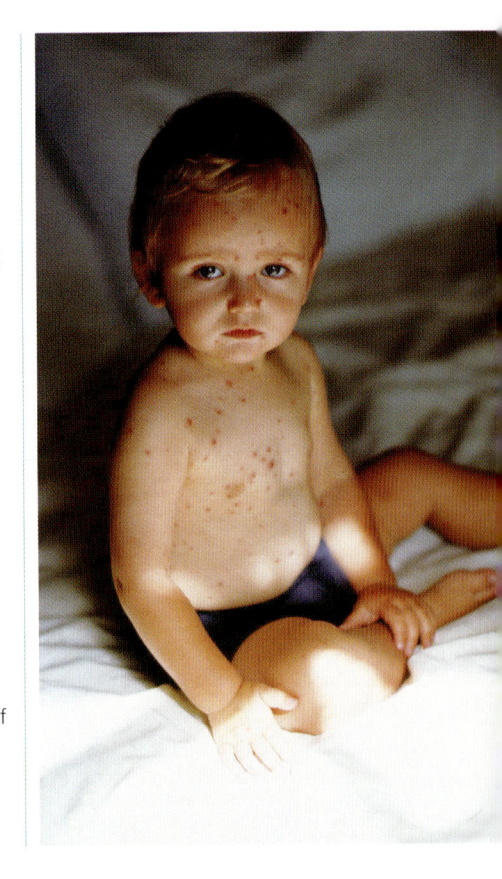

- **Phytolacca decandra** When there are swollen glands in the neck and swollen tonsils.
- **Sulphur** For swollen tonsils that touch each other. The child is hot.

chicken pox

Although chicken pox usually occurs in a mild form in children it can be more of a problem in adults. It is highly contagious and should be reported to your doctor.

- **Aconite** To be given in the early stages of onset. The child will be fretful, fearful and nervous. This will soothe the symptoms.
- **Antimonium tartaricum** For irritable, vexatious children who crave attention.
- **Belladonna** For chicken pox with fever, sore throat and flushed skin where the child is hot, thirstless and has a throbbing headache.
- **Pulsatilla** For weepy, clingy children who are fretful.

Homeopathy can help a child cope with the itching that accompanies chicken pox.

- **Rhus toxicodendron** To be used when the blisters are forming, Rhus toxicodendron also helps with all the signs of irritability that accompany this illness.
- **Sulphur** Give to hot children who are thirsty with no appetite.

measles

This highly contagious illness can sometimes have complications and should be reported to your doctor immediately.

- **Aconite** Use this remedy in the first stages of measles.
- **Apis mellifica** Good for high temperatures and sore eyes. The child is worse from fever and being too warm but they are not thirsty.
- **Belladonna** For high fevers, redness and restlessness. Good for a severe cough that is worse at midnight.

- **Bryonia alba** Good for painful coughs that are worse for movement. Bryonia alba will bring a fever down and help the patient to absorb water. The patient is worse for moving around and wants to stay in bed with their back to the door.
- **Chamomilla** For a child who is irritable and cranky, demanding and difficult. Chamomilla calms, soothes and eases the tension of being confined.
- **Gelsemium** For the exhausted, listless child who has a high temperature and who cannot keep warm.
- **Pulsatilla** Us this remedy after the illness; it is good for cleaning up the croupy symptoms that follow measles.

rubella (German measles)

German measles is dangerous to the unborn child if contracted by a pregnant woman, so it is important not to allow a child with the illness to come into contact with a woman who is pregnant.

- **Aconite** For first stages of illness with cold symptoms, chill and fever.
- **Belladonna** For a pink-red rash, swollen glands and both cheeks flushed.
- **Chamomilla** For irritable children who demand constant attention, and then reject it when given.

mumps

Although usually mild in children, mumps can be serious in adults. It is highly contagious and should be reported to your doctor straight away.

- **Aconite** Use in the early stages of mumps to help the respiratory symptoms that accompany this disease.
- **Belladonna** For red, hot, swollen glands that are worse for touch.
- **Calcarea carbonica** For pale, plump, children who sweat on their heads.
- **Pulsatilla** For mild, weepy and clingy children. They have no thirst with a fever. It is also useful for testicular pain associated with mumps.

- **Rhus toxicodendron** When the patient is restless and constantly moving. The salivary glands are worse on the left side and are dark, swollen and painful.

whooping cough

This illness is highly contagious and can be dangerous. It should be reported to your doctor immediately.

- **Antimonium tartaricum** Use to treat the post-fever stage of whooping cough if the patient has a wet, rattling cough.
- **Belladonna** For an acute fever that accompanies the disease
- **Drosera rotundifolia** Use if the symptoms are worse after midnight.
- **Ipecac** For coughing that induces vomiting and gagging.
- **Kali carbonicum** Use if the patient is exhausted from coughing.
- **Spongia tosta** Use if the patent is suffering from barking coughs.

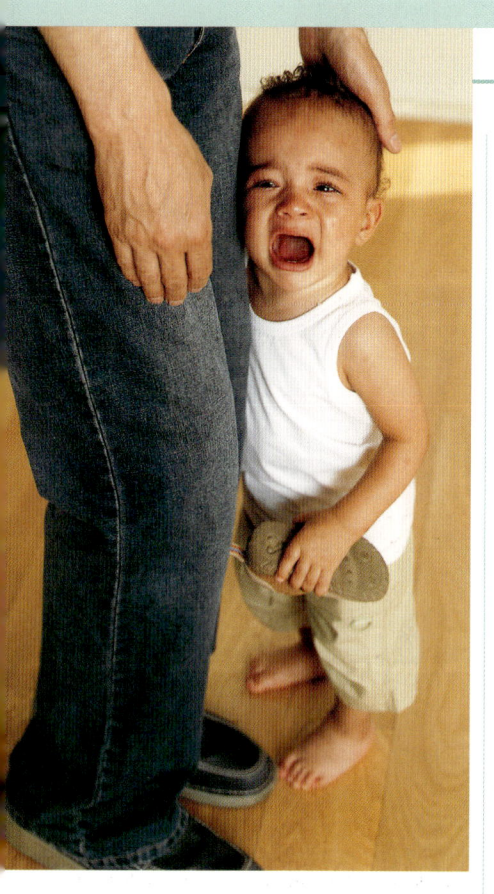

Whooping cough is potentially dangerous. Vomiting can accompany coughing.

immunization side effects

Homeopathy can help restore the body's natural balance after immunization. If you or your child suffer any serious side effects after immunization you should seek medical advice.

- **Apis mellifica** For allergic histamine reactions with swelling, or hot dry hives and welts over the body.
- **Belladonna** For a hot, red, throbbing swelling with high fever after immunization.
- **Hepar sulphuricum** Where there is a failure to heal after injection, including pus and hypersensitivity to touch.
- **Hypericum perforatum** Where there are sharp, shooting pains at the injection site. The site may be infected with red streaks that are beginning to move up the arm.
- **Ledum palustre** For bruising that occurs at the injection site
- **Pulsatilla** For weeping and sobbing after immunization, especially after having received vaccines for measles, mumps or rubella.

High pollen counts mean that summer can be uncomfortable for hayfever sufferers.

- **Silica** For children who lose energy and are unable to play or keep up with their peers after vaccination.
- **Thuja occidentalis** For symptoms after a smallpox vaccine.

allergies

A number of allergies can respond well to homeopathy. These remedies can help to alleviate symptoms but you should consult a homeopath for help with the underlying cause of the allergy.

- **Allium cepa** Used for episodic sneezing and tears. Cold compresses improve symptoms.
- **Arsenicum album** Sneezing and burning in the nose, eyes and throat. Symptoms are better for hot compresses and hot drinks.
- **Euphrasia** For eye irritation with burning and a watery discharge.
- **Hydrastis** For allergies that have a thick yellow discharge from the nose.

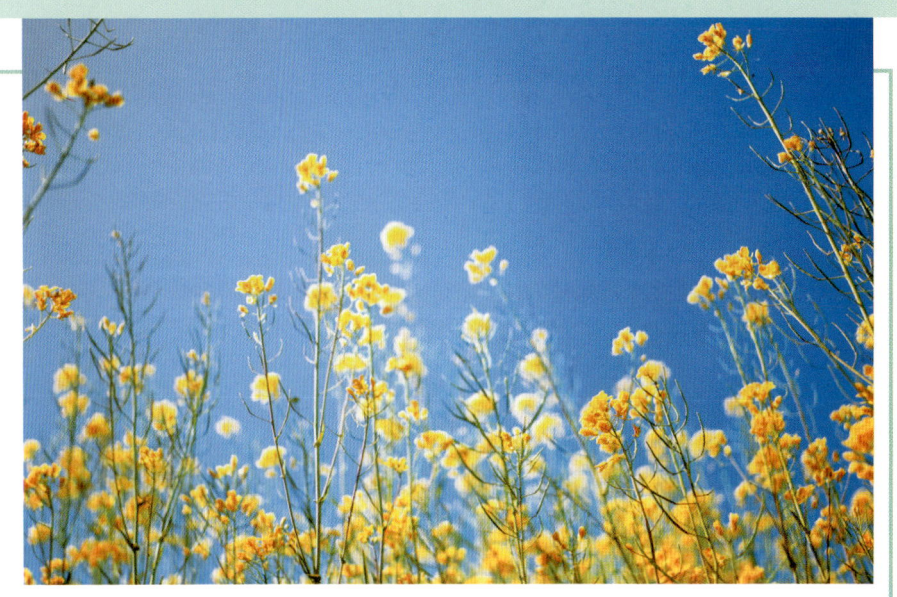

- **Pulsatilla** For stuffed-up noses with green discharge. Good for sinus infections and stuffy ears caused by flying.
- **Silica** An excellent allergy remedy especially where the patient is allergic to grasses and wheat. Good also for digestive disturbances caused by food allergies.

hayfever

When pollen counts are high hayfever sufferers can be extremely uncomfortable. The following remedies can help.

- **Euphrasia** For burning and watery eyes.
- **Pulsatilla** When all symptoms are better for being outdoors.
- **Silica** For people who are prone to being chilly, sedentary and weak.

bedwetting

If your child is wetting the bed this can be a sign of stress and anxiety. Try talking to them about any problems they may be currently facing.

- **Arsenicum album** For nervous children who are restless, and who toss and turn, and who feel unsure of themselves and are afraid of the night and being alone.
- **Benzoic acid**** For children with strong-smelling urine where the odour fills the bedroom.
- **Causticum** For children who wet the bed immediately on going to sleep and who are also unable to control their bladder during the day.
- **Cina** For irritable children with big appetites, who may be affected by worms as well.
- **Equisetum**** For children with pale, profuse amounts of urine.
- **Lycopodium** For frightened children who express their passive-aggressive anger by wetting their bed. They hold their urine in all day and go to sleep and relax, then their bladder empties.
- **Natrum muriaticum** For children who feel rejected and neglected. They will not urinate outside of their homes or in public washrooms. They hide their bedwetting.
- **Phosphorus** For children who are thirsty at night and drink before bedtime.
- **Pulsatilla** Give to a child who has a weak bladder and who is clingy and seeks company.
- **Sepia** For bedwetting in the first hours of sleep when the body is relaxed.
- **Thuja occidentalis** For multiple flooding at night; as many as five or six episodes.

fever

If a fever reaches a temperature higher than 39.5°C/103°F please consult your doctor immediately.

- **Aconite** For the beginnings of a fever, cold or flu. The child will be restless and frightened, and will be chilly.
- **Arsenicum album** For a fever that is worse after midnight. The patient is better for being cooled down with cold applications. They are anxious and restless.

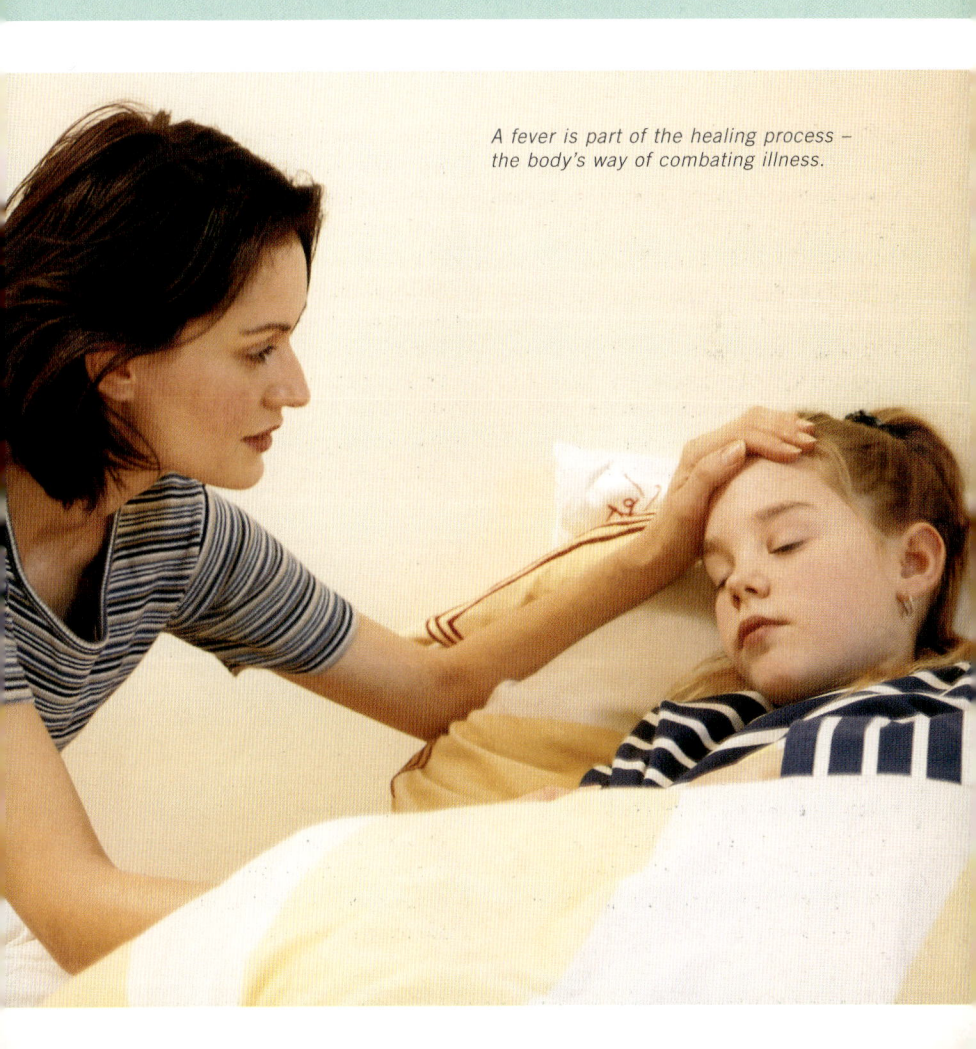

A fever is part of the healing process – the body's way of combating illness.

- **Belladonna** For high fevers where the child is dry, thirstless and even delirious. Pupils are dilated, eyes are glassy and the child is hot to the touch. They do not want to drink.
- **Chamomilla** For treatment of fevers associated with teething. One cheek will be red, the other white.
- **Ferrum phosphate** Use this cell salt to help a fever pass. The patient will be exhausted and apathetic.
- **Gelsemium** For fever accompanied by aches and pains, heavy eyelids and laziness.

impetigo

The skin infection impetigo usually occurs around the nose and mouth and is most likely to occur in children and teenagers. It is highly contagious and you should consult your doctor.

- **Antimonium crudum** For treatment of impetigo where there are cases of thick, yellow crusting lesions around the face. Washing and bathing only make the condition worse.
- **Arsenicum album** Use in cases where the skin eruption has dark, offensive pus with pain and irritation.
- **Calcarea carbonica** For an infection that comes with teething and forms dry crusts.
- **Graphites** For lesions that discharge and spread around the mouth and nose.
- **Hepar sulphuricum** For ulcerated, discharging lesions that are very tender and smell.
- **Lycopodium** To treat itching eruptions on the face and head that ooze and smell.
- **Sulphur** For skin lesions that have thick, yellow scabs and discharge.
- **Thuja occidentalis** Where there are eruptions all over the body that itch and shooting pains which are worse at night.

lice

Head lice commonly affect children and can be persistent, so should be treated quickly and thoroughly.

- **Lycopodium** For use as a rinse on the hair and scalp in the treatment of body lice.

Banishing head lice

Children can catch head lice (nits) from each other repeatedly, regardless of how clean their hair is. Use the remedy above in conjunction with the following:

- *Shampoo and rinse the hair.*
- *Work in large amounts of hair conditioner (a cheap version is fine).*
- *Comb through the hair, from the roots to the ends, using a nit comb and rinsing it each time to remove any nits or eggs.*
- *Rinse.*
- *Repeat this every three days for two weeks until all the nits' eggs have hatched and been removed.*

Head lice are now probably the most common parasite, and most children will be infected at some time.

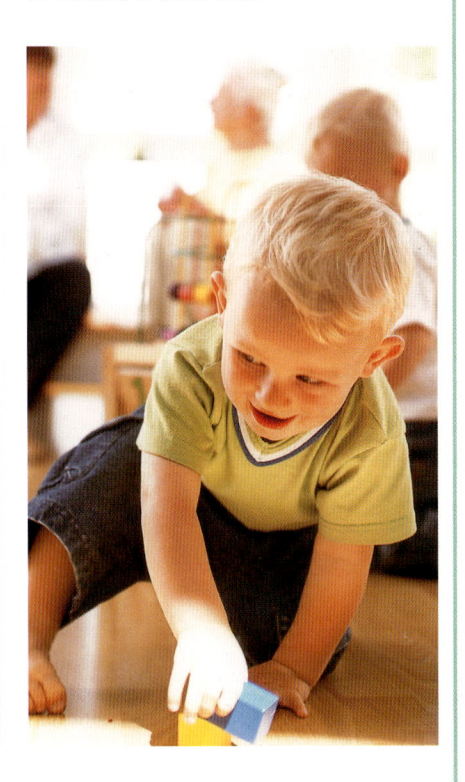

threadworms (pinworms)

Tiny worms, called threadworms, primarily affect children and cause anal itching and scratching.

- **Cina** This is a specific remedy for threadworms. Give the remedy three times a day for four days.

scabies

The skin complaint scabies is a skin infestation that is caused by a mite. It is highly contagious and should be reported to your doctor.

- **Arsenicum album** Used for scabies tracks that are filled with pus and occur at the back of the knee, causing burning and itching.
- **Carbo vegetabilis** For children who have a total body reaction to scabies when it appears as a fine, dry rash all over the body with much itching.
- **Lycopodium** Used for an infection that erupts, with deep scabies tracks and itching that is unbearable when the patient is covered and warm.
- **Mercurius solubilis**** Used for scabies in the elbow creases with itching that is so bad it is impossible to sleep.
- **Psorinium** Used to prevent repeated outbreaks of solitary eruptions after the main infection has been treated.
- **Sulphur** For use after the infection has cleared, on scruffy skin that is not clean. The child cannot stop scratching.

roseola

This is a contagious but mild viral illness that mainly affects children between six months and two years old. It is extremely common and can cause several days of high fever, which are followed by a rash as the fever breaks.

- **Aconite** Use in first stages of any illness in children. Aconite treats a body rash that extends to the hands.

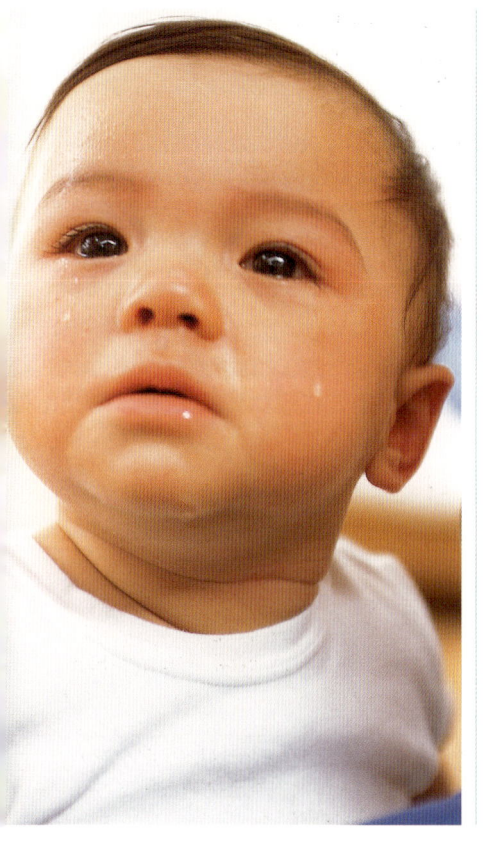

- **Belladonna** For a high fever with dilated pupils. It treats itchy, bright-red spots on the face and body.
- **Bryonia alba** For a skin rash that burns, itches, stings and is worse for movement.
- **Mercurius solubilis**** For raised rashes that have red blotches. The skin is wet with perspiration.
- **Pulsatilla** Used to treat an itchy measle-like rash that is worse for the heat of bed.

The mild viral illness, roseola, is common among young children and causes a high fever which can be treated with Belladonna.

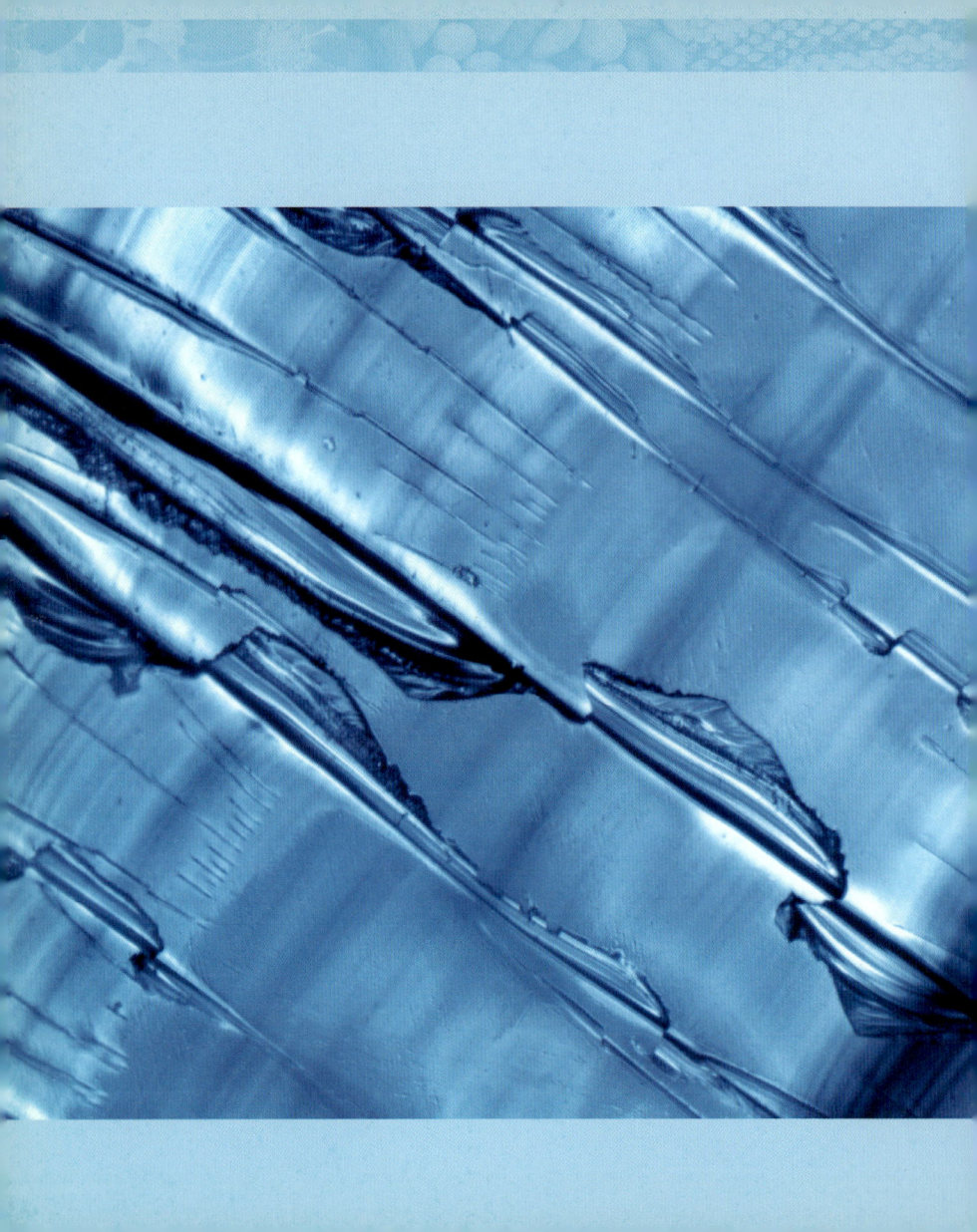

PART FOUR

support therapies and essences

cell salts

Some homeopaths use preparations called cell salts, which are are low-potency mineral salts that are found in the human body. These preparations come in small, easily dissolvable pellets. They treat many physical conditions and work where there is a biochemic insufficiency in the body. They help build tissues, regulate fluids in the body, purify the blood and build natural vitality.

These salts, originally prepared by Dr Schuessler of Germany, are known as the biochemic cell salts. They duplicate, in salt form, the vital building materials essential for growth, balance and healing in the physical body. When there is a lack of one of these salts, abnormal conditions will develop and lead to chronic illnesses. The theory is that health is maintained when the body is properly supplied with the cell salts it needs.

There are 12 salts in the biochemic cell salt remedies. Using these salts during pregnancy, for example, helps the fetus to develop strong bones, healthy blood and a strong cell structure. When a person suffers from chronic disease the cell salts help to rejuvenate their system. The salts work on the mucous membranes, the nerves, the fluids, hair, bones, nails and also on the crystalline lenses of the eyes.

An effective sore-throat cure comes from mixing two homeopathically prepared cell salts of Natrum phosphoricum 6X and Kali sulphuricum 6X. If this preparation is taken at the onset of a sore throat it can bring instant relief and stop it from developing further.

CALCAREA FLUORICA

This salt gives tissues their elasticity. It works on connective tissue and the surface of the bones as well as the enamel of teeth, where it is deficient or discoloured. Whenever there is a weakening or an overly relaxed condition, this salt is indicated. It is good for sluggish circulation, cracks in the skin, loose teeth and muscular weakness caused by overstraining or overstretching muscles, ligaments and joints, especially in active, loose-limbed people such as gymnasts or athletes.

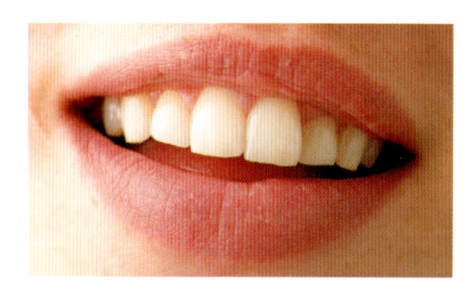

Calcarea fluorica helps to improve the enamel and condition of the teeth.

CALCAREA PHOSPHORICA

This salt works on growth and nutrition. It is used to restore weakened organs and tissues. It is also used for bones and teeth and is particularly appropriate when a child is not growing or is slow to develop. It also aids absorption and digestion of food in the body.

CALCAREA SULPHURICA

This tissue salt is a blood purifier. It cleans out accumulated non-functional, organic matter in the tissues and throws off decaying organic matter. It is used for all blood impurities.

FERRUM PHOSPHATE

This is the pre-eminent cell salt first-aid remedy. It is the oxygen carrier and is the remedy primarily used to quell fever. It is good for congestion, pain, high temperatures and a quickened pulse. It can also be given in the early stages of acute disorders and should be administered frequently until the inflammation subsides. It is good for illness in old age and in young children and it is a useful first-aid cell salt for muscular strains and sprains.

KALI MURIATICUM

This cell salt is for sluggish conditions. It works on skin problems, such as eczema and warts, on mucous membranes and wherever pus occurs. It is also used to cleanse and purify the blood. Use Kali muriaticum when the tongue has a white coating and when the liver is torpid and dysfunctional. It is also effective in the treatment of colds, sore throats, coughs, tonsillitis, bronchitis and in all children's illnesses such as measles, chicken pox and mumps.

KALI PHOSPHORICUM

This is the nerve nutrient. It is a wonderful remedy for nervous people, or for those under stress and faced with intense demands. It also helps to keep school children contented, happy and sharp witted. When children are fretful, ill humoured, bashful or lazy this remedy helps restore balance. Good for nervous headaches, sleeplessness, lowered vitality, depression, weariness, grumpiness and other conditions where vitality is low.

KALI SULPHURICM

This remedy helps respiration when a person feels they cannot get enough air. It is also indicated when there is a sticky, yellowish discharge on the skin or mucous membrane. It works on eruptions on the skin and scalp accompanied by scaling. It will help eliminate a sore throat.

MAGNESIA PHOSPHORICA

This remedy is an anti-spasmodic. It works with the nervous system when there is pain. It is indicated for neuralgia, neuritis, sciatica and headaches with shooting, darting pains or that start in the nape of the neck. It will relieve muscular twitching, heartburn, cramps, hiccups, convulsive coughing and sharp twinge-like pains. It works best when the pellets are taken with a sip of hot water.

NATRUM MURIATICUM

This remedy works on water distribution. It maintains the proper balance of moisture in the cell wall. Excessive moisture or excessive dryness in any part of the system can lead to a deficiency in salt, which is what Natrum muriaticum is.

Take these cell salts for low spirits, despair, depression, headaches with constipation, colds with discharges of mucus and sneezing, a dry painful nose, and throat symptoms. Also good for heartburn, a tremendous thirst, toothache and facial neuralgia with a flow of tears, weak eyes, hayfever, muscular weakness, unrefreshed sleep and the after-effects of alcohol.

NATRUM PHOSPHORICUM

This remedy is known as the acid neutralizer. It is good for a wide group of ailments arising from too much acid in the blood. This remedy controls the assimilation of fats and has an affinity with the digestive system. It is indicated for dyspepsia, pain after eating, highly coloured urine, worms and nervous irritability. It also works for sleeplessness from nervous indigestion, and for rheumatism, lumbago, fibrositis (inflammation of the fibrous connective tissue, usually affecting the back) and associated ailments.

NATRUM SULPHURICUM

This remedy helps eliminate excessive water. It controls the healthy functioning of the liver by promoting the free flow of bile and is indicated for biliousness and sandy deposits in the urine. It is the principal agent for treating flu, humid asthma, malaria and other conditions associated with humidity. A few doses will help dispel the languid feeling experienced during humid weather.

SILICA

This remedy is the cleanser. It throws off non-functional organic matter. It can initiate the healing process by promoting suppuration, which is one way the body releases toxins, and by breaking down pathological debris in the blood. It is good for abscesses, skin and nail weakness, and for strong bones. It acts as a nerve insulator and is good for toothache and other forms of acute pain. Use Silica for offensive perspiration of the feet and armpits, and for when pus forms or there are abscesses, boils or styes. It can also be used to treat tonsillitis.

> *Note: Many homeopaths also work with a number of non-homeopathic remedies and give advice on nutrition, supplements, lifestyle, relaxation techniques and kinesiology. The following are just some of the possible support therapies that can be useful.*

flower essences

Although not homeopathic remedies, flower essences can be used to help support your health and well-being in conjunction with homeopathy and a healthy lifestyle. Flower essences are tinctures of elixir made from distilled water in which the buds and blooms of various flowers are placed and left to diffuse in natural sunlight. They have not been potentized in the homeopathic fashion and remain in their natural state, known as mother tincture form. The stock is preserved in alcohol, which acts as a preservative, and it contains the essence of the flower that has leached into the water. Contained within the essence are healing properties that work on the emotions and create stability and balance.

HEALING FROM FLOWERS

Everything in nature has healing qualities. Finding the essential qualities of flowers, trees and shrubs is the work of people who create

Honeysuckle is one of many flowers used to provide healing essences. This essence is taken to ease homesickness.

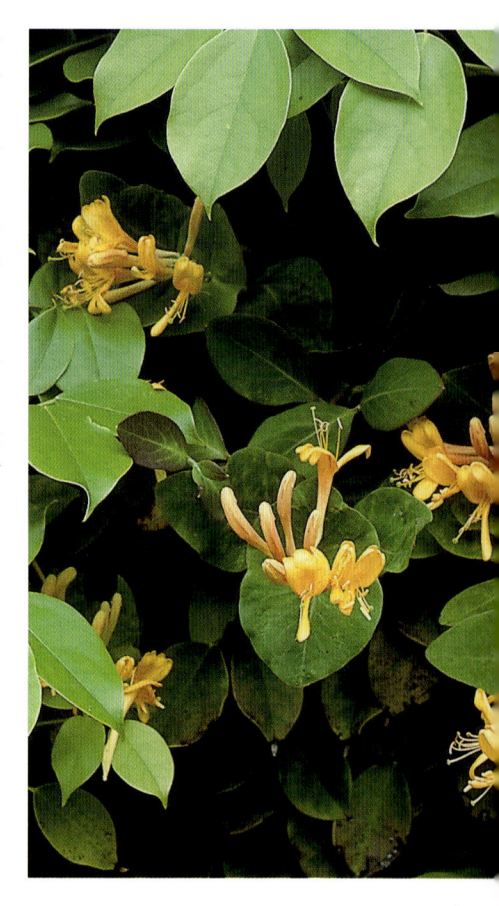

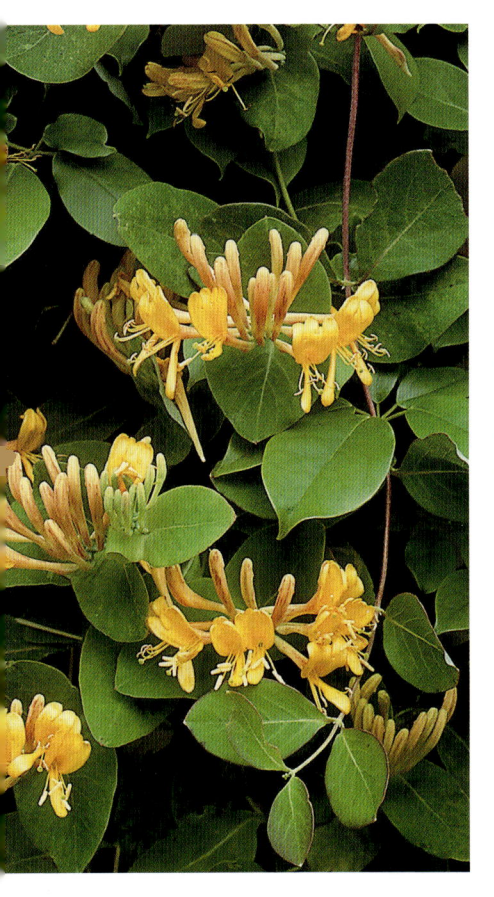

flower essences. There are many different brands and types of flower essences on the market today and they all have similar healing properties.

Whether they are used as herbal tinctures, potentized homeopathic remedies or flower essences, the healing benefit of the plant is expressed and experienced as medicine. Each works at its own unique level for healing different aspects of imbalance.

Flower essences work directly on our emotions, balancing distraught emotions and creating peace, harmony and inner balance. They are superb for taking the edge off homeopathic aggravations that have occurred through taking a high potency homeopathic remedy. Flower essences help deal with suppressed emotions that rise to the surface of consciousness and may be challenging to deal with until they pass away from the conscious mind. You can use flower essences as a significant part of emotional healing. Do not rely on them, however, to transform physical ailments. That is not their purpose.

A deep-acting constitutional homeopathic remedy can stir up long-buried and suppressed emotions. These unexpressed feelings can block the vital life forces and affect health. The emotions rising out of the realm of the unconscious can be experienced as anger, anxiety, grief or joy. A flower essence will help move the patient from a negative emotional state to a positive one and create greater emotional equilibrium. They do not affect physical health, but because so much of well-being depends on how a person feels emotionally these remedies work to increase health and vitality.

BACH FLOWER ESSENCES

There are many brands of flower essences available, and some people enjoy making their own essences from flowers that grow in their own gardens. The first person to develop flower essences was Edward Bach, a British homeopath who lived in the mid 1900s. He was a deeply sensitive person who felt the impact of a harsh and violent world and discovered the healing to be found in flower essences. A popular brand of flower essences is named after him and these are widely available in many countries.

RESCUE REMEDY

Bach harnessed the healing power of plants to work directly on stabilizing the emotions, and the world is indebted to him for his research. One of his premier remedies is a combination of five flowers called Rescue Remedy. This works for just what it says: it rescues us whenever we need relief from the grip of strong emotions.

Rescue Remedy can be purchased in most health-food stores today. A dose consists of two drops neat on the tongue or mixed with a small amount of water and sipped. It can relieve strong emotions that have become burdensome. It is also found in cream form and is excellent for skin irritations that itch or burn. You can also buy it in spray form, which works well in helping children and pets settle down quickly.

You will probably find it is worthwhile having a bottle of Rescue Remedy close at hand, in your handbag, your car, briefcase or on the kitchen shelf. Use it to take away fear and anxiety. Give your pet a drop of the remedy before you take it to the vet, as Rescue Remedy is calming for frightened animals. It can also help in any fraught and difficult situation to de-stress and bring core energy back to the surface of life.

If you are interested in making your own flower essences you will find plenty of information about the healing property of the flowers from several books now on the market.

Rescue Remedy is intended to be used for immediate situations; it is not a replacement for homeopathic or medical treatment.

Take two drops of Rescue Remedy after an accident, upset or shock to help lessen the immediate unpleasant effects.

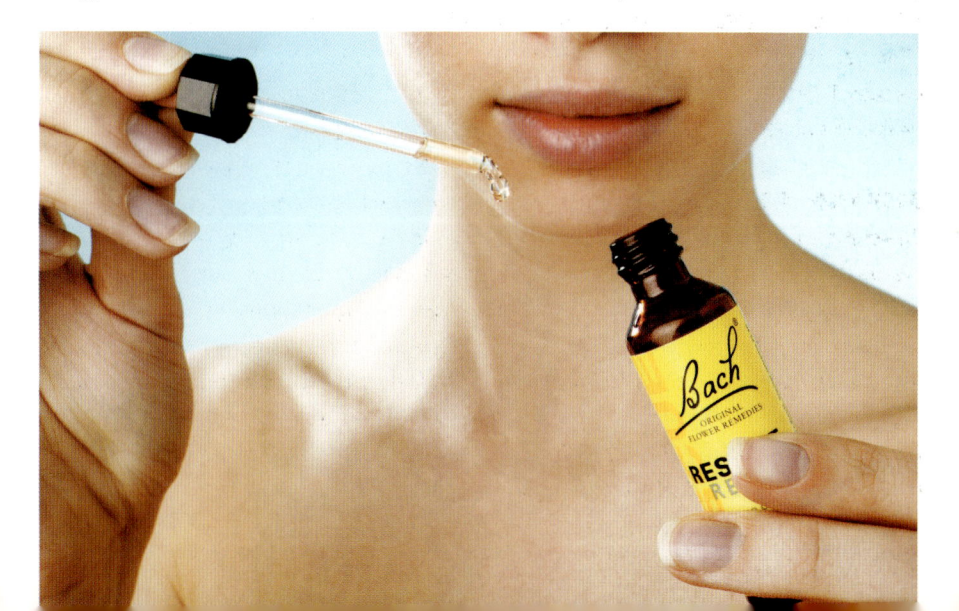

hormonal remedies

Hormonal remedies are quite different from homeopathic remedies. They are part of a treatment known as isopathy, which uses identicals rather than similars to heal. Hormonal remedies are not prescribed holistically or on an individualised basis so many homeopaths do not support their use. Hormonal remedies should never be used for home treatment.

When human hormones are potentized in the homeopathic fashion they become hormonal remedies. Although they no longer contain the original hormonal substance they carry its quintessential energetic pattern in the same way that all other remedies do. Hormonal remedies work energetically; because they are in potency they stimulate the ductless glands to rebalance themselves. This section explains the place of these remedies in homeopathy, but they are not intended to be used for self-prescribing, as complex physical problems like the ones that follow need professional guidance in conjunction with consulting your doctor.

HORMONAL IMBALANCE

When there is imbalance with hormones a serious condition can occur that creates havoc in the system. Although hormonal remedies are useful stimulants to redress imbalance they are best used as a support for deeper constitutional homeopathic remedies. For example, if a person suffered a thyroid imbalance it would be appropriate to give them homeopathic thyroid along with their particular constitutional remedy.

A constitutional remedy addresses the underlying cause of imbalance in the body. This may be emotional and connected to life issues or it can be part of one's genetic predisposition. For example, a deficient or overactive thyroid might register imbalance in a routine blood test and an allopathic doctor would treat this with synthetic thyroid hormones. The homeopath might want to know about the patient's ability to speak up for themselves, communicate their world view and express themselves, as these aspects of a person's make-up are relevant for prescribing the correct remedy. The homeopath may also ask the patient a variety of questions about their mind and emotions as well as physical problems they have had over the years to see what symptoms might have been suppressed that would have caused the function of the thyroid to be compromised.

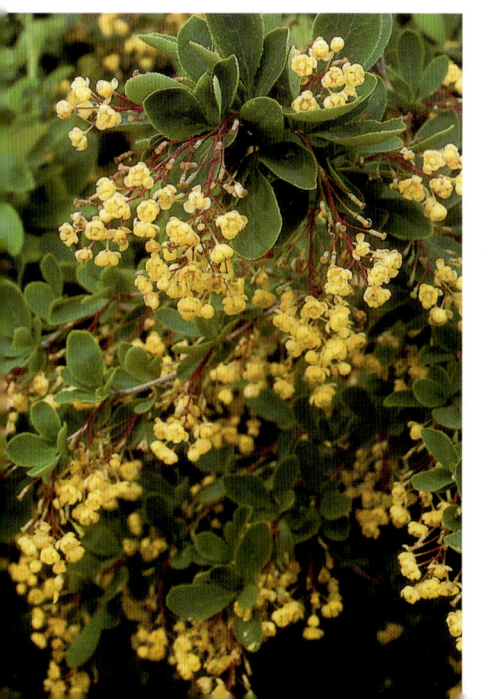

A hormonal remedy, such as Thyroid, can support the action of the deeper-acting constitutional remedy and can help the thyroid readjust to normal levels of performance.

TONIFYING THE KIDNEYS

In recent years homeopaths have observed that adrenal insufficiency is a common problem as a result of excess stress. The adrenal gland is found at the top of the kidneys, and homeopathy finds that the kidneys carry ancestral energy and can be easily taxed by shock and stress. There are therefore many support remedies to revitalize the metabolism and stimulate kidney function.

Tonifying the kidneys requires the use of several different remedies. In this case hormones of the adrenal cortex are not used, but plant remedies such as *Berberis vulgaris* in low potency work to regenerate kidney

The plant Berberis vulgaris *is used to prepare a tonic that will help improve poor kidney function induced by stress.*

function. Colour remedies can also help to stimulate kidney action; the colour orange works particularly well. Tonifying the kidneys should not be done at home.

MALE AND FEMALE HORMONES

In the case of sexual hormones homeopaths use remedies made from the inner lining of the human ovary, which is called Folliculinium as well as Oophorinum, made from the lining of the uterus, to help women who have had hysterectomies. Some homeopaths also recommend taking this hormone to help increase fertility. These two remedies have an affinity to the female body. They also have an emotional counterpart.

Male sexual hormones are also used in homeopathy. Testosterone is used for the male menopause, when the sex drive slows down and various dysfunctions appear, including enlarged prostates, frequent urination and other problems, psychological and chemical, that respond to constitutional treatment as well as hormonal stimulation.

STIMULATING OTHER GLANDS IN THE BODY

If the pancreas is not functioning properly this can lead to diabetes. Potentized Pancreas gland works well as a remedy and helps to keep this organ functional. Plant remedies such as Szygizum are also used to stimulate the pancreas, and are given in low potency.

Thymus gland is a homeopathic remedy used to build up the immune system. The thymus gland is very important in early years of childhood development but shrinks as the person grows older. Stimulating the vital force increases the chance of boosting immune responses to stress and shock. Again, this is given in low potencies and repeated regularly for several weeks.

Homeopathic Thyroid is used to assist both an underactive and overactive thyroid. It creates balance where there has been weakness, as well as alleviating sugar cravings, sleep irregularities and confusion. Where a person is treated with deeper-acting constitutional remedies by a homeopath, it may be possible for allopathic synthetic thyroid preparations to be substituted with the homeopathic Thyroid. However, never consider changing from allopathic treatment to solely homeopathic treatment without consulting your doctor, and always consult a qualified homeopath if you think that these remedies might be appropriate.

Anterior and Posterior Pituitary gland are also used as support remedies in homeopathy to assist people during times of change and stress in their lives. They can be helpful in treating tumours to the pituitary gland and also various physical and emotional functions of this gland.

Homeopathy has assisted people with many health-related problems that are connected to hormonal imbalance. However, colour and plant remedies rather than hormonal remedies are considered the best to use to stimulate the function of the pineal gland, which is responsible for the production of melatonin. Deep-acting remedies are used to treat dysfunction of this gland.

Homeopaths believe that alcoholism, epilepsy and brain disorders respond best to gentle stimulation, so colour and traditional homeopathic remedies are more appropriate than the hormonal ones here.

SENSIBLE USE

Hormonal remedies have an important place in homeopathy. It is ill advised, however, to take them without consulting a homeopath. Besides the expertise involved in diagnosing and prescribing there is always the question of support. This means that while you are taking the treatment you will have a professional to assist you in making the best choices if you encounter an aggravation or a problem. It is essential that you also consult your doctor before taking any of these remedies.

homeopathic colour remedies

A different, and sometimes controversial, branch of homeopathy uses colours to stimulate the energy centres in the body. To make these remedies, coloured light is transformed into homeopathic remedies in low potency dilutions. The colour remedies work directly on the energy system to stimulate, balance and tonify the chakras, which are energy centres in the body. The chakras reside in the spiritual body and control the vitality of the body; they also determine how energy functions.

There are eight major chakras in the human energy system that stimulate and regulate the flow of hormones. They are all associated with a certain colour and resonate with sounds and mental attitudes.

'Chakra' means 'wheel of light' and comes from ancient Sanskrit. It refers to life energy centres that run along the spine directing the flow of energy into the physical body. When a person is in balance the chakras spin in a positive flow bringing life energy into the system and discharging negative energy. They act as a subtle hydraulic system for moving energy through the entire human system.

The chakras respond to coloured light, both through physical application and in homeopathic preparations. Colour remedies are made in 6X, 12C and 30C potency. Each colour stimulates a particular chakra. They resonate with and affect the physical body, emotional well-being and mental clarity. The warm and hot colours can be taken when there is a lack of energy in the system, and the cooler colours can be used when the system needs sedating from too much energy.

Colour remedies can be used alone or in conjunction with deep-acting constitutional remedies. They can stimulate, tone and sedate the energy field according to what is needed and bring healing at a deep level. If a person has too much energy and is prone to inflammation, the colour remedies cool them and sedate their animal forces, bringing more spiritual energy into play and allowing them to find balance. If a person is too detached and disembodied in a spiritual sense, the colour

The chakras, the main energy points in the body, spin when the body is in balance.

remedies charge their physical forces and help them connect to the earth plane making them more grounded.

Many homeopaths find that a number of the life issues that relate to the chakras are resolved by using the colour remedies. For example, one of the problems that can result from moving house or changing jobs or relationships, is becoming ungrounded. The chakra that governs grounding is called the root chakra and it is located base of the spine.

Crown chakra
Third eye chakra
Throat chakra
Heart chakra
Solar plexus chakra
Sacral chakra
Base chakra

RED

The base chakra feeds energy into the legs and feet, the rectum and cervix. It governs one's sense of belonging to a family, tribe and community. If a person is cut off from their clan or separated from the flow of mother love and nurturing the homeopathic colour remedy red supports them in their healing and helps them find where they belong.

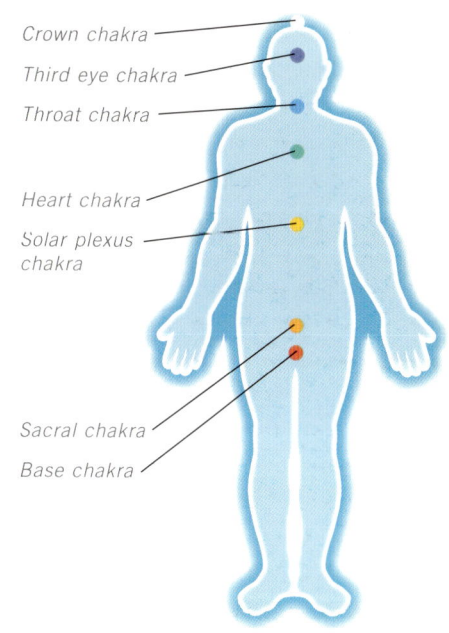

ORANGE

This is the colour of vitality and supplies the sacral chakra, located just below the navel. This colour rejuvenates and revitalizes the life force. It can be used if someone is recovering from an illness or is weakened by too much stress or hard work.

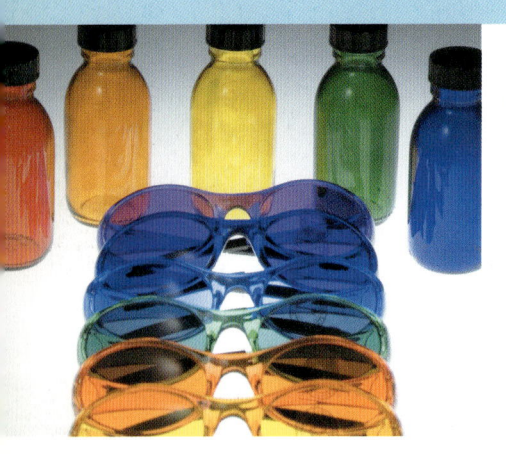

Solarized water, for remedies, and coloured spectacles are used in colour therapy.

YELLOW

Yellow has an affinity to the solar plexus chakra, and is located in the area of the stomach. It feeds energy into the vital organs of the liver, gallbladder, pancreas and stomach. At an emotional level it governs self-worth and personal identity. When our egotistic forces need to be fortified, for whatever reason, this colour remedy assists the spirit in staying strong and helps us find our inner power.

GREEN

This colour works on the heart chakra, along with pink, which is the colour of mother love. These two colours nourish the heart centre; first, by bringing peace and balance to the physical heart and stabilizing and nurturing the emotional heart. If you need to take the rough edges off your emotions, a dose of pink restores love and joy. Green is a calming and stabilizing force.

PINK

Pink is a colour that relates to the heart chakra. It is connected to mother love and is a gentle colour that stimulates kindness, self-love and gentleness.

TURQUOISE

This colour works on the throat chakra. This centre holds suppressed feelings and unexpressed thoughts, and it is here that a person may develop addictive behaviour. Many people encounter so much negativity each day and seem to be unable to be true to themselves in their daily lives that this can lead to an inability to express themselves creatively. This colour supports personal expression and creative flow. It works on the thyroid gland and helps with sore throat, toothache and gum problems.

INDIGO BLUE

Indigo blue works on the brow chakra, which controls pituitary functions and stimulates the mind. Without the stimulation of this centre we become like zombies, following the dictates of other people and never making the best choices for ourselves. A dose of indigo blue helps us to find objectivity and detachment from emotional dramas. It also helps us to form clear thoughts and to see the bigger picture when we are caught up in too much mental activity.

VIOLET

Violet works on the crown chakra and corresponds to the pineal gland. This is where we reflect on our relationship with beauty, bliss and our eternal connection with God, or with the Source or our Creator, depending on our own personal beliefs. We use this colour to help release physical pain and to calm the spirit if it becomes agitated. It has helped many people who suffer from chronic pain.

MAGENTA

This colour is made from red, green and violet. It works on the alta major chakra. It helps people garner insight into their true spiritual nature and helps them to sort out their needs on a human level. Magenta brings together the heat of red, the calmness of green and the softness of violet.

SPECTRUM

This is made of all colours and is an energy booster. We use it for auto-immune deficiency and weakened states of physical health and mental fatigue. It stabilizes low energy levels and supports people when they require more energy. It can also be used to help treat Seasonal Affective Disorder and depression.

gemmotherapy

Used by some homeopaths alongside traditional homeopathy, gemmotherapy is a support system of tinctures made from trees, which provides a high level of physical energy to help in the healing of physical problems. The name comes from the Latin *gemma* meaning 'bud', as most of the tinctures are derived from buds. All the tinctures are freshly harvested from growing plants.

Gemmotherapy is used to treat many conditions including anti-inflammatory problems, osteoporosis, asthma, infections, heart problems and colitis. They are liquid remedies in an alcohol and glycerine base and are potentized to a 1X dilution. They work best in conjunction with deep-acting homeopathic constitutional remedies, and their main function is to drain toxins out of the body.

This low-potency medicine works well for drainage and for increasing the energy in the body. The plant tinctures can be combined into specific formulas that are taken two times a day for several weeks. They are useful for conditions of stagnation and congestion in the body, where the body becomes sluggish so that nothing works efficiently; the person will become constipated, angry and lazy. Together with constitutional remedies, gemmotherapy tinctures are capable of improving a variety of health problems. They support healing and are useful in serious cases to help eliminate toxins, break down calcification and treat inflammation.

You can consult a homeopath to find out more about gemmotherapy. Tinctures are widely available on the Internet or from a homeopathic pharmacy.

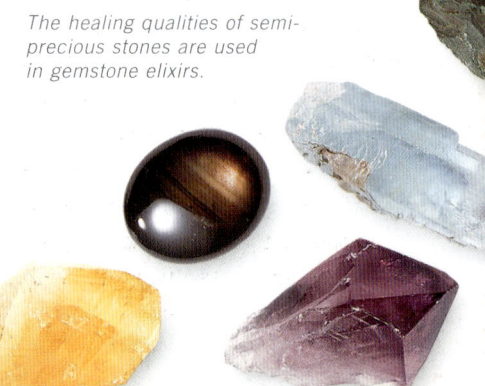

The healing qualities of semi-precious stones are used in gemstone elixirs.

gemstone elixirs

Another therapy that can be used alongside homeopathy are gemstones elixirs. These are made from gems that have been found to have an affinity with the individual chakras (see page 382–384), which are energy centres along the spine, each one responsible for different areas of the body. Various gems have been converted into homeopathic remedies through a process of immersion then potentization. They support healing by stimulating the body's energy centres to release more energy into the physical body.

Remedies made from diamond immersion have been useful for deep chronic depression, whereas emerald is used to stimulate the thymus gland for building immunity. Both of these gems are potentized into various strengths and used to treat a variety of conditions.

Aquamarine focuses energy on the throat chakra and is a support remedy for speaking truth and receiving the wisdom to see the truth. It also stimulates the thyroid gland.

Rose quartz in homeopathic potency is used to heal the heart. It brings peace, love and calmness, and supports people in finding their own inner forces of love. When given together with pink homeopathic colour remedy, this helps people with serious heart conditions find strength and peace.

The other gemstones that have been used successfully in homeopathic dilutions are tiger's eye, cornelian, bloodstone, hematite, citrine, peridot, jade, sapphire and amethyst. These gemstones all correspond to specific chakras and their respective life issues and challenges, as well as to their physical counterparts, which are the ductless glands that secrete hormones. Gemstone elixirs resonate with the chakras as well as adding to the body the mineral content from the gem itself, which aids healing.

Gemstone elixirs should be taken only under the advice of a qualified homeopath.

glossary

Acute illnesses An illness that is described as acute is a condition that generally begins quickly and will usually clear of its own accord, although some acute illnesses are very serious. Acute conditions include childbirth, accidents and illnesses such as colds and flu. The home user can prescribe remedies to alleviate the symptoms of acute illnesses such as colds and flu as well as helping in childbirth and for emergency relief for accidents, although serious illnesses such as pneumonia need to be referred to your doctor.

Aggravations After giving a patient a remedy a homeopathic aggravation can occur. According to Samuel Hahnemann's theory, the remedy is so closely matched to the patient's own symptoms that its effect can be mistaken for an aggravation of the patient's natural disease. In fact, an aggravation is a sign that the body is responding to the treatment. Aggravations are normally short-lived.

Cell salts Preparations called cell salts are low-potency mineral salts that are found in the human body. They were first identified in the 19th century by Dr W. H. Schuessler, a German physiological chemist and physicist. They can be used alongside homeopathic remedies to treat many physical conditions. They help to build tissues, regulate fluids in the body, purify the blood and build natural vitality.

Chronic illness An illness that is chronic is an ongoing illness that generally takes a long time to develop and tends to degenerate over time. Examples of chronic illnesses are arthritis and heart disease. Chronic illnesses should not be prescribed for at home.

Constitutional remedy A constitutional remedy is prescribed by a qualified homeopath to cover a range of conditions that a person displays that are part of their deep underlying character and are specific to them. These will be physical, emotional and mental symptoms and the homeopath will need to take a full and detailed case history before prescribing.

Contraindications There are a few instances when you should consult your doctor before using homeopathic remedies, such as if you are pregnant, have recently had surgery or are on medication from your doctor.

Dilution Remedies are made from substances that have been diluted so that the original toxins no longer exist, or only traces of them remain.

Flower essences The buds and blooms of various flowers can be added to distilled water and left to diffuse in sunlight to form flower essences. They are not potentized, as is the case for homeopathic remedies, but are used in their natural state to bring healing and balance to the body. Although not homeopathic remedies, flower essences can be used alongside them.

Gemmotherapy This is a low-potency support system of tinctures made from the buds of trees that are prescribed to help heal physical problems. The name comes from the Latin '*gemma*' meaning 'bud'. The tinctures work best in conjunction with deep-acting homeopathic constitutional remedies and their main function is to drain toxins out of the body.

Gemstone elixirs Made from gems, gemstone elixirs are potentized remedies that can be used alongside homeopathic remedies as prescribed by a qualified homeopath.

Hahnemann The German doctor Samuel Hahnemann began working on the development of homeopathic remedies after he closed his medical practice in 1790. He based his alternative therapy on the Law of Similars.

Hormonal remedies Remedies made from hormones are potentized in the same way as usual remedies and are used to balance the ductless glands.

Materia Medica Dr Samuel Hahnemann devised a comprehensive list of remedies, called the Materia Medica, which includes the emotional symptoms and physical complaints that can be helped by using them.

Miasms Dr Samuel Hahnemann believed that certain people held taints in their constitution, which might be handed down through the generations, and these would actually block remedies from working so that the patient could not get well. It is commonly believed by homeopaths that there are five miasms: the psoric miasm, tubercular miasm, scycotic miasm, cancer miasm and the syphilitic miasm. If a homeopath believes a patient has a miasmic block they will treat the problem accordingly over a period of several months.

Minimum dose Rather than taking a course of medication, as in conventional medicine, homeopathic remedies are taken one at a time and repeated only if necessary. They are stopped immediately improvement occurs.

Potency Remedies are used in various potencies, which relate to the amount of times they have been diluted and shaken. A centesimal potency is diluted in the ratio of 1 part to 99 parts of water or alcohol. It is then shaken and diluted again 3, 6, 30 or more times until the final potency is reached. These potencies will be labelled 3C, 6C, 30C, and so on. Where the substances have been diluted 1 part to 9 parts of water or alcohol these are called decimal potencies. They are labelled 6X and 30X, and so on. Dilutions of 6C or 30C are the most commonly used by the home prescriber.

Potentization Homeopathic remedies are made from substances (derived from a plant, animal or mineral) that have been diluted and shaken many times. The shaking is very important to the efficacy of the resulting remedy and is known as succussion. The process of dilution and succussion is known as potentization. A remedy can be prepared in different potencies according to the number of times it has been diluted. The more times the solution has been diluted and shaken, the greater and deeper its effect, so although a 30C remedy is more diluted than a 6C the 30C is the remedy with the stronger potency.

Remedy Homeopathic medicines are substances (from a plant, animal or mineral) that have been diluted in water and shaken. In the higher potencies, from 12C onwards, none of the original substance is present. The dilution, however, holds a kind of blueprint of the original substance. Hahnemann, who first developed the remedies, discovered that a substance that produced a shock-like reaction in the body, such as the poisonous plant aconite, when prepared as a remedy would be able to alleviate those same reactions in a body that was suffering from a similar shock-like condition.

Suppression When a person's life force has been slowed down, damaged or diverted by something externally, this is known in homeopathy as suppression. Suppression can be caused on a physical level through drugs that have pushed the symptoms deeper into the body instead of allowing them to work their way out from the inside. In homeopathy, the remedies kick-start the body's own immune system to cure the illness, and as a result other symptoms might be experienced until the core problem is reached and cured. Suppression also has an emotional aspect. We may suppress our feelings about an event or situation, such as denying anger, fear or grief. As a result we stop feeling alive, creative or even able to make a wise decision. In today's world homeopaths believe that suppression is the cause of many conditions, both physical and emotional. Homeopathy addresses both the mind and the body when prescribing remedies so these suppressed conditions can be alleviated.

The Law of Similars Hippocrates first came up with the idea that Hahnemann then called 'The Law of Similars', which states 'let likes be cured with likes' and this was adopted as the basis for homeopathy when Hahnemann first developed it in the 18th century. Hahnemann believed that if a toxic substance created a particular reaction in a person in its natural state it could cure a similar reaction in a person in its diluted and potentized state.

Vital force A kind of balancing mechanism, the vital force is a presence in all living things and it controls the physical, emotional and mental aspects of a person's well-being or illness and relates to their spirit. The vital force can be disturbed by emotional problems or large doses of medication. By choosing homeopathic remedies that harmonize with the vital force these disturbances can be healed.

index

Figures in *italics* indicate captions.
Main references to remedies and symptoms are indicated in **bold** type.

abdominal problems 60, 121, 131, 135, 150, 233, *306*, **306**, 307, 310, 311, *311*, *312*, **312**
abrasions **333**
abscesses **331**
accidents 39, 58, 87, 96, **351**
acid neutralizer 373
acid reflux **306–7**
acne **331**
Aconitum napellus (Aconite) 16, *17*, 58, **64–5**, 298–301, 309, 312, 317, 321, 323, 324, 325, 327, 328, 344, 345, 351, 353, 354, 357, 358, 362, 366
Actaea racemosa 325
addictions 37
adenoids (for children only) **355–6**
adolescence 76
Aethusa 311, 354
Agaricus muscarius **66–7**
ageing 57, 250
air-travel sickness **325**
alcohol
  abuse 60, 381
  after-effects 372
allergies 337, 339, **360–1**
Allium cepa **68–9**, 301, 360
allopathic medicine 39, *42*
Aloe socotrina **70–1**
Alumina **72–3**, 308
Anacardium oriental **74–5**
anaemia 47, *297*, **297**
anger 57, 76, 117, 144, 167, 218, 261, 308, 328, 354, 362, 386
ankles, weak 211
Anterior Pituitary gland 381
anti-ageing remedies 57
anti-inflammatory problems 386
antibiotics 29, *29*, 42
antidepressants 42
Antimonium crudum **76–7**, 312, 364
Antimonium tartaricum **78–9**, 298, 311, 357, 359
anxiety 57, 83, 104, 107, 115, 119, 139, 160, 204, 249, 256, 277, 301, 354, 362
see also apprehension
apathy 301, 364
Apis mellifica *59*, **80–1**, 309, 317, 319, 321, 332–5, 347, 357, 360
appendicitis 307
appetite 19
  excessive *307*, **307**
  loss of **305**, 307, 357
apprehension *343*, **343**
Argentum nitricum **82–3**, 309, 337, 339, 343, *343*, 345
Aristolochia clematis **84–5**
Arnica montana 58, 61, **86–7**, 315, 316, 317, 319, 321, 323, 325, 326, 328, 333, 334, 336, 340, 351
Arnica tincture 332
aromas, strong 41
Arsenicum album 58, **88–9**, 298, 299, 301, 305, 307, 310, 311, 313, 315, 323, 327, 328, 333, 337, 345, 360, 362, 364, 366
arthritis 36, 190, 278, 319, **319**
asthma 8, 28, 58, 149, 179, 222, 255, **298**, 373, 386
Aurum metallicum **90–1**
Australian Homeopathic Association 45
Avena sativa 328
avoiding common illnesses 50–53

babies
  colic 307
  diarrhoea 126
  problems with milk 135, 311, 354
  remedies for 57
  taking a remedy 41
  and vomiting 53
  see also teething
Bach, Edward 376
Bach flower essences 376
Bacillinum 335
back problems 61, 99, 155, 184, 244, 277, **315**
bad breath (halitosis) *305*, **305**
bad temper 95, 203
Baptisia tinctoria 336
Baryta carbonica **92–3**, 356
bedwetting 193, **362**
Belladonna *12*, 59, **94–5**, 301, 309, 319, 321, 322, 324–7, 329, 331, 340, 347, 349, 353, 354, 357–60, 364, 367, **367**
Bellis perennis **96–7**, 322, 351
Benzoic acid 362
Berberis vulgaris **98–9**, 379–80, *379*
bereavement **344**, *345*
bile, biliousness 180, 306, 373
birth control pill 253
bites 59, **332**
black eye 165, **334**
bladder problems 115, 362
bleeding 42, 247, 249, 297, 308, 317, 318, 323, 326
blisters 125, **331**, 353, 357
bloating 121, 131, 143, 222, 306, 311
blood pressure 42
blood sugar 52, 323
body
  attitude to own 171
  illnesses felt on left side 197
  stiffness 215
boils 34, 59, **333**
bone problems 34, 35, 93, 155, 301, 302, 315
Borax **100–1**, 336

bowel problems 275, 308
brain disorders 381
breast problems 96, 347
breastfeeding 101, 297
breathing problems 35, 42, 152, 183, 298, 300, 301, 372
bronchitis 32, **298**, 301, 371
bruising, feeling bruised 58, 87, 96, 239, 315, 319, **319**, 321, 327, 333, 334, *336*, **336**
Bryonia alba 59, **102–3**, 298, 299, 301, 306, 308, 309, 311, 319, 325, 326, 327, 349, 358, 367
burning 67, 95, 309, 313, 335, 339, 360, 366, 367
burns 50, 125, **340**

Cactus grandiflorus **104–5**
Calcarea carbonica **106–7**, 297, 299, 307, 318, 322, 324, 334, 337, 339, 347, 353, 356, 358, 364
Calcarea fluorica **108–9**, 299, 318, **370**, *371*
Calcarea phosphorica **110–111**, 347, 356, **371**
Calcarea sulphurica **112–13**, 333, **371**
calcification 386
Calendula ointment 331
Calendula tincture 317, 331, 332, 333, 335, 338
cancer 13, 36–7, 241, **340**
cancer miasm 34, 37, *37*
Cantharis vesicatoria **114–15**, 332, 340, 347
Capsicum **116–17**
Carbo animalis **118–19**
Carbo vegetabilis 60, **120–21**, 303, 309, 310, 311, 366
carers 187
case studies 20–23
catarrh 36, **299**

Caulophyllum **122–3**
Causticum **124–5**, 331, 340, 362
cell production 35, 37, *37*
cell salts 370–73
centesimal potencies 24
chakras 382–5, 387
Chamomilla **126–7**, 313, 318, 321, 322, 347, 353, 354, 358, 364
chamomilla granules 53
Chelidonium majus **128–9**, 301, 334
chest complaints 32, 42, 79, 104, 256, 298, 299
chicken pox *357*, **357**, 371
chilblains 67
childbirth 57, 122, 132, 184, 189, 225, 247, 323
children
 behavioural problems 149
 convulsions 321
 coughing 298, 299
 difficult 135, 358
 earache 285, 322
 easily frightened 101
 failure to thrive 256, 297
 growing pains 111, 152
 high temperature *44*, 57
 monitoring 295, *295*
 motion sickness 324
 nosebleeds 326, *326*
 over-rapid growth 111
 overexcited 135
 pneumonia 301
 poor nutrition 297
 problems at school 233
 remedies for 57
 ringworm 335
 slow development 93, 107
 slow pulse 42
 styes 334
 taking a remedy 41
 tooth decay 318
 and vomiting 53
 weak memory 233
chilliness 72, 107, 163, 167, 193, 222, 236, 273, 286, 290, **299**, 309, 311, 324, 328, 334, 361
chills 64, 299, 300, 311, 358
China officinalis **130–31**, 302, 313, 323
cholera 28, 313
choosing a remedy 38–9
 the correct dose 38–9
 finding the appropriate remedy 38
 how many to take 39
 useful remedies 39
 using the Materia Medica 38
Cimacifuga 132–3
Cina **134–5**, 354, 362, 366
cinchona bark *11*
circulation 370
cirrhosis of the liver 37
clamminess 249, 356
clumsiness 81
Coca **136–7**
Cocculus indicus **138–9**, 325
Coffea cruda **140–41**, 323
Colchicum autumnale **142–3**
cold compresses 360
cold sores 243
cold sweats 298
coldness 249, 281
colds 8, 26, *26*, 30, *30*, 32, 50–51, 57, 58, 59, 61, 255, 256, 299, **301–2**, *302*, 309, 326, 327, 337, 362, 371, 372
colic 144, 306, 307, **354**, *355*
colitis 37, 386
Colocynthis **144–5**
complexes 30–31, *30*
concentration problems 68, 163
concussion **321**
confusion 72, 324
congestion 70

Conium maculatum **146–7**
conjunctivitis (pink eye) **337**
constipation 21, 46, 56, 57, 60, 72, 107, 169, 218, 221, 262, 273, 275, **308**, 328, 348, 372, 386
contraindications 42–5
conventional medicine 28–9
convulsions 42, 149, **321**, 353
cortisone 42
coughs 50–51, *51*, 57, 58, 59, 136, 152, 157, 171, 259, 298, **299**, 300, 301, 302, 354, 357, 371, 372
cradle cap **354–5**
cramps 218, 281, 282, 347, 372
 muscle **315**, 324
 stomach 241, 324
croup **354**
Cullen, William 10
Cuprum metallicum **148–9**, 299, 315, 321, 324, 340
cuts 8, **333**
cystitis 306, **347**
cysts 35

danger signs 294
degenerative conditions 169
dehydration 53, 301, 327
delirium 42, 59, 321, 364
dental problems 108, 255, **316–17**
 see also teeth; teething; toothache
dentistry, post- 87, 169
depression 45, 91, 132, 233, 235, 241, 286, 321, 347, 372, 385, 387
dermatitis 84
desire for company 88, 253
desire to be alone 79, 119, 136, 159
destructive behaviour 37
detoxification process *26*, 27, 42
diabetes 37, 268, 309, 380
diagnosis 18–19
diarrhoea 26, 51, 56, 57, 58, 144, 159, 235, 290, 294, 297, 306, *306*, 308, 310, 311, *311*, **313**, 343, 353
 in babies 126
diet 20, 21, *21*, 22, 46–7
digestive problems 76, 103, 119, 121, 144, 180, 183, 211, 236, 288, 335
 see also gastro-intestinal problems
dilution 24, *24*
 discovery of 11
Dioscorea villosa **150–51**
disappointment 175, 225
discharges 26, 68, 112, 169, 183, 187, 190, 193, 215, 228, 277, 299, 301, 302, 303, 322, 334, 337, 356, 360, 361, 364, 372
discomfort 155, 301, 319
dizziness 271, 297, 325, 328
dose, correct 38–9
dreams 290
drinks
 coffee 115
 cold 155, 281, 309, 318
 excessive drinking 311
 hot 128, 360
 tea 150
driving 323
drops 40
Drosera rotundifolia **152–3**, 299, 359
drowsiness 79
dryness 72, 103
ductless glands 387
Dulcamara 302
dullness 324
dyspepsia **309**, 373
 see also indigestion

ear problems 57, 117, 187, 285, *322*, **322**
eating disorders 45
eczema 8, 28, 84, **339**, 371
emotional problems 22–3, *23*, 26, 28, 39, 60, 321, 323
 see also anxiety; depression

energy levels 19, 21
epilepsy 381
Equisetum 362
Eupatorium perfoliatum **154–5**, 302
Euphrasia **156–7**, 321, 337, 360, 361
exams
 nerves 160
 study 323
excitability 222
exercise 20, 21, *21*, 23, 48, *48*, 302
exhaustion 187, 189, 203, 225, 233, 253, 256, 288, 302, **323**, 327, 364
eye problems 44, 83, 91, 157, 227, 262, 265, 266, 299, 321, 357, 361, 364
eye strain 244, **321**

face, flushed 159, 326
faintness 60, 301, 311, *323*, **323–4**, 325
fatigue 18, 301, 327, 385
fear 57, 64, 83, 88, 104, 107, 206, 227, 241, 256, 262, 290, 301, 310, 313, 317, 325, 343, **345**, 353, 354
 see also fright
feet, cold 190
female sexual conditions 57, 230
Ferrum metallicum **158–9**, 297
Ferrum phosphate 301, 302, 307, 322, 326, 364, **371**
fertility 380
fever 56, 58, 59, 61, 64, 87, 155, 160, 239, 250, 294, 298–301, 321, 324, 347, 354, 357, 358, 359, *362*, **362**, 364, **364**, 367, *367*
fibrositis 373
fibrous tissue growth 36
fidgeting 81
fingers, crushed **315**
first aid remedies 39, 56, 58–61
flatulence 60, 121, 201, 241
flower essences 374–7
 Bach flower essences 376

healing from flowers 374–6
Rescue Remedy 376–7, *377*
flu *see* influenza
fly agaric *9*
Folliculinium 378
food
  aversion to 305, 311
  highly seasoned 227, 348
  hot 201
  juicy 247
  organic 47
  pungent 195
  refreshing 225, 247
  rich 215, 306, 311, 312, 313, 327, 328, 348
  sour 247
  strongly flavoured 215
food poisoning 53, 58, **310**, 311, *311*
forgetfulness 250
fractures 266, *319*, **319**
Fragaria tincture 317
freckles 35
fresh air craving 83, 273, 309
fried food craving 215
fright 298, 299, 321, 328
  see also fear
fruit 46, 47, *47*, 281, 290, 313, 336
fullness 70

gastro-intestinal problems 201
  see also digestive problems
Gelsemium **160–61**, 302, 309, 313, 324, 326, 327, 343, *343*, 358, 364
gemmology 386
gemstone elixirs *386*, 387
general remedies 57
general symptoms 18, 19
genetic predisposition 32–3, *32*
giddiness 324
ginger tea 53
glandular problems 147, 176, 209, 228, 255, 256, 356, 357, 358

Glonine 327
gonorrhoea 33
goose pimples 299
gout 143, 198, 278
Graphites **162–3**, 334, 339, 364
grief 60, *60*, 125, 175, 225, 315, 321
  see also bereavement
growths 277
gum problems 317, 353, 385
gumboils 318

haemorrhage 165
Hahnemann, Samuel
  development of homeopathy 10–11
  genetic predisposition 32, *32*
  Homeopathic Materia Medica 11
  and the Law of Similars 10, 12
  and 'like cures like' principle 8, 10
  and miasms 33, 34, *34*, 37, *37*
  The Organon of Medicine 11, 14
  potentization 24
  and the vital force 14, 16, 17
Hamamelis virginiana **164–5**, 321, 326
hands
  cold 190, 225, 299
  sore 61
  swelling of left hand 104
  wringing/moving 171
hangover 60
hayfever *360*, **361**, 372
head
  injury 217, 221, 321
  sharp pains 321
  tight feeling in 285
headaches 21, 26, 30, 44, 48, 51–2, 56, 59, 64, 70, 103, 104, 111, 131, 180, 206, 213, 235, 244, 265, 271, 285, 286, 298, 301, 306, 321, 324, 325, **327–8**, 347, 357, 372
health: keeping healthy 46–9
heart problems 236, 386, 387

heartburn 13, 306, 372
heat exhaustion (heatstroke) **324**
hectic lifestyle 20–21, *21*
Helleborus niger 321
Hepar sulphuricum **166–7**, 298, 299, 301, 302, 322, 331, 333, 334, 340, 354, 356, 360, 364
Hering, Constantine 27, *27*
Hering's Laws of Cure 27, *27*
hiccups **310–311**, 372
Hippocrates 10, *12–13*
hives 278, 360
hoarseness 83, 259, 299, *303*, **303**, 354
holism 9, 28
homeopathic aggravation 26–7, 38
homeopathic colour remedies 382–5
Homeopathic Materia Medica 38, *39*, 54–291
homeopaths, qualified 45
homeopathy
  definition 8
  history of 10–11
  the practice of 30–31
  the remedies 8–9
homesickness 117, *374*
hormonal remedies 378–81
  hormonal imbalance 378–9
  male and female hormones 380
  sensible use 381
  stimulating other glands in the body 380–81
  tonifying the kidneys 379–80
Hydrastis **168–9**, 360
Hyoscyamus niger **170–71**
Hypericum cream 333
Hypericum perforatum **172–3**, 315, 318, 321, 331, 332, 334, 336, 360
hysteria 310, 344

ice cream 312, *312*
  craving 227

Ignatia 22, 23, *23*, 60, *60*, **174–5**, 299, 305, 310, 311, 315, 321, 323, 329, 344
immune system 29, *29*
immunization side effects **360**
impetigo **364**
indigestion 103, 307, 373
see also dyspepsia
infections 112, 239, 243, 255, 309, 322, 334, 335, 337, 349, 354, 355, 356, 364, 386
infectious diseases 28–9, 33
inflammation 59, 143, 316, 317, 332, 334, 356, 386
influenza 8, 26, 30, 50–51, 56–9, 155, 256, 299, **301–2**, *302*, 326, 327, 362, 373
injuries 16, 39, 56, 58, 64, 87, 96, 165, 172, 266, 277, 316, 321, 351
insects 59, *59*, 332, *332*
insomnia 30, *30*, 37, 58, 117, 139, 261, 286, **328–9**, *329*, 372, 373, 380
intestinal worms 135
involuntary/exaggerated movements 67
Iodine tincture 335
Iodum **176–7**
Ipecacuanha (Ipecac) **178–9**, 298, 311, 325, 348, 359
Iris tenax 307
Iris versicolor **180–81**
irritation, irritability 21, 117, 126, 144, 159, 167, 179, 218, 243, 301, 308, 311, 313, 322, 325, 328, 335, 353, 354, 357, 358, 373
isopathy 378
itching 67, 265, 268, 313, 335, 339, 364, 366, 367

jealousy 81, 171, 197, 218
jerking 67, 149, 273, 329

joint problems 61, 108, 143, 243, 244, 316, 319, **319**, 370

Kali bichromicum **182–3**, 298, 299, 302, 303, 340, 354
Kali carbonicum **184–5**, 315, 359
Kali muriatum **186–7**, 337, **371**
Kali phosphoricum **188–9**, 305, 323, **372**
Kali sulphuricum **190–91**, **372**
Kent, Dr James Tyler: *Repertory to the Homeopathic Materia Medica* 11
kidney problems 99, 379–80, *379*
Kreosotum **192–3**, 318

Lac caninum **194–5**
Lachesis **196–7**
lack of confidence 75, 93, 195, 201, 255
lactose 24
laryngitis **303**
lavender, essential oil of 50
Law of Similars 10, 12–13
laziness 190, 364, 386
leadership qualities 36
Ledum palustre **198–9**, 315, 332, 334, 337, 338, 360
legs, tired and restless 286
lethargy 321
lice **364–5**, *365*
ligaments 61, 316, 370
light aversion 321
'like cures like' principle 8, 10, 33
liver ailments 143, 217
loners 198
lumbago 373
lung conditions 32, 34, 35, 217, 300, 305
Lycopodium **200–201**, 306–9, 334, 347, 362, 364, 366

Magnesia carbonica **202–3**, 336, 354
Magnesia muriatica **204–5**, 347
Magnesia phosphorica **206–7**, 307, 311, **372**
malaria 373
male sexual conditions 57
manipulativeness 36
mastitis 59, *349*, **349**
materia medica 38, *39*, 54–291
first aid remedies 58–61
understanding the *materia medica* 56–7
measles 285, **357**, 360, 371
melatonin 381
memory 233, 285
meningitis 44
menopause 57, 84, 132, 141, 197, 253
menstruation 57, 132, 193, 204, 230, 247, 282, 306, *306*, 311, **347**
mental confusion 44
mental exertion 75, 111, 250, 328
mental regression 93
Mercurius solubilis 318, 322, 331, 333, 339, 353, 366, 367
Mercurius vivus (Mercury) **208–9**, 305
mercury 37
metabolism 305
Mezerium 339
miasms 33, 34–7
migraine 213, 325, 326
milk
allergy 311, 354
craving 309
miscarriage 122, 247
moles 32, 35
monitoring improvement 294–5
mood swings 159
morning sickness 139, *348*, **348**
mother tincture form 374
motion sickness *324*, **324–5**

mouth
  abscesses 331
  bitter taste 305
  dry 309
  infection 305
  metallic taste 305
  ulcers (apthae) **336**
mucus, excess 35, 51, 157, 217, 259, 298, 299, **299**, 301, 302, 303, 313, 354, 372
mumps **358–9**, 360, 371
muscle
  ache 301, 302
  coordination problems 160
  pain 56, 125
  strain 108, 370, 371
  weakness 370, 372

nail problems 76, 255
nappy rash **355**
nasal congestion 302, 361
nasal discharge 68
Natrum carbonicum **210–211**
Natrum muriaticum **212–13**, 302, 303, 309, 311, 321, 326, 327–8, 337, 344, 347, 362, **372**
Natrum phosphoricum **214–15**, **373**
Natrum sulphuricum **216–17**, 321, **373**
nausea 53, 57, 119, 128, 179, 225, 271, 282, 298, 303, 311, **311**, 324, 325, 328, 348
neck problems 44, 52, 111, 132
negative thoughts 286
nerve injury 172
nervousness 101, 206, 282, 336, 362, 372
neuralgia 144, **325–6**, 372
neuritis 372
nightmares 329
Nitric acid 308
North American Society of Homeopaths, The (NASH) 45

nosebleeds 165, *326*, **326**
numbness 230, 332
nursing mothers 57
Nux vomica 21, 42, 60, **218–19**, 302, 306, 308, 311, 315, 324, 325, 328, 348

observation 19
Oophorinum 380
Opium **220–21**
oral hygiene *305*, *317*
osteoporosis 386
over-excitement 323
overactive mind 197, 281
overeating 306, *306*, 309, 311
oversensitivity 91, 286
overweight 20, 297, 324, 334, 356

pain 239, 241, 319
  abdominal *306*, **306**, 307, 310, 311, *311*
  burning 81, 88, 227, 278, 332, 334
  chest 42, 298
  chronic 385
  cramping 206
  dental 317
  face and head 303
  general 203
  head 321
  joint **319**
  left-sided 275
  with nausea and perspiration 128
  pricking 266
  radiating 99
  right-sided 128
  sensitivity to 167, 347
  severe 144, 150
  sharp, cutting 184
  sharp, darting 318
  sharp, sticking 334
  shooting 172, 206, 228, 360, 364, 372
  stabbing 167
  stinging 81, 278, 332, 340
  stitching 206, 266, 327
  and sudden spasms 286
  testicular 358
  wandering 228
pallor 297
panic attacks 64, 72, 298
Paracelsus 13, *13*
paralysis 233
particular symptoms 18–19
Passiflora incarnata 328
periods *see* menstruation
perspiration 107, 126, 128, 203, 209, 221, 275, 281, 311, 324, 356, 367, 373
Petroleum **222–3**, 325, 339
phlegm 244, 298, 300, 301
Phosphoric acid **224–5**, 344
Phosphorus **226–7**, 299, 303, 309, 313, 318, 325, 326, 329, 345, 351, 354, 362
Phytolacca decandra **228–9**, 334, 349, 357
Phytolacca tincture 349
Pilates 48, 51
pills 40, *40*
pimples 268
pineal gland 381, 385
pituitary gland 381, 385
Platina **230–31**
pleurisy 301
plug-like sensation 75
Plumbum **232–3**
PMS (pre-menstrual syndrome) 328
pneumonia 32, 61, **300–301**, *301*
Podophyllum **234–5**, 313
poison ivy *61*
poisons *9*, 11, *17*
Posterior Pituitary gland 381
potency 294
  high 24, 26–7, *26*
  low 24, 40

potentization 16, 24, *24*, 387
poverty, fear of 103, 108
pregnancy 42, 84, 119, 122, 297, *297*, 307, 348, *348*, 358
prickly heat 268
psoriasis 34, *34*
psoric miasm 33, 34–7, *34*
Psorinium 366
Pulsatilla **236–7**, 298, 299, 301, 302, 309, 311, 312, *312*, 313, 319, 322, 324, 328, 331, 334, 347, 348, 354, 357, 358, 360, 361, 362, 367
pulse rate 42
puncture wounds 198, 337
pupils, dilated 301, 321, 364, 367
pus 112, 331, 333, 360, 364, 366
Pyrogen **238–9**

qualified homeopaths 45

radiation 13, 241
Radium bromatum **240–41**
rashes 34, *34*, 52, 59, 61, 329, 358, 366, 367
relationship problems 230
Rescue Remedy 376–7, *377*
respiration *see* breathing problems
restlessness 18, 34–5, 58, 64, 88, 115, 152, 155, 176, 249, 273, 281, 282, 298, 301, 302, 313, 325, 327, 328, 336, 357, 362
rheumatism 36, 61, 143, 183, 198, 241, 278, 319, 373
Rhus toxicodendron 61, *61*, **242–3**, 302, 309, 315, 316, *316*, 319, 329, 357, 359
ringworm *335*, **335**
ritalin 13
roseola **366–7**, *367*
rubella (German measles) **358**, 360
Ruta graveolens 61, **244–5**, 315, 316, 319, 336

Sabina **246–7**
sadness 230, 247, 253
safe keeping of remedies 41
safety first 42, 44, *44*
salivation 139, 180, 325
salt
 craving 195, 213, 281, 309
 loss 324
scabies 33, **366**
scalds 50
scalp
 dry 265
 shingles 329
Schuessler, Dr 370
sciatica **318**, 372
seasickness 271, **325**
Season Affective Disorder 385
Secale cornutum **248–9**
sedentary lifestyle 60, 218, 361
Selenium **250–51**
self-control problems 209
self-hatred 195
self-medication 20, 294–5
sense of duty 91
sensitivity 206, 247, 261, 336
 to cold 93, 209
 to heat 209
 to pain 318
 to temperature 19
 to touch 95, 332, 360
Sepia **252–3**, 299, 348, 362
sexual hormones 380
sexual problems 115, 147, 193, 230, 253
shellfish 278
shingles **329**
shivering 299
shock 16, *17*, 39, 57, 58, 64, 221, 310, 315, 319, 321, 336, 340, 344, 351, 380
Silica **254–5**, 303, 322, 331, 338, 353, 360, 361, **373**

sinusitis 302, **303**, 305
skin
 burning 265, 313, 339, 367
 cancer *340*
 cracked 163, 222, 339, 355, 370
 dry 324, 339, 354
 flushed 357
 growths 277
 infections 34, *34*, 354, 355, 364
 inflammation 59
 irritations 243, 355
 itching 265, 313, 339, 364, 367
 pale 299
 problems 76, 183, **339**
 sensitivity 331, 339
 yellowing 44
sleep patterns 19
sleepiness 68
sleeplessness *see* insomnia
slowness 72
smallpox vaccine 360
Society of Homeopaths, The 45
soft tissue problems 96
solarized water *384*
soreness 165, 167, 239, 319, 337
spasms 281, 282, 286, 299, 311, 321
spectacles, coloured *384*
splinters 52, *338*, **338**
Spongia tosta **256–7**, 299, 354, 359
sprains 56, 61, 244, *316*, **316**, 371
stage fright 160
Stahl, Georg Ernst 13
Stanum metallicum **258–9**
Staphysagria **260–61**, 334
stiff neck 44, 52, 111
stiffness 230, 302, 319
stings 59, *59*, *332*, **332**
stomach problems *see* abdominal problems
stools 44, 70, 297, 308, 313, 353
strain(s) 96, 242, 244
Stramonium **262–3**

stress 21, 37, 51, 57, 239, 309, 311, 327, *329*, 339, 362, *379*, 380, 381, 383
styes *334*, **334**
sudden/violent onset of symptoms 95
sugar craving 380
  see also sweet foods craving
suicidal tendencies 91
sulkiness 76
Sulphur 42, **264–5**, 298, 301, 308, 313, 329, 331, 333, 335, 339, 355, 356, 357, 364, 366
sunburn 53, *340*, **340**
suppuration 373
surgery, post- 42, 87, 96, 169, 351
Swan, Dr 34
sweating see perspiration
sweet foods craving 83, 180, 201, 261
  see also sugar craving
swellings 81, 96, 143, 309, 317, 319, 332, 334, 347, 360
  glands 176, 209, 228, 256, 356, 357, 358
sycotic miasm 33, 34, 35–6
Symphytum **266–7**, 319, 334
symptoms, differentiating 18–19, *19*
syphilis 33, 37
syphilitic miasm 33, 34, 37
Syzygium **268–9**
Syzygizum 380

Tabacum **270–71**, 325
taking a remedy 40–41, *40*
Tarantula cubensis **272–3**
Taraxacum **274–5**
teeth 370, *371*
  see also dental problems; teething; toothache
teething 53, 126, 193, 235, 313, 321, *353*, **353**, 364
temperature 42, *44*, 57, 309, 357, 358
  sensitivity 19
tendons 61, 93, 316
tension 57, 218, 285, 301
testicular pain 358
testosterone 380
thirst 19, 44, 59, 65, 103, 126, 139, 268, 273, 290, 301, 302, 308, *308*, **309**, 327, 357, 362, 364, 372
  lack of 160, 179, 301, **309**, 311, 357, 358
threadworms (pinworms) **366**
throat
  burning 265
  dry 309
  sore 57, 195, 302, 357, 370, 371, 372, 385
  swollen 309
Thuja occidentalis **276–7**, 337, 355, 360, 362, 364
thymus gland 380, 387
Thyroid, homeopathic 379, 380–81
thyroid gland 378–9, 385, 387
timidity 93, 160
tiredness 131, 139, 297
tobacco 60, 175, 271, 325
toes, crushed **315**
tongue 79, 275, 348, 371
tonsillitis 187, **356–7**, 371
toothache 255, 316, 318, 372, 385
  see also dental problems; teeth; teething
toxins 26, 386
travel sickness 53, 139
trembling 67, 343
tubercular miasm 34–5
tumours 35, 36, 381
twitching 67, 149, 273, 329, 372
typhoid 28

urinary tract problems 46–7, 84, 115, 218, 221, 261, 262, 347, 362, 373
Urtica urens **278–9**, 340
uterus: bearing-down feeling 253

vegetables 46, 47, *47*, 290, 336
Veratrum album **280–81**, 298, 351
vertigo 136
Vertrum viride 311
Viburnum opulus **282–3**
Viola tricolor **284–5**
viral infection 299
Viscum album **286–7**
vital force 14, *14*, 16–17
  a fine balance 14
  maintaining harmony 16
  the minimum dose 17
  replicating reactions 16
voice loss 299, 303
vomiting 44, 53, 58, 180, 233, 298, 310–313, *311*, **311**, 324, 325, 327, 328, 359, *359*
  projectile 294

warts 32, 35, 277, **337**, 371
water
  drinking 46, 115, 310, 311, 312
  solarized *384*
weakness 44, 79, 111, 131, 225, 244, 249, 250, 297, 301, 361
weather
  changes in 217
  cold 163, 228, 244, 271, 302, 303, 318
  damp 319
  warm/hot 160, 190, 213, 235, 236, 250, 271
weight loss 21
wheezing 44, 298
whooping cough 321, *359*, **359**
worms 135, 362, 373
wounds 112, 198, 266, *337*, **337**

yoga 48, 51

Zincum metallicum **288–9**
Zingiber officinale **290–91**

AUTHOR'S ACKNOWLEDGEMENTS

My thanks to the School of Spiritual Homeopathy and the Institute of Life Energy Medicine in Tucson, Arizona for their willingness to take homeopathy to a deeper level of treatment. I want to thank the students of the School of Spiritual Homeopathy who made and prepared the homeopathic sound remedies in 2004. I want to thank Ian Townsens, who has shared his knowledge and wisdom so graciously. To Jude Creswell in Sydney, Australia, who believes in healing the heart and mind. To Susan Nemcek for being a true spiritual homeopath. To the spirit of my grandmother, who taught me to love a garden and explore its healing nature. Blessings to all who love homeopathy.

PICTURE ACKNOWLEDGEMENTS

Alamy 85; /AAA Photostock 209; /Applestock 302; /Arco Images 114; /bildagentur-online.com/th-foto 17; /Juniors Bildarchiv 58–59; /blickwinkel 60, 142, 170, 174–175, 246–247; /Paul Bradforth 120–121; /Christopher Burrows 234; /Scott Camazine 242–243; /Luca DiCecco 109; /Dynamic Graphics/Photis 305; /Florida Images 161; /GC Minerals 78; /Jane Gould 252; /Chris Howes/Wild Places Photography 257; /Kevin Lang 269; /mediacolor's 34; /Profimedia CZ s.r.o. 39, 300; /Bengt Sall/Pixonnet.com 199; /David Sanger Photography 324; /Lynne Siler 49; /Trevor Sims/ GardenWorld Images 260; /TH Foto 130; /Libby Welch 40. **BananaStock** 110, 295, 353, 355. **Kristopher Bigos** 384. **Corbis UK Ltd** 29, 224–225; /Niall Benvie 153; /Vincent Besnault 185; /Bettmann 10; /Emely/Zefa 80–81; /Envision 20; /Jack Fields 158; /William Gottlieb 106; /Philip Gould 200; /Rob Lewine 32; /LWA-Dann Tardif 202; /Roy Morsch 89; /Steve Prezant 189; /Anthony Redpath 215; /Stapleton Collection 13; /Stock4B 205. **DigitalVision** 6, 97, 248, 322. **DK Images** 27; /Andy Crawford and Steve Gorton 52, 338. **Frank Lane Picture Agency**/Robin Chittenden 146; /Foto Natura Stock 219. **Garden Picture Library**/Rich Pomerantz 61. **Getty Images** 344–345; /Christopher Bissell 356; /Christoph Burki 332–333; /Alan Danaher 77; /Donna Day 307; /Ghislain & Marie David de Lossy 303; /Ken Lucas 232–233; /John Millar 306; /Laurence Monneret 348; /Martine Mouchy 177; /Neo Vision 101; /White Packert 226, 341; /Jeremy Samuelson 35; /T. Schmidt 65; /Harry Taylor 231; /Luis Veiga 141; /Mel Yates 74. **ImageSource** 113, 196, 264, 343. **Masterfile**/Steve Prezant 323. **Octopus Publishing Group Limited** 9 left, 66, 69, 117, 229, 237, 267; /Colin Bowling 2, 30, 31, 54, 71, 86, 123, 135, 151, 154–155, 156–157, 165, 168–169, 336; /Michael Boys 374–375; /Stephen Conroy 312; /Frazer Cunningham 191; /Philip Dowell 172–173, 181, 221, 245, 263, 279, 287, 386 bottom right, 386 bottom centre, 387 bottom left; /Jerry Harpur 62, 98–99, 105, 133, 280, 283, 379; /Andy Komorowski 148–149; /William Lingwood 291; /Adrian Pope 359; /Mike Prior 73, 387 centre left; /Peter Pugh-Cook 166, 192; /William Reavell 46–47, 102–103, 212–213, 329; /Guy Ryecart 386 bottom centre right, 386 centre right top; /Russell Sadur 129, 365, 367; /Gareth Sambidge 207; /Niki Sianni 124; /Roger Stowell 127, 274–275; /Ian Wallace 241; /George Wright 284–285. **PhotoDisc** 4, 9 right, 15, 23, 26, 43, 44, 50, 93, 118, 216, 238, 273, 296, 297, 308, 314, 316, 317, 318, 320, 330, 337, 342, 346, 349, 350, 352, 361. **Photolibrary Group** 304; /Chassnet 310, 371; /Alice Garik 195; /David Johnston 25; /Laurent 326; /Natalia Laurent 292, 363; /Novastock 210; /TH Foto-Werbung 276. **Science Photo Library**/AJ Photo 182; /John Clegg 145; /Mauro Fermariello 377; /Astrid & Hanns-Frieder Michler 36; /Bob Gibbons 12; /John Hadfield 335; /Martin Land 162–163; /BSIP, Laurent 186; /Jerry Mason 94; /Steve Percival 138; /Dr. Morley Read 137; /Francoise Sauze 334; /Stephen A. Skirius 82; /Shiela Terry 254, 368; /TH Foto-Werbung 11, 178, 270; /Rich Treptow 258–259; /U. S. Dept. of Energy 223; /Dirk Wiersma 91; /Charles D. Winter 251, 289; /Hattie Young 19.

Executive Editor: Sandra Rigby
Executive Art Editor: Sally Bond
Editors: Alice Bowden, Lisa John
Picture Researcher: Sophie Delpech
Production Controller: Simone Nauerth
Designer: Annika Skoog for Cobalt Id